Computers in the Medical Office

Sixth Edition

Susan M. Sanderson

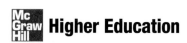
Higher Education

Boston   Burr Ridge, IL   Dubuque, IA   New York   San Francisco   St. Louis
Bangkok   Bogotá   Caracas   Kuala Lumpur   Lisbon   London   Madrid   Mexico City
Milan   Montreal   New Delhi   Santiago   Seoul   Singapore   Sydney   Taipei   Toronto

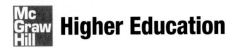

Higher Education

COMPUTERS IN THE MEDICAL OFFICE, SIXTH EDITION

Published by McGraw-Hill, a business unit of The McGraw-Hill Companies, Inc., 1221 Avenue of the Americas, New York, NY, 10020. Copyright © 2009 by The McGraw-Hill Companies, Inc. Previous editions © 1995, 1999, 2002, 2005, and 2007. All rights reserved. No part of this publication may be reproduced or distributed in any form or by any means, or stored in a database or retrieval system, without the prior written consent of The McGraw-Hill Companies, Inc., including, but not limited to, in any network or other electronic storage or transmission, or broadcast for distance learning.

Some ancillaries, including electronic and print components, may not be available to customers outside the United States.

This book is printed on acid-free paper.

4 5 6 7 8 9 0 DOW/DOW 0 9

ISBN   978-0-07-340199-7
MHID   0-07-340199-4

Vice President/Editor in Chief: *Elizabeth Haefele*
Vice President/Director of Marketing: *John E. Biernat*
Senior sponsoring editor: *Debbie Fitzgerald*
Managing developmental editor: *Patricia Hesse*
Executive marketing manager: *Roxan Kinsey*
Lead media producer: *Damian Moshak*
Media producer: *Marc Mattson*
Director, Editing/Design/Production: *Jess Ann Kosic*
Project manager: *Marlena Pechan*

Senior production supervisor: *Janean A. Utley*
Designer: *Marianna Kinigakis*
Senior photo research coordinator: *Lori Hancock*
Media project manager: *Mark A. S. Dierker*
Outside development house: *Wendy Langerud*
Cover design: *Jon Resh*
Typeface: *11/13.5 Palatino*
Compositor: *Aptara®, Inc.*
Printer: *R. R. Donnelley*

Codeveloped by McGraw-Hill Higher Education and Chestnut Hill Enterprises, Inc. chestnuthl@aol.com

The Student Data Template file, illustrations, instructions, and exercises in *Computers in the Medical Office* are compatible with the Medisoft™ Advanced Version 14 Patient Accounting software available at the time of publication. Adaptations may be necessary for use with subsequent versions of the software. Text changes will be made in reprints when possible.

All brand or product names are trademarks or registered trademarks of their respective companies.

CPT five-digit codes, nomenclature, and other data are copyright 2007 American Medical Association. All rights reserved. No fee schedules, basic unit, relative values, or related listings are included in the CPT. The AMA assumes no liability for the data contained herein.

CPT codes are based on CPT 2008.

ICD-9-CM codes are based on ICD-9-CM 2008.

All names, situations, and anecdotes are fictitious. They do not represent any person, event, or medical record.

Library of Congress Cataloging-in-Publication Data

Sanderson, Susan M.
    Computers in the medical office/Susan M. Sanderson.—6th ed.
        p. ; cm.
    Includes indexes.
    ISBN-13: 978-0-07-340199-7 (alk. paper)
    ISBN-10: 0-07-340199-4 (alk. paper)
    1. Medical offices—Automation. 2. MediSoft. I. Title.
    [DNLM: 1. MediSoft. 2. Office Automation—Problems and Exercises. 3. Practice Management, Medical—Problems and Exercises. 4. Office Management—Problems and Exercises. 5. Software—Problems and Exercises. W 18.2 S216c 2009]
    R864.S26 2009
    651'.9610285—dc22
                                                2008020249

The Internet addresses listed in the text were accurate at the time of publication. The inclusion of a Web site does not indicate an endorsement by the authors or McGraw-Hill, and McGraw-Hill does not guarantee the accuracy of the information presented at these sites.

www.mhhe.com

Contents

Preface   x
    Your Career in Medical Billing   x
    Overview   xi
    Computer Supplies and Equipment   xi
    To the Student   xii
    What Every Instructor Needs to Know   xii
      What's New in the Sixth Edition?   xii
    Teaching and Learning Supplements   xiii
      For the Instructor   xiii
    About the Author   xiv
What Every Student Needs to Know   xv
Acknowledgments   xviii
How Can I Succeed In This Class?   xix

PART 1   INTRODUCTION TO COMPUTERS IN THE MEDICAL OFFICE   1

CHAPTER 1   The Medical Office Billing Process   3

    Step 1 Preregister Patients   4
    Step 2 Establish Financial Responsibility for Visit   5
    Step 3 Check in Patients   7
    Step 4 Check Out Patients   10
    Step 5 Review Coding Compliance   14
    Step 6 Check Billing Compliance   14
    Step 7 Prepare and Transmit Claims   15
    Step 8 Monitor Payer Adjudication   15
    Step 9 Generate Patient Statements   17
    Step 10 Follow up Patient Payments and Handle Collections   18

CHAPTER 2   Information Technology and HIPAA   23

    Medical Office Applications   24
      Electronic Medical Records   24
      Electronic Prescribing   25
      Practice Management   26
      Advantages of Computer Use   30
      A Note of Caution: What Computers Cannot Do   31
    HIPAA and Electronic Exchange of Information   32
      HIPAA Electronic Transaction and Code Sets Standards   33
      Privacy Requirements   35
      Security Requirements   37

CHAPTER 3   **Introduction to Medisoft**   **45**

What is Medisoft?   46
How Medisoft Data are Organized and Stored   46
   Medisoft Databases   46
The Student Data Template   47
The Medisoft Menu Bar   47
   Exercise 3-1   51
The Medisoft Toolbar   51
   Exercise 3-2   53
Entering and Editing Data   53
   Changing the Medisoft Program Date   53
   Exercise 3-3   57
Saving Data   58
Deleting Data   58
Using Medisoft Help   59
   Exercise 3-4   60
   Exercise 3-5   62
Exiting Medisoft   63
   Making a Backup File While Exiting Medisoft   63
   Exercise 3-6   64
   Restoring the Backup File   65
File Maintenance Utilities   66
   Rebuilding Indexes   67
   Packing Data   68
   Purging Data   69
   Recalculating Patient Balances   71

CHAPTER 4   **Entering Patient Information**   **77**

How Patient Information is Organized in Medisoft   78
Entering New Patient Information   79
   Name, Address Tab   80
   Exercise 4-1   81
   Other Information Tab   82
   Payment Plan Tab   85
   Exercise 4-2   86
   Adding an Employer to the Address List   86
   Exercise 4-3   89
Editing Patient Information   90
Searching for Patient Information   90
   Search for and Field Option   91
   Exercise 4-4   93
   Locate Buttons Option   93
   Exercise 4-5   95
On Your Own Exercises   95
On Your Own Exercise 1 Entering a New Patient   95

CHAPTER 5   **Entering Insurance, Account, and Condition Information**   **103**

Working with Cases   104
  When to Set Up a New Case   104
  Case Command Buttons   105
Creating a New Case for a New Patient   106
  Personal Tab   108
  Exercise 5-1   110
  Account Tab   111
  Exercise 5-2   113
  Diagnosis Tab   114
  Exercise 5-3   115
  Policy 1 Tab   115
  Exercise 5-4   117
  Policy 2 Tab   118
  Policy 3 Tab   119
  Condition Tab   119
  Exercise 5-5   121
  Miscellaneous Tab   122
  Medicaid and Tricare Tab   123
  Comment Tab   125
  EDI Tab   125
  Editing Case Information on an Established Patient   129
  Exercise 5-6   129
  On Your Own Exercise 2 Creating a Case for a New Patient   130

CHAPTER 6   **Entering Charge Transactions and Patient Payments**   **135**

Transaction Entry Overview   136
Patient/Account Information   136
  Chart   136
  Case   138
  Totals and Charge Tabs   138
Charge Transactions   140
  Buttons in the Charges Area of the Transaction Entry Dialog Box   143
  Saving Charges   145
  Editing Transactions   146
  Color Coding in Transaction Entry   146
  Exercise 6-1   148
  Exercise 6-2   149
Payment/Adjustment Transactions   149
  Entering Payments Made During Office Visits   150
  Saving Payment Information   153
  Exercise 6-3   154
  Exercise 6-4   155
  Printing Walkout Receipts   156
  Exercise 6-5   158
  Entering Adjustments   158
  Exercise 6-6   161
  On Your Own Exercise 3 Enter Procedure Charges and a Patient Payment 162
  On Your Own Exercise 4 Print a Walkout Receipt   162

CHAPTER 7	**Creating Claims**	**167**
	Introduction to Health Care Claims	168
	Creating Claims	168
	Create Claims Dialog Box	172
	Exercise 7-1	174
	Claim Selection	175
	Editing Claims	176
	Carrier 1 Tab	177
	Carrier 2 and Carrier 3 Tabs	178
	Transactions Tab	178
	Comment Tab	179
	Exercise 7-2	180
	Electronic Claims	180
	Steps in Submitting Electronic Claims	181
	Sending Electronic Claim Attachments	185
	Changing the Status of Claims	186
	Exercise 7-3	186
	On Your Own Exercise 5 Create Insurance Claims	186

CHAPTER 8	**Posting Insurance Payments and Creating Patient Statements**	**191**
	Third-Party Reimbursement Overview	192
	Indemnity Plan Example	192
	Managed Care Plan Example	192
	Medicare Participating Example	193
	Remittance Advice Processing	194
	Steps for Processing a Remittance Advice	196
	Entering Insurance Carrier Payments in Medisoft	197
	Entering Insurance Payments	200
	Applying Insurance Payments to Charges	201
	Exercise 8-1	206
	Exercise 8-2	208
	Exercise 8-3	209
	Entering Capitation Payments and Adjustments	211
	Exercise 8-4	215
	Exercise 8-5	216
	Creating Statements	217
	Statement Management Dialog Box	217
	Create Statements Dialog Box	218
	Exercise 8-6	220
	Editing Statements	220
	General Tab	220
	Transactions Tab	221
	Comment Tab	221
	Exercise 8-7	222
	Printing Statements	222
	Selecting a Format	223
	Selecting the Filters and Printing Statements	224
	Exercise 8-8	225
	On Your Own Exercise 6 Enter Insurance Payments	226
	On Your Own Exercise 7 Create Statements	226

CHAPTER 9   Printing Reports   231

Reports in the Medical Office   232
  Day Sheets   232
  Exercise 9-1   238
  Exercise 9-2   239
  Exercise 9-3   242
  Analysis Reports   242
  Exercise 9-4   245
  Aging Reports   248
  Exercise 9-5   249
  Collection Reports   250
  Patient Ledger Reports   251
  Exercise 9-6   252
  Standard Patient Lists   252
  Custom Reports   253
  Exercise 9-7   254
  Exercise 9-8   254
Using Report Designer   255
  Exercise 9-9   256
  On Your Own Exercise 8 Print a Patient Day Sheet   258
  On Your Own Exercise 9 Print a Practice Analysis Report   259

CHAPTER 10   Collections in the Medical Office   263

The Importance of Collections in the Medical Practice   264
  The Patient Collection Process   264
  Laws Governing Timely Payment of Insurance Claims   268
Using a Practice Management Program for Collections Activities   268
  Exercise 10-1   269
  Using the Collection List   269
  Entering a Tickler Item   274
  Exercise 10-2   276
  Creating Collection Letters   277
  Exercise 10-3   280
  Printing a Collection Tracer Report   281
  Exercise 10-4   282
  On Your Own Exercise 10 Print a Patient Aging Applied Payment Report 282
  On Your Own Exercise 11 Add an Item to the Collection List   282
  On Your Own Exercise 12 Create a Collection Letter   282

CHAPTER 11   Scheduling   287

Introduction to Office Hours   288
  Overview of the Office Hours Window   288
  Program Options   290
  Entering and Exiting Office Hours   290
Entering Appointments   291
  Looking for a Future Date   294
  Exercise 11-1   295
  Exercise 11-2   295
  Exercise 11-3   296

Exercise 11-4   297
Searching for Available Appointment Time   297
Exercise 11-5   297
Exercise 11-6   298
Entering Appointments for New Patients   299
Exercise 11-7   299
Booking Repeated Appointments   299
Exercise 11-8   300
Changing or Deleting Appointments   301
Exercise 11-9   302
Creating a Recall List   303
Adding a Patient to the Recall List   304
Exercise 11-10   306
Creating Breaks   306
Exercise 11-11   308
Previewing and Printing Schedules   308
Exercise 11-12   309
On Your Own Exercise 13 Enter an Appointment   310
On Your Own Exercise 14 Change an Appointment   310
On Your Own Exercise 15 Print a Physician Schedule   310

PART 3   APPLYING YOUR KNOWLEDGE   **317**

CHAPTER 12   Handling Patient Records and Transactions   319

Exercise 12-1: Inputting Patient Information   320
Exercise 12-2: An Emergency Visit   324
Exercise 12-3: Inputting Transaction Data   325
Exercise 12-4: Entering a New Patient and Transactions   325
Exercise 12-5: Entering and Applying an Insurance Carrier Payment   326

CHAPTER 13   Setting Up Appointments   327

Exercise 13-1: Scheduling Appointments   328
Exercise 13-2: Making an Appointment Change   328
Exercise 13-3: Juggling Schedules   329
Exercise 13-4: Adding Patients to the Recall List   329
Exercise 13-5: Diane Hsu and Michael Syzmanski   330
Exercise 13-6: Changing a Transaction Record   331

CHAPTER 14   Printing Lists and Reports   333

Exercise 14-1: Finding a Patient's Balance   334
Exercise 14-2: Printing a Schedule   335
Exercise 14-3: Printing Day Sheet Reports   335
Exercise 14-4: Creating a Patient Aging Applied Payment Report   336
Exercise 14-5: Adding Items to the Collection List   337
Exercise 14-6: Creating a Practice Analysis Report   338
Exercise 14-7: Stewart Robertson   338
Exercise 14-8: Michael Syzmanski   339

CHAPTER 15   **Putting It All Together**   **341**

    Exercise 15-1: Scheduling Appointments   342
    Exercise 15-2: Creating Cases   342
    Exercise 15-3: Entering Transactions   342
    Exercise 15-4: Creating Claims   343
    Exercise 15-5: Entering Insurance Payments   343
    Exercise 15-6: Creating Patient Statements   343
    Exercise 15-7: Printing Reports   343
    Exercise 15-8: Adding Items to the Collection List   344
    Exercise 15-9: Creating Collection Letters   344

PART 4   SOURCE DOCUMENTS   345

GLOSSARY   386

INDEX   390

Preface

Welcome to the sixth edition of *Computers in the Medical Office*. This text/workbook introduces you to the concepts and skills you will need for a successful career in medical office billing. Medical biller is one of the 10 fastest-growing allied health occupations. This employment growth is the result of the increased medical needs of an aging population, advances in technology, and the growing number of health practitioners.

YOUR CAREER IN MEDICAL BILLING

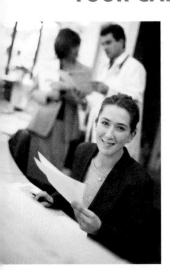

Medical billers play important roles in the financial well-being of every health care business. Billing for services in health care is more complicated than in other industries. Government and private payers vary in payment for the same services, and healthcare providers deliver services to beneficiaries of several insurance companies at any one time. Medical billers must be familiar with the rules and guidelines of each health care plan in order to submit the proper documentation so that the office receives maximum appropriate reimbursement for services provided. Without an effective billing staff, a medical office would have no cash flow!

Administrative duties in medical offices are becoming more dependent on technology. Computers are now used in almost all medical practices, for a variety of administrative and clinical functions. Anyone who seeks a job in medical billing will find that an understanding of the billing process and hands-on experience with billing software are often prerequisites to being hired. Although this text/workbook features Medisoft Advanced Version 14 Patient Accounting, its concepts are general enough to cover most administrative software intended for health care providers. Students who complete *Computers in the Medical Office* should be able to use other medical administrative software with a minimum of training.

In addition to specialized knowledge about medical billing and computer skills, you will also need to possess excellent customer service skills to succeed in this field. Even though they are not involved in the actual process of providing medical care, medical billers come in contact with clients, insurance companies, and patients. For example, incoming calls from patients who have questions regarding a charge are often directed to the billing staff, who must be able to communicate effectively with all types of people.

Medical billing is a challenging, interesting career, where you are compensated according to your level of skills and how effectively you put them to use. Those with the right combination of skills and abilities may have the opportunity to advance to management positions, such as patient account managers, physician office supervisors, and medical office managers. The more education the individual has, the more employment options and advancement opportunities are available. Individuals who have practical experience using computers and patient billing software will find themselves well prepared to enter this ever-changing field.

OVERVIEW

Computers in the Medical Office is divided into four parts.

Part 1, "Introduction to Computers in the Medical Office," covers the general flow of information in a medical office and the role that computers play. Instructors may wish to use the first part as a review or, if students have had other courses in computers, they may wish to start directly with Part 2. A test has been provided in the Instructor's Manual to determine the level of students' familiarity with computers.

Part 2, "Medisoft Advanced Training," teaches students how to start, input data, and use Medisoft to bill patients, file claims, record data, print reports, and schedule appointments. The sequence takes the student through Medisoft in a clear, concise manner. Each chapter includes a number of exercises that are to be done at the computer. These exercises give the student realistic experience using an administrative medical software program.

Part 3, "Applying Your Knowledge," completes the learning process by requiring the student to perform a series of tasks using Medisoft. Each task is an application of the knowledge required in the medical office.

Part 4, "Source Documents," gives the student the data needed to complete the exercises. These forms, including patient information forms and encounter forms, are similar to those used in medical offices.

COMPUTER SUPPLIES AND EQUIPMENT

The Student Data Template found on the Online Learning Center *www.mhhe.com/cimo6e*, provides a base of case study information. Other equipment and supplies needed are as follows:

◆ PC with 500 MHz or greater processor speed

◆ 256 MB RAM

◆ 500MB available hard disk space (if saving data to hard disk)

◆ CD-ROM 2X or faster disk drive

◆ Color display

◆ External storage device for storing backup copies of the working database

◆ Mouse or compatible pointing device

◆ Windows Vista Business 32-bit version (Medisoft 14 will not work on the 64-bit system), Windows XP Professional, or Windows 2000 Professional

Medisoft™ Advanced Version 14 Patient Accounting is available to schools adopting *Computers in the Medical Office*. Information on ordering and installing the software is located in the Instructor's Manual that accompanies the text/workbook.

TO THE STUDENT

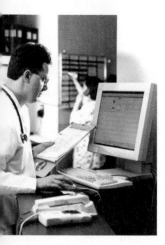

Computers in the Medical Office includes a tutorial and a simulation. Once you learn how to operate the Medisoft™ Advanced Version 14 program by completing the tutorial, you can practice those skills by working through the simulation. Both the tutorial and the simulation use a medical office setting, Family Care Center, to provide a realistic environment in which you can learn how to use the software.

Medisoft is a popular patient billing and accounting software program. It enables health care practices to maintain their billing data as well as to generate report information. The software handles all the basic tasks that a medical biller needs to effectively perform his/her job. As such, Medisoft is an excellent training tool for anyone interested in working as a medical biller. Even if you do not use Medisoft on the job, the skills you learn here will be similar to those skills needed to use almost any medical accounting program. You will learn how to perform the following tasks:

- Input patient information
- Enter patient transactions
- Create insurance claims
- Produce patient statements
- Enter payments and adjustments
- Produce reports
- Create collections letters

The prerequisite for successful completion of *Computers in the Medical Office* is an understanding of the concepts and procedures for medical coding, billing, and reimbursement. This background can be obtained by studying McGraw-Hill's related insurance titles, the briefer, focused *From Patient to Payment* (Newby) or the longer, comprehensive *Medical Insurance* (Valerius/Bayes/Newby/Seggern). Students must also possess basic computer skills, and familiarity with the Windows operating system.

After completing *Computers in the Medical Office*, students can build on their skills and enhance their qualifications for employment by studying *Case Studies for the Medical Office*, an excellent "internship in a box." *Case Studies for the Medical Office* contains a simulation covering two weeks of work in a medical office using Medisoft. In addition to providing activities through which students can practice and reinforce their basic Medisoft skills, the text/workbook introduces new Medisoft training topics which expand their knowledge.

WHAT EVERY INSTRUCTOR NEEDS TO KNOW

What's New in the Sixth Edition?

- **Medisoft™ Advanced Version 14** patient billing software, a full-featured software program, is available to adopters.

◆ Coverage of **processing refunds for patients** provides information for creating an adjustment that refunds money to a patient.

◆ **Electronic Medical Record Exchange** feature explores how billing programs and electronic health records share data and improve productivity.

◆ **Student Worksheet** feature was created in response to instructors' requests for an easier way to measure students' performance on Medisoft exercises. The Worksheets contain objective questions that require students to accurately complete the computer exercises in chapters 4-11.

◆ CIMO 6/e is written for Medisoft V14 which **includes the updated version of CMS 1500 that prints NPI information** in fields 17B and 24J.

◆ Medisoft V14 provides an option to **export reports to a PDF file** that students can email to their instructors.

Computers in the Medical Office provides your students with the opportunity to learn and perform the duties of a medical biller, using Medisoft Advanced Version 14 Patient Accounting, a computerized patient billing program. Teaching students how to use a software application such as Medisoft can be a challenging endeavor. For that reason, this text/workbook is accompanied by several teaching and learning supplements.

TEACHING AND LEARNING SUPPLEMENTS

For the Instructor

Instructor's Software Medisoft™ Advanced Version 14 CD-ROM This full working version allows a school to place the live software on the laboratory or classroom machines (only one copy needs to be sent per campus location).

Instructor's Manual includes:

◆ course overview.

◆ information on ordering Medisoft Advanced Version 14 software.

◆ lesson plans

◆ software troubleshooting tips.

◆ answer keys for the worksheets, end-of-chapter questions, and software exercises

◆ correlation tables: SCANS, AAMA Role Delineation Study Areas of Competence (2003), and AMT Registered Medical Assistant Certification Exam Topics.

After you install the software and are ready for your students to begin using the Medisoft Advanced Version 14 program, you can rely on the manual for important information that you can use to help your students work through the exercises in the book.

Instructor Productivity Center (IPC) CD-ROM (packaged with the Instructor's Manual) includes:

◆ instructor's PowerPoint® presentation of Chapters 1–11.

◆ electronic testing program featuring McGraw-Hill's EZ Test. This flexible and easy-to-use program allows instructors to create tests from book specific items. It accommodates a wide range of question types and instructors may add their own questions. Multiple versions of the test can be created and any test can be exported for use with course management systems such as WebCT, Blackboard, or PageOut.

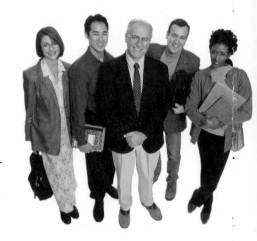

◆ Instructor's Manual.

◆ end-of-chapter Medisoft backup files for Chapters 4–15. These backup files can be used to help teachers evaluate students' work at the end of each chapter. By restoring the backup file for a given chapter, the instructor has easy access to the current state of the database when the exercises for that chapter have been completed. The backup files can also be provided to students who misplace or damage their Medisoft data file during the course of the semester.

Online Learning Center (OLC), *www.mhhe.com/cimo6e,* Instructor Resources include:

◆ Student Data Template file (contains database to be used with exercises in the book)

◆ Instructor's Manual in Word and PDF format.

◆ PowerPoint® files for each chapter.

◆ links to professional associations.

◆ Medisoft tips and frequently asked questions.

◆ Medisoft Advanced Version 14 installation instructions.

◆ Medisoft Newsletter.

◆ PageOut link.

For the Student

Student-at-Home Medisoft Advanced Version 14 This version is an option for distance education or students who want to practice with the software at home.

Student Data Template is available for download from the Online Learning Center, *www.mhhe.com/cimo6e.* The data template provides the patient database to complete Medisoft Advanced, Version 14 simulation exercises.

Online Learning Center (OLC), *www.mhhe.com/cimo6e.*

ABOUT THE AUTHOR

Susan M. Sanderson, senior technical writer for Chestnut Hill Enterprises, Inc., has developed successful products for McGraw-Hill for more than ten years. She has authored all Windows-based editions of *Computers in the Medical Office.* She has also written *Patient Billing, Case Studies for the Medical Office, Electronic Health Records for Allied Health Careers,* and Medisoft simulations for other medical office/insurance programs. Susan has worked with instructors to site-test materials and has provided technical support to McGraw-Hill customers. Susan has experience in business training, instructional design, and computer-based presentations. She is a graduate of Drew University, with further study at Columbia University.

What Every Student Needs To Know

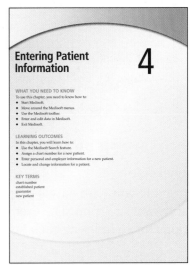

Many tools to help you learn have been integrated into your text.

CHAPTER FEATURES

What You Need To Know

lets you check whether you understand and recall the information you learned in previous chapters. Mastery of the information listed here is necessary to complete the current chapter.

Learning Outcomes

present a list of the key points you should focus on in the chapter.

Shortcuts

suggest ways to be a more efficient user of the software.

Screen Captures

show how the concepts described in the book actually appear in the medical billing software.

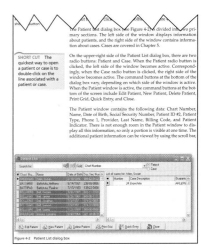

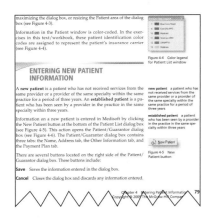

Key Terms

are introduced in the chapter opener and defined in the margin, so you will become familiar with the terms necessary to perform medical billing tasks.

Tips

provide helpful suggestions about using the medical billing software effectively.

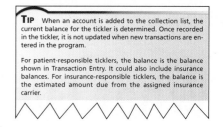

TIP When an account is added to the collection list, the current balance for the tickler is determined. Once recorded in the tickler, it is not updated when new transactions are entered in the program.

For patient-responsible ticklers, the balance is the balance shown in Transaction Entry. It could also include insurance balances. For insurance-responsible ticklers, the balance is the estimated amount due from the assigned insurance carrier.

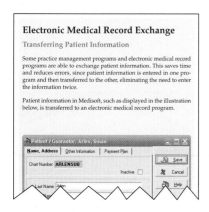

Figures

illustrate the concepts in the chapter in a visual format.

Electronic Medical Records Exchange

explores how billing programs and electronic medical records share data and improve productivity.

COMPUTER PRACTICE

Exercises

provide you with hands-on practice using a medical billing software program. The exercises offer step-by-step instructions for completing each task.

On Your Own Exercises

let you see how well you have learned the medical billing tasks in the chapter. In the On Your Own exercises, you perform tasks in the software without the help of step-by-step instructions.

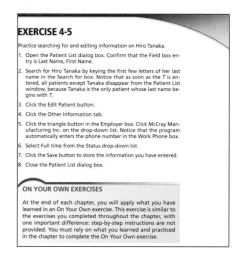

Student Worksheet

contains objective questions that require students to accurately complete the computer exercises in each chapter.

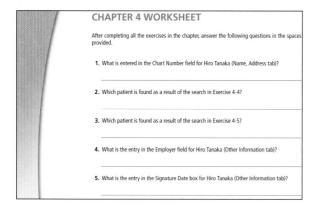

CHAPTER REVIEW

Vocabulary Review

questions check your mastery of the key terms presented in the chapter.

Checking Your Understanding

questions confirm that you understand the main topics in the chapter.

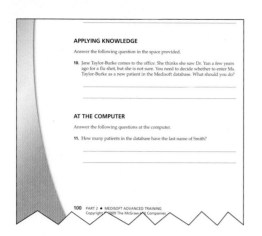

Applying Knowledge

Applying Knowledge

questions ask you to use critical thinking skills to apply what you learned in the chapter to different situations.

At The Computer

At The Computer

activities offer you a chance to demonstrate the software skills you learned on the computer.

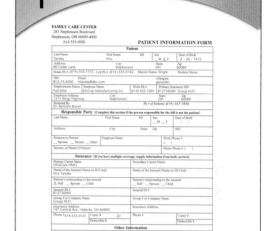

SOURCE DOCUMENTS

Source Documents

are facsimiles of typical documents and forms you would work with in a medical practice. These documents provide you with the information you need to complete the software exercises in the book.

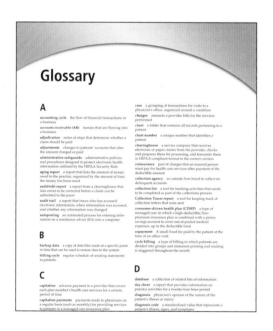

THE GLOSSARY

Glossary

at the back of the book makes it easy to find a definition of a term.

ONLINE LEARNING CENTER (OLC)

www.mhhe.com/cimo6e

The OLC offers additional learning and teaching tools.

In addition to the Student Data Template file, the site includes additional chapter quizzes, flash cards, and installation instructions for Medisoft Advanced Version 14 at home software.

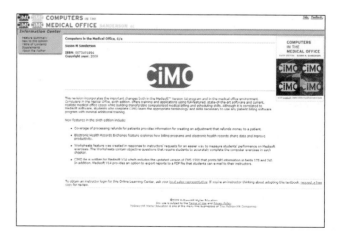

Acknowledgments

For insightful reviews, criticisms, helpful suggestions, and information, we would like to acknowledge the following:

Sixth Edition Reviewers

Katie Barton, BA, LPN
Director of Allied Health
Savannah River College

Nia J. Bullock, PhD
Miller-Motte College

Denise Carsillo, MS, BS, AS, RMA
Lincoln College of Technology

Patricia Casey, BBE
Trident Technical College

Stephanie Cox, BS
YTI - Career Institute

Darlene K. Edwards, AA, BS, MEd
Bellingham Technical College

Anita Ferguson
Paris Junior College

Daniel F. Gant, BS, M. Div.
Savannah River College

Jim Irwin, MS, BS
Everest College

Colleen A. King, CPC, CCP
National College of Business

Jamie Leigh, BA
Assistant Professor
Bluegrass Community and Technical College

Loreen W. MacNichol, CMRS, RMC
Andover College

Krista Mahan, MA
Walla Walla Community College

Elizabeth W. McKinley, BBA, MS, JD
San Jacinto Community College

Mrs. Bronna McNeely, MBA
American Commercial College

Darlene Owen
S.E. School for Career Development

Pamela K. Roemershauser, CPC
MedVance Institute

Nina Thierer, CMA, BS, CPC, CCAT
Ivy Tech Community College of Indiana

Carole A. Zeglin, MS, BS, RMA
Director Medical Assistant Program
Westmoreland County Community College

Sixth Edition Focus Group

Yvonne Alles
Davenport University
Grand Rapids, MI

Stacey Ashford
Remington College
Cleveland, OH

Stacey Burks-Bradley
Everest Institute
Eagan, MN

Dorothea Cabral
Keiser University
Fort Lauderdale, FL

Christina Conklin, AA, RMA, CPEd.
Keiser University
Lakeland, FL

Anne Fielden
Medix School—Education Affiliates
Smyrna, GA

Emma Hill, CMA
Everest Institute
Southfield, MI

Kelley Lamb
Everest Insitute
Kalamazoo, MI

Tanjya Thomas
Everest Institute
Eagan, MN

Marta Urdaneta, PhD.
Keiser University
Fort Lauderdale, FL

Lisa Wallis, BS, RMA
Keiser University
Tampa, FL

Fifth Edition Reviewers

Marion Bucci
Delaware Technical and Community College

Kelley Fazzone
Blair College

Nona Stinemetz
Vatterott College

Geiselle Thompson
Quality Staffing Specialists
Cary, NC

Valeria D. Truitt
Craven Community College

Terri D. Wyman, CMRS
Sanford Brown Institute

Symposium Participants

Kelli Batton
Career Technical College

Gladys Hamic
McLennon Community College

Denise Harris
Georgia Medical Institute

Amy Lee
Valencia Community College

Samantha Lopez
Career Point Institute

Wilsetta McClain
Baker College

Angela Parmley
Sanford Brown Institute

Cari McPherson
Ross Medical Education Center

Elaine Miyamoto
Robert Morris College

Yolanda Savoy
Medical Career Institute

Lillia Torres
Florida Career College

How Can I Succeed In This Class?

An important step in effective learning begins with a solid study strategy. Many students feel overwhelmed when learning new concepts and a new software program at the same time. The following study tips will help ensure your success in this course.

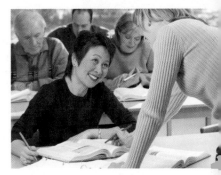

"You are the same today that you are going to be five years from now except for two things: the people with whom you associate and the books you read."
—Charles Jones

Right now, you're probably leafing through this book feeling just a little overwhelmed. You're trying to juggle several other classes (which probably are equally as intimidating), possibly a job, and on top of it all, a life.

It's true—you are what you put into your studies. You have a lot of time and money invested in your education. Don't blow it now by only putting in half of the effort this class requires. Succeeding in this class (and life) requires:

◆ A commitment—of time and perseverance
◆ Knowing and motivating yourself
◆ Getting organized
◆ Managing your time

This special introduction has been designed specifically to help you learn how to be effective in these areas, as well as offer guidance in:

◆ Getting the most out of your lecture
◆ Thinking through—and applying—the material
◆ Getting the most out of your textbook
◆ Finding extra help when you need it

MAKING A COMMITMENT—OF TIME AND PERSEVERANCE

Learning—and mastering—takes time. And patience. Nothing worthwhile comes easily. Be committed to your studies and you will reap the benefits in the long run.

Consider this: your accounting courses are building the foundation for your future—a future in your chosen profession. Sloppy and hurried craftsmanship now will only lead to ruins later.

> **SIDE NOTE:** A good rule of thumb is to allow 2 hours of study time for every hour you spend in lecture.

KNOWING AND MOTIVATING YOURSELF

What type of a learner are you? When are you most productive? Know yourself and your limits and work within them. Know how to motivate yourself to give your all to your studies and achieve your goals. Quite bluntly, you are the one that benefits most from your success. If you lack self-motivation and drive, you are the first person that suffers.

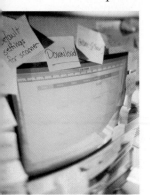

Knowing yourself—There are many types of learners, and no right or wrong way of learning. Which category do you fall into?

◆ **Visual learner**—You respond best to "seeing" processes and information. Particularly focus on the text's figures and tables.

◆ **Auditory learner**—You work best by listening to—and possibly tape recording—the lecture and by talking information through with a study partner. Be sure not to miss any lectures.

◆ **Tactile/Kinesthetic Learner**—You learn best by being "hands on." You'll benefit by applying what you've learned during lab time. Think of ways to apply your critical thinking skills in application ways. Be sure to complete all the computer exercises in the textbook.

Identify your own personal preferences for learning and seek out the resources that will best help you with your studies. Also, learn by recognizing your weaknesses and try to compensate/work to improve them

GETTING ORGANIZED

It's simple, yet it's fundamental. It seems the more organized you are, the easier things come. Take the time before your course begins to look around and analyze your life and your study habits. Get organized now and you'll find you have a little more time—and a lot less stress.

◆ **Find a calendar system that works for you.** The best kind is one that you can take with you everywhere. To be truly organized, you should integrate all aspects of your life into this one calendar—school, work, leisure. Some people also find it helpful to have an additional monthly calendar posted by their desk for "at a glance" dates and to have a visual of what's to come. If you do this, be sure you are consistently synchronizing both calendars as not to miss anything. *More tips for organizing your calendar can be found in the time management discussion on the next page.*

◆ **Keep everything for your course or courses in one place**—and at your fingertips. A three-ring binder works well because it allows you to add or organize handouts and notes from class in any order you prefer. Incorporating your own custom tabs helps you flip to exactly what you need at a moments notice.

◆ **Find your space.** Find a place that helps you be organized and focused. If it's your desk in your dorm room or in your home, keep it clean. Clutter adds confusion, stress, and wastes time. Or perhaps your "space" is at the library. If that's the case, keep a backpack or bag that's fully stocked with what you might need—your text, binder or notes, pens, highlighters, Post-its, phone numbers of study partners

(hint: a good place to keep phone numbers is in your "one place for everything calendar").

MANAGING YOUR TIME

Managing your time is the single most important thing you can do to help yourself. And, it's probably one of the most difficult tasks to successfully master.

> **A HELPFUL HINT**
> add extra "padding" into your deadlines to yourself. If you have an assignment due on Friday, set a goal for yourself to have it done on Wednesday. Then, take time on Thursday to look over your work again, with a fresh eye. Make any corrections or enhancements and have it ready to turn in on Friday.

You are taking this course because you want to succeed in life. You are preparing for a career. You are expected to work much harder and to learn much more than you ever have before. To be successful you need to invest in your education with a commitment of time.

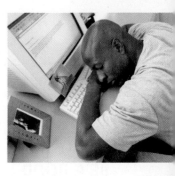

How Time Slips Away

People tend to let an enormous amount of time slip away from them, mainly in three ways:

1. **procrastination,** putting off chores simply because we don't feel in the mood to do them right away
2. **distraction,** getting sidetracked by the endless variety of other things that seem easier or more fun to do, often not realizing how much time they eat up
3. **underestimating the value of small bits of time,** thinking it's not worth doing any work because we have something else to do or somewhere else to be in 20 minutes or so.

We all lead busy lives. But we all make choices as to how we spend our time. Choose wisely and make the most of every minute you have by implementing these tips.

Know Yourself and When You'll Be Able to Study Most Efficiently

When are you most productive? Are you a late nighter? Or an early bird? Plan to study when you are most alert and can have uninterrupted segments. This could include a quick 5-minute review before class or a one-hour problem solving study session with a friend.

Create a Set Study Time for Yourself Daily

Having a set schedule for yourself helps you commit to studying, and helps you plan instead of cram. Find—and use—a planner that is small enough that you can take with you—everywhere. This can be a $2.50 paper calendar or a more expensive electronic version. They all work on the same premise—**organize *all* of your activities in one place.**

Less is more. Schedule study time using shorter, focused blocks with small breaks. Doing this offers two benefits:

1. You will be less fatigued and gain more from your effort, and
2. Studying will seem less overwhelming and you will be less likely to procrastinate.

Plan Time For Leisure, Friends, Family, Exercise, and Sleep

Studying should be your main focus, but you need to balance your time—and your life.

Try to complete tasks ahead of schedule. This will give you a chance to carefully review your work before you hand it in (instead of at 1 a.m. when you are half awake). You'll feel less stressed in the end.

Prioritize!

In your calendar or planner, highlight or number key projects; do them first, and then cross them off when you've completed them. Give yourself a pat on the back for getting them done!

Try to resist distractions by setting and sticking to a designated study time (remember your commitme and perseverance!) Distractions may include friends and surfing the Internet . . .

Multitask When Possible

You may find a lot of extra time you didn't think you had. Review material or organize your ter your head while walking to class, doing laundry, or during "mental down time." (Note—menta does NOT mean in the middle of lecture.)

GETTING THE MOST OUT OF LECTURES

Believe it or not, instructors want you to succeed. They put a lot of effort into helping yc their lectures. Attending class is one of the simplest, most valuable things you can d doesn't end there. . . . getting the most out of your lectures means being organize'

xxii

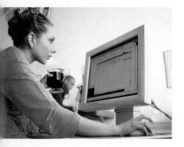

PREPARE BEFORE YOU GO TO CLASS

Really! You'll be amazed at how much more comprehensible the material will be when you preview the chapter before you go to class. Don't feel overwhelmed by this already. One tip that may help you—plan to arrive to class 5-15 minutes before lecture. Bring your text with you and skim the chapter before lecture begins. This will at the very least give you an overview of what may be discussed.

BE A GOOD LISTENER

Most people think they are good listeners, but few really are. Are you?

Obvious, but important points to remember:

1. You can't listen if you are talking.

2. You aren't listening if you are daydreaming.

3. Listening and comprehending are two different things. If you don't understand something your instructor is saying, ask a question or jot a note and visit the instructor after hours. Don't feel dumb or intimidated; you probably aren't the only person who "doesn't get it."

TAKE GOOD NOTES

1. Use a standard size notebook, and better yet, a three-ring binder with loose leaf notepaper. The binder will allow you to organize and integrate your notes and handouts, integrate easy-to-reference tabs, etc.

2. Use a standard black or blue ink pen to take your initial notes. You can annotate later using a pencil, which can be erased if need be.

3. Start a new page with each lecture or note taking session (yes—you can and should also take notes from your textbook).

4. Label each page with the date and a heading for each day.

5. Focus on main points and try to use an outline format to take notes to capture key ideas and organize sub-points.

6. Review and edit your notes shortly after class—at least within 24 hours—to make sure they make sense and that you've recorded core thoughts. You may also want to compare your notes with a study partner later to make sure neither of you have missed anything.

GET A STUDY PARTNER

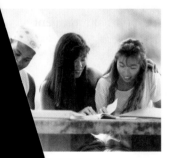

Having a study partner has so many benefits. First, he/she can help you keep your commitment to this class. By having set study dates, you can combine study and social time, and maybe even make it fun! In addition, you now have two sets of eyes and ears and two minds to help digest the information from lecture and from the text. Talk through concepts, compare notes, and quiz each other.

An obvious note: Don't take advantage of your study partner by skipping class or skipping study dates. You obviously won't have a study partner—or a friend— much longer if it's not a mutually beneficial arrangement!

INTRODUCTION TO COMPUTERS IN THE MEDICAL OFFICE

Chapter 1
The Medical Office Billing Process

Chapter 2
Information Technology and HIPAA

The Medical Office Billing Process

1

LEARNING OUTCOMES

When you finish this chapter, you will be able to:

◆ Describe the billing and reimbursement cycle in a medical office.

◆ Discuss the type of information collected from patients.

◆ Identify the major types of health plans.

◆ Describe the information recorded about a patient's office visit.

◆ Discuss the process of adjudication.

◆ Discuss the process required to balance a medical office's accounts.

◆ Explain the importance of collections in the medical office.

KEY TERMS

accounting cycle
accounts receivable (AR)
adjudication
billing cycle
capitation
coding
coinsurance
consumer-driven health plan (CDHP)
copayment
diagnosis
diagnosis code
encounter form
explanation of benefits (EOB)
fee-for-service
health maintenance organization (HMO)

health plan
managed care
medical coder
medical necessity
modifier
patient information form
payer
policyholder
practice management program (PMP)
preferred provider organization (PPO)
premium
procedure
procedure code
remittance advice (RA)
statement

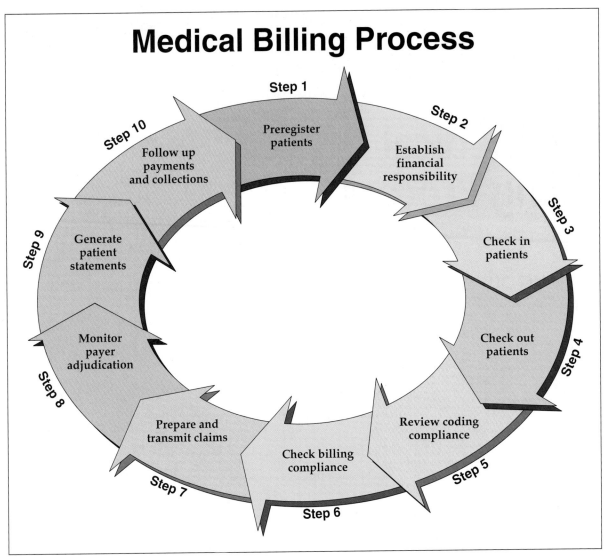

Medical Billing Process

Step 1 Preregister patients

Step 2 Establish financial responsibility

Step 3 Check in patients

Step 4 Check out patients

Step 5 Review coding compliance

Step 6 Check billing compliance

Step 7 Prepare and transmit claims

Step 8 Monitor payer adjudication

Step 9 Generate patient statements

Step 10 Follow up payments and collections

Figure 1-1 Billing and reimbursement cycle.

From a business standpoint, the key to the financial health of a medical practice is billing and collecting fees for services. Without a steady flow of money coming in, payrolls cannot be met; supplies cannot be ordered; and utility bills cannot be paid. To maintain a regular cash flow, specific billing tasks must be completed on a regular schedule. The billing process consists of ten steps that result in timely payment for patients' medical services (see Figure 1-1).

STEP 1: PREREGISTER PATIENTS

The first step in the billing and reimbursement process is to gather information so patients can be preregistered before their office visit. This information includes the patient's name, contact information, reason for visit, and whether the patient is new to the practice. The information is obtained over the telephone or via the Internet, if the practice has a web site.

STEP 2: ESTABLISH FINANCIAL RESPONSIBILITY FOR VISIT

Many patients are covered by some type of insurance. It is important to ask whether the patient has insurance and, if so, to find out the specific type of coverage. This should be done before the patient arrives for the appointment. Physicians usually participate in some insurance plans and not in others; this information must be provided to the patient before the office visit, since it will affect the amount the patient will pay. For example, if the physician does not participate in an insurance plan, the patient may be liable for all charges.

Medical insurance represents an agreement between a person, known as the **policyholder,** and a **health plan.** A health plan is any plan, program, or organization that provides health benefits; it may be an insurance company, also called a carrier, a government program, or a managed care organization (MCO). Payments made to the health plan by the policyholder for insurance coverage are called **premiums.** In exchange for the payments, the health plan agrees to pay for the insured's medical services according to the terms of the insurance policy or agreement.

policyholder a person who buys an insurance plan; the insured.

health plan a plan, program, or organization that provides health benefits.

premium the periodic amount of money the insured pays to a health plan for insurance coverage.

OVERVIEW OF MEDICAL INSURANCE

There are many sources of medical insurance in the United States. Most policyholders are covered by group policies, often through their employers. Some people have individual plans. Insurance coverage may be supplied by a private company, such as CIGNA, or by a government plan. CMS—Centers for Medicare and Medicaid Services—runs the Medicare and Medicaid programs. The most common government plans are:

◆ **Medicare** Medicare is a federal health plan that covers persons aged sixty-five and over, people with disabilities, and dependent widows.

◆ **Medicaid** People with low incomes who cannot afford medical care are covered by Medicaid, which is cosponsored by federal and state governments. Qualifications and benefits vary by state.

◆ **TRICARE** TRICARE is a government program that covers medical expenses for dependents of active-duty members of the uniformed services and for retired military personnel. Formerly known as CHAMPUS, it also covers dependents of military personnel who were killed while on active duty.

◆ **CHAMPVA** The Civilian Health and Medical Program of the Veterans Administration is for veterans with permanent service-related disabilities and their dependents. It also covers surviving spouses and dependent children of veterans who died from service-related disabilities.

◆ **Workers' compensation** People with job-related illnesses or injuries are covered under workers' compensation insurance. Workers' compensation benefits vary according to state law.

Whether it is a private company or a government program, the health plan is called a **payer.** The term *third-party payer* is also used, because the primary relationship is between the provider and the patient, and the health plan is the third party.

payer private or government organization that insures or pays for health care on the behalf of beneficiaries.

Different types of medical insurance can be purchased. In a **fee-for-service** plan, which was the first type of plan to be widely used, policyholders are repaid for costs of health care due to illnesses and accidents. The policy lists the medical services that are covered and the amounts that are paid. The benefit may be for all or part of the charges. For example, the policy may indicate that 80 percent of charges for surgery are covered and that the policyholder is responsible for paying the other 20 percent. The portion of charges that an insured person must pay is known as **coinsurance.**

fee-for-service health plan that repays the policyholder for covered medical expenses.

coinsurance part of charges that an insured person must pay for health care services after payment of the deductible amount.

Another type of insurance is known as **managed care.** Most people who are insured through their employers are covered by some form of managed care. Managed care organizations control both the financing and the delivery of health care to policyholders. The managed care organization establishes contracts with physicians and other health care providers that control fees.

managed care a type of insurance in which the carrier is responsible for both the financing and the delivery of health care.

In some managed care plans, providers are paid a fixed amount per month to provide necessary, contracted services to patients who are plan members. This fixed payment is referred to as **capitation.** The rate the provider is paid is based on several factors, including the number of plan members in the insured pool and their ages. The capitated rate per enrollee is paid to the provider even if the provider does not provide any medical services to the patient during the time period covered by the payment. Similarly, the provider receives the same capitated rate if a patient is treated more than once during the time period. In other plans, negotiated per-service fees are paid. These fees are less than the regular rate for a service that the provider normally charges.

capitation advance payment to a provider that covers each plan member's health care services for a certain period of time.

The most common type of managed care health plan is a **preferred provider organization (PPO).** A PPO is a network of providers under contract with a managed care organization to perform services for plan members at discounted fees. Usually, members may choose to receive care from other doctors or providers outside the network, but they pay a higher cost.

preferred provider organization (PPO) managed care network of health care providers who agree to perform services for plan members at discounted fees.

Another common type of managed care system is a **health mainte-nance organization (HMO)**. In an HMO, providers are paid fixed rates at regular intervals, such as monthly, that cover any services they need for that period. In some HMOs, a patient also pays a **copayment**—a small fixed fee, such as $20—at the time of an office visit. Usually, patients in an HMO must choose from a specific group of health care providers. If they seek services from a provider who is not in the health plan, the payer does not pay for the care.

A **consumer-driven health plan** (CDHP) is a type of managed care insurance in which a high-deductible/low-premium insurance plan is combined with a pretax savings account to cover out-of-pocket medical expenses, up to the deductible limit. These plans typically include three elements. The first is an insurance plan, usually a PPO, with a high deductible (such as $1,000) and low premiums.

The second element is a designated "savings account" that is used to pay medical bills before the deductible has been met. The savings account, similar to an Individual Retirement Account (IRA), lets people set aside untaxed wages to cover their out-of-pocket medical expenses. Some employers contribute to employees' accounts as a benefit. If money is left in the account at the end of a plan year, it rolls over to help cover the next year's health expenses.

The third element of a CDHP is access to informational tools that help consumers make informed decisions about their healthcare, such as plan-sponsored websites. Since the patient is purchasing health care services directly, both insurance companies and employers believe that paying for medical services causes patients to be educated, efficient consumers of health care.

health maintenance organization (HMO) a managed health care system in which providers agree to offer health care to the organization's members for fixed periodic payments from the plan.

copayment A small fixed fee paid by the patient at the time of an office visit.

consumer-driven health plan (CDHP) a type of managed care in which a high-deductible/low-premium insurance plan is combined with a pretax savings account to cover out-of-pocket medical expenses, up to the deductible limit.

STEP 3: CHECK IN PATIENTS

When a patient arrives in the office, additional information is collected. If they have not already done so via the Internet, patients asked to complete a patient information form. The **patient information form** contains the personal, employment, and medical insurance information needed to collect payment for the provider's services. This form, illustrated in Figure 1-2, becomes part of the patient's medical record and is updated when the patient reports a change, such as a new address or different medical insurance. Most offices ask all patients to update these forms periodically to ensure that the information is current and accurate.

The patient information form requires the patient's signature or a parent's or guardian's signature if the patient is a minor, mentally incapacitated, or incompetent. The signature authorizes the health

patient information form form that includes a patient's personal, employment, and insurance data needed to complete an insurance claim.

FAMILY CARE CENTER
285 Stephenson Boulevard
Stephenson, OH 60089-4000
614-555-0000

PATIENT INFORMATION FORM

Patient				
Last Name	First Name	MI	Sex __ M __ F	Date of Birth / /
Address	City		State	Zip
Home Ph # ( )	Cell Ph # ( )	Marital Status		Student Status
SS#	Email		Allergies	
Employment Status	Employer Name	Work Ph # ( )	Primary Insurance ID#	
Employer Address	City		State	Zip
Referred By		Ph # of Referral ( )		

Responsible Party (Complete this section if the person responsible for the bill is not the patient)

Last Name	First Name	MI	Sex __ M __ F	Date of Birth / /
Address	City	State Zip		SS#
Relation to Patient __ Spouse __ Parent __ Other	Employer Name		Work Phone # ( )	
Spouse, or Parent (if minor):			Home Phone # ( )	

Insurance (If you have multiple coverage, supply information from both carriers)

Primary Carrier Name	Secondary Carrier Name
Name of the Insured (Name on ID Card)	Name of the Insured (Name on ID Card)
Patient's relationship to the insured __ Self __ Spouse __ Child	Patient's relationship to the insured __ Self __ Spouse __ Child
Insured ID #	Insured ID #
Group # or Company Name	Group # or Company Name
Insurance Address	Insurance Address
Phone #	Copay $	Phone #	Copay $
	Deductible $		Deductible $

Other Information

Is patient's condition related to:	Reason for visit:
__ Employment __ Auto Accident (if yes, state in which accident occurred: ___) __ Other Accident	
Date of Accident: / / Date of First Symptom of Illness: / /	

Financial Agreement and Authorization for Treatment

I authorize treatment and agree to pay all fees and charges for the person named above. I agree to pay all charges shown by statements, promptly upon their presentation, unless credit arrangements are agreed upon in writing.

I authorize payment directly to FAMILY CARE CENTER of insurance benefits otherwise payable to me. I hereby authorize the release of any medical information necessary in order to process a claim for payment in my behalf.

Signed: _____   Date: _____

Figure 1-2 Patient information form.

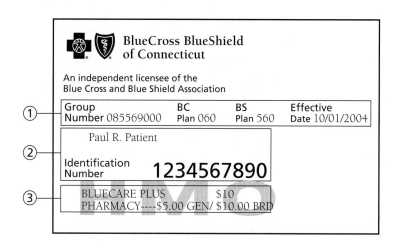

1. **Group identification number**
   The 9-digit number used to identify the member's employer.

   Blue Cross Blue Shield plan codes
   The numbers used to identify the codes assigned to each plan by the Blue Cross Blue Shield Association: used for claims submissions when medical services are rendered out-of-state.

   Effective date
   The date on which the member's coverage became effective.

2. **Member name**
   The full name of the cardholder.

   Identification number
   The 10-digit number used to identify each Anthem Blue Cross and Blue Shield of Connecticut or BlueCare Health Plan member.

3. **Health plan**
   The name of the health plan and the type of coverage; usually lists any copayment amounts, frequency limits or annual maximums for home and office visits; may also list the member's annual deductible amount.

   Riders
   The type(s) of riders that are included in the member's benefits (DME, Visions).

   Pharmacy
   The type of prescription drug coverage; lists copayment amounts.

Figure 1-3 Sample insurance identification card.

plan or government program to send payments directly to the provider rather than to the patient. The signature also indicates that the patient accepts responsibility for payment of all charges not paid by the health plan, and authorizes the release of information required to process an insurance claim.

During check-in, it is also common practice to photocopy the patient's insurance identification card (see Figure 1-3). Once the insurance information is obtained, the patient's current eligibility and benefits are verified with the payer. Verification may be done by telephone; it can also be checked via the Internet. At this time, it is also important to make sure that the health plan's conditions for payment, such as preauthorization requirements, are met before treatment is provided.

Payments may be collected from the patient during check-in. Payments may be made by cash, check, or credit/debit card. When a payment is made, a receipt is given to the patient. Copayments are routinely collected during check-in. In addition, if a patient owes a balance to the practice, this amount is also collected, or arrangements for payment are made. New patients receive information about the practice's financial policy, so they understand that they are responsible for payment of charges that are not paid by their health plans.

While physician practices have always expected patients to pay copayments when they come in for care, some medical offices are now asking patients for partial payment of the office visit charges during check-in. The amount of the partial payment is the estimated patient responsibility for the procedure. For example, if the fee for a procedure is $80.00, and the patient is responsible for 20 percent of charges, the patient may be asked to pay $16.00 at check-in. Since it is not always possible to accurately estimate a patient's financial obligation at check-in, offices usually base the patient's share on the average charge for the scheduled service. The prepayments are usually low enough that few patients overpay.

STEP 4: CHECK OUT PATIENTS

encounter form a list of the procedures and charges for a patient's visit.

During an office visit, a physician evaluates and treats a patient's condition. This information about the evaluation and treatment is documented on an **encounter form,** also known as a superbill (see Figure 1-4). The information may also be recorded electronically, on a tablet or laptop computer, or on a personal digital assistant (PDA). Whether captured via paper or an electronic device, the information collected is the same: the patient's diagnosis and the services performed by the physician.

diagnosis physician's opinion of the nature of the patient's illness or injury.

procedure medical treatment provided by a physician or other health care provider.

coding the process of assigning standardized codes to diagnoses and procedures.

The **diagnosis** is the physician's opinion of the nature of the patient's illness or injury, and the **procedures** are the services performed. When diagnoses and procedures are reported to health plans, code numbers are used in place of descriptions. **Coding** is a way of translating a description of a condition into a shorter, standardized code. Standardization allows information to be shared among physicians, office personnel, health plans, and so on, without losing the precise meaning.

diagnosis code a standardized value that represents a patient's illness, signs, and symptoms.

A patient's diagnosis is communicated to a health plan as a **diagnosis code,** a code found in the *International Classification of Diseases,*

ENCOUNTER FORM

DATE _____   TIME _____

PATIENT NAME _____   CHART # _____

OFFICE VISITS - SYMPTOMATIC

NEW

99201	OF--New Patient Minimal	
99202	OF--New Patient Low	
99203	OF--New Patient Detailed	
99204	OF--New Patient Moderate	
99205	OF--New Patient High	

ESTABLISHED

99211	OF--Established Patient Minimal	
99212	OF--Established Patient Low	
99213	OF--Established Patient Detailed	
99214	OF--Established Patient Moderate	
99215	OF--Established Patient High	

PREVENTIVE VISITS

NEW

99381	Under 1 Year	
99382	1 - 4 Years	
99383	5 - 11 Years	
99384	12 - 17 Years	
99385	18 - 39 Years	
99386	40 - 64 Years	
99387	65 Years & Up	

ESTABLISHED

99391	Under 1 Year	
99392	1 - 4 Years	
99393	5 - 11 Years	
99394	12 - 17 Years	
99395	18 - 39 Years	
99396	40 - 64 Years	
99397	65 Years & Up	

PROCEDURES

12011	Simple suture--face--local anes.	
29125	App. of short arm splint; static	
29425	App. of short leg cast, walking	
50390	Aspiration of renal cyst by needle	
71010	Chest x-ray, single view, frontal	

PROCEDURES

71020	Chest x-ray, two views, frontal & lateral	
71030	Chest x-ray, complete, four views	
73070	Elbow x-ray, AP & lateral views	
73090	Forearm x-ray, AP & lateral views	
73100	Wrist x-ray, AP & lateral views	
73510	Hip x-ray, complete, two views	
73600	Ankle x-ray, AP & lateral views	

LABORATORY

80019	19 clinical chemistry tests	
80048	Basic metabolic panel	
80061	Lipid panel	
82270	Blood screening, occult; feces	
82947	Glucose screening--quantitative	
82951	Glucose tolerance test, three specimens	
83718	HDL cholesterol	
84478	Triglycerides test	
85007	Manual differential WBC	
85018	Hemoglobin	
85651	Erythrocyte sedimentation rate--non-auto	
86580	TB Mantoux test	
87072	Culture by commercial kit, nonurine...	
87076	Culture, anaerobic isolate	
87077	Bacterial culture, aerobic isolate	
87086	Urine culture and colony count	
87430	Strep test	
87880	Direct streptococcus screen	

INJECTIONS

90471	Immunization administration	
90703	Tetanus injection	
90772	Injection	
92516	Facial nerve function studies	
93000	Electrocardiogram--ECG with interpretation	
93015	Treadmill stress test, with physician...	
96900	Ultraviolet light treatment	
99070	Supplies and materials provided	

FAMILY CARE CENTER
286 Stephenson Blvd.
Stephenson, OH 60089
614-555-0000

☐ DANA BANU, M.D.
☐ ROBERT BEACH, M.D.
☐ PATRICIA MCGRATH, M.D.

☐ JESSICA RUDNER, M.D.
☐ JOHN RUDNER, M.D.
☐ KATHERINE YAN, M.D.

NOTES

REFERRING PHYSICIAN   NPI   AUTHORIZATION #

DIAGNOSIS

PAYMENT AMOUNT

Figure 1-4 Encounter form.

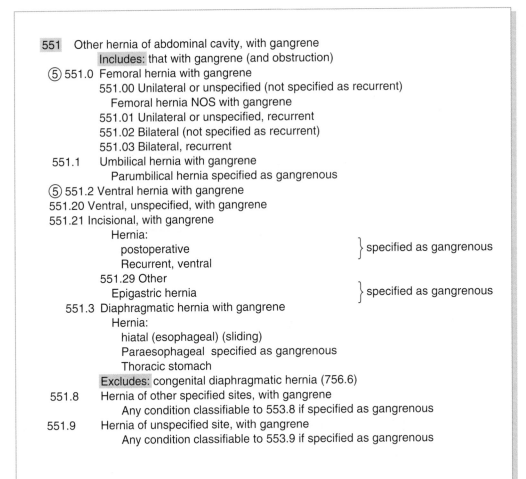

| 551 | Other hernia of abdominal cavity, with gangrene |
| | Includes: that with gangrene (and obstruction) |

⑤ 551.0 Femoral hernia with gangrene
   551.00 Unilateral or unspecified (not specified as recurrent)
      Femoral hernia NOS with gangrene
   551.01 Unilateral or unspecified, recurrent
   551.02 Bilateral (not specified as recurrent)
   551.03 Bilateral, recurrent
551.1 Umbilical hernia with gangrene
   Parumbilical hernia specified as gangrenous
⑤ 551.2 Ventral hernia with gangrene
551.20 Ventral, unspecified, with gangrene
551.21 Incisional, with gangrene
   Hernia:
      postoperative   } specified as gangrenous
      Recurrent, ventral
   551.29 Other
      Epigastric hernia   } specified as gangrenous
551.3 Diaphragmatic hernia with gangrene
   Hernia:
      hiatal (esophageal) (sliding)
      Paraesophageal specified as gangrenous
      Thoracic stomach
   Excludes: congenital diaphragmatic hernia (756.6)
551.8 Hernia of other specified sites, with gangrene
   Any condition classifiable to 553.8 if specified as gangrenous
551.9 Hernia of unspecified site, with gangrene
   Any condition classifiable to 553.9 if specified as gangrenous

Figure 1-5 Sample of ICD codes.

Ninth Revision, *Clinical Modification* (ICD-9-CM) (see Figure 1-5). Diagnosis codes provide health plans with very specific information about the patient's specific illness(es), sign(s), and symptom(s). For example, the code for Alzheimer's disease is 331.0, and the code for influenza with bronchitis or with a cold is 487.1.

procedure code   a code that identifies a medical service.

Similarly, each procedure the physician performs is assigned a **procedure code** that stands for the particular service, treatment, or test. This code is selected from the *Current Procedural Terminology* (CPT) (see Figure 1-6). A large group of codes cover the physician's evaluation and management of a patient's condition during office visits or visits at other locations, such as nursing homes. Other codes cover groups of specific procedures, such as surgery, pathology, and radiology. For example, 99431 is the CPT code for the physician's examination of a newborn infant, and the code for a total hip replacement is 27130. Codes can also be followed by one or more modifiers. A CPT **modifier** is a two-digit character that is appended to a CPT code to report special circumstances involved with a procedure or service.

modifier   a two-digit character that is appended to a CPT code to report special circumstances involved with a procedure or service.

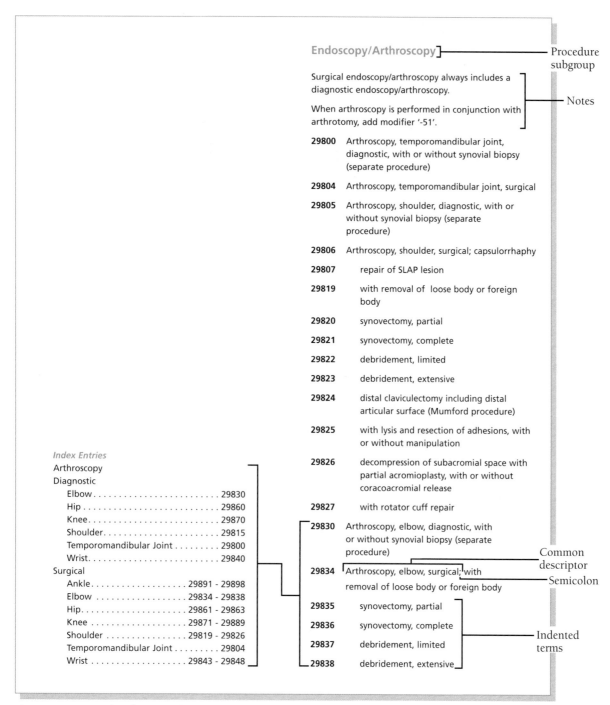

Figure 1-6 Sample of CPT codes.

Procedure and diagnosis codes are entered into a **practice management program (PMP),** which is a software program that automates many of the administrative and financial tasks required to run a medical practice. For example, the PMP is used to process the financial transactions that result from patients' appointments. The program calculates charges for the office visit, estimates patient and insurance financial responsibilities, and creates insurance claims. The software is also used to record patients' payments, provide

practice management program (PMP) a software program that automates many of the administrative and financial tasks required to run a medical practice.

receipts, and compute patients' outstanding account balances. Later, when insurance payments are received, those payments are posted to patients' accounts, reducing the balance that the patients owe.

STEP 5: REVIEW CODING COMPLIANCE

Whether physicians are paid by health plans for treating patients depends in part on the diagnosis and procedure codes assigned to the office visit. The medical office staff member who does the coding must have specialized knowledge. In some medical practices, the physicians assign these codes; in others, a **medical coder** or a medical insurance specialist handles this task.

medical coder a person who analyzes and codes patient diagnoses, procedures, and symptoms.

In the area of coding, compliance involves following official guidelines of the American Hospital Association and the American Medical Association when codes are assigned. After they are selected, diagnosis and procedure codes must be checked for errors. Also, the diagnosis and the medical services that are documented in the patient's medical record should be logically connected, so that the **medical necessity** of the charges is clear to the insurance company.

medical necessity treatment provided by a physician to a patient for the purpose of preventing, diagnosing, or treating an illness, injury, or its symptoms in a manner that is appropriate and provided in accordance with generally accepted standards of medical practice.

Medical necessity is defined differently by different insurance plans. The American Medical Association (AMA) has defined medical necessity as "services or products that a prudent physician would provide to a patient for the purpose of preventing, diagnosing, or treating an illness, injury, or its symptoms in a manner that is: (1) in accordance with generally accepted standards of medical practice; (2) clinically appropriate in terms of type, frequency, extent, site, and duration; and (3) not primarily for the convenience of the patient, physician, or other health care provider." If medical necessity is not met, the physician will not receive payment from the health plan.

STEP 6: CHECK BILLING COMPLIANCE

Each charge, or fee, for a visit is related to a specific procedure code. The provider's fees for services are listed on the medical practice's fee schedule. Most medical practices have a standard fee schedule listing their usual fees. However, the fees listed on the master fee schedule are not necessarily the amount the provider will be paid. Many providers enter into contracts with insurance plans that require a discount from standard fees.

In addition, although there is a separate fee associated with each code, each code is not necessarily billable. Whether it can be billed depends on the payer's particular rules. Following these rules when preparing claims results in billing compliance. Some payers include particular codes in the payment for another code. Medical insurance specialists apply their knowledge of payer guidelines to analyze what can be billed on health care claims.

STEP 7: PREPARE AND TRANSMIT CLAIMS

To receive payment, medical practices must produce documents for health plans and patients. One kind of document is an insurance claim. For a health plan to pay a claim, certain information about the patient must be shared. For example, a health plan needs to know the procedures the provider performed while the patient was in the office, as well as the date and location of the visit.

Health plans also require basic information about the provider who is treating the patient, including the provider's name and identification number. Beyond the basic information requirements that are common to all payers, there are differences in what information is required on an insurance claim. A payer lists the required information in a provider's manual that is available to the medical office.

In general, the information needed to create a claim is found on two documents—the patient information form and the encounter form. For the most part, health care claims are created using practice management programs and are sent electronically to health plans.

STEP 8: MONITOR PAYER ADJUDICATION

When the claim is received by the payer, it is reviewed following a process known as **adjudication**—a series of steps designed to judge whether it should be paid. Claims may be paid in full, partially paid, or denied. The results of the adjudication process are explained in a document that is sent to the provider along with the payment. This document is called a **remittance advice (RA)** or **explanation of benefits (EOB)** (see Figure 1-7). The remittance advice provides details about each patient transaction, such as:

◆ Date of service

◆ Services provided

◆ Patient insurance identification number

adjudication series of steps that determine whether a claim should be paid.

remittance advice (RA) an explanation of benefits transmitted electronically by a payer to a provider.

explanation of benefits (EOB) paper document from a payer that shows how the amount of a benefit was determined.

EAST OHIO PPO
10 CENTRAL AVENUE
HALEVILLE, OH 60890

PROVIDER REMITTANCE

FAMILY CARE CENTER
285 STEPHENSON BLVD.
STEPHENSON, OH 60089

PAGE:	1 OF 1
DATE:	11/12/2010
ID NUMBER:	4679323

PROVIDER: PATRICIA MCGRATH, M.D.

PATIENT: BROOKS LAWANA   CLAIM: 234567890

FROM DATE	THRU DATE	PROC CODE	UNITS	AMOUNT BILLED	AMOUNT ALLOWED	DEDUCT	COPAY/ COINS	PROV PAID	REASON CODE
10/29/10	10/29/10	99212	1	54.00	48.60	.00	20.00	28.60	
10/29/10	10/29/10	73600	1	96.00	86.40	.00	.00	86.40	
	CLAIM TOTALS			150.00	135.00	.00	20.00	115.00	

PATIENT: HSU DIANE   CLAIM: 345678901

FROM DATE	THRU DATE	PROC CODE	UNITS	AMOUNT BILLED	AMOUNT ALLOWED	DEDUCT	COPAY/ COINS	PROV PAID	REASON CODE
10/29/10	10/29/10	99213	1	72.00	64.80	.00	20.00	44.80	
10/29/10	10/29/10	80048	1	50.00	45.00	.00	.00	45.00	
	CLAIM TOTALS			122.00	109.80	.00	20.00	89.80	

PROVIDER: DANA BANU, M.D.

PATIENT: PATEL RAJI   CLAIM: 567890123

FROM DATE	THRU DATE	PROC CODE	UNITS	AMOUNT BILLED	AMOUNT ALLOWED	DEDUCT	COPAY/ COINS	PROV PAID	REASON CODE
10/29/10	10/29/10	99212	1	54.00	48.60	.00	20.00	28.60	
	CLAIM TOTALS			54.00	48.60	.00	20.00	28.60	

PATIENT: SYZMANSKI MICHAEL   CLAIM: 678901234

FROM DATE	THRU DATE	PROC CODE	UNITS	AMOUNT BILLED	AMOUNT ALLOWED	DEDUCT	COPAY/ COINS	PROV PAID	REASON CODE
10/29/10	10/29/10	99212	1	54.00	48.60	.00	20.00	28.60	
	CLAIM TOTALS			54.00	48.60	.00	20.00	28.60	

PAYMENT SUMMARY		TOTAL ALL CLAIMS		EFT INFORMATION	
TOTAL AMOUNT PAID	262.00	AMOUNT CHARGED	380.00	NUMBER	4679323
PRIOR CREDIT BALANCE	.00	AMOUNT ALLOWED	342.00	DATE	11/12/10
CURRENT CREDIT DEFERRED	.00	DEDUCTIBLE	.00	AMOUNT	262.00
PRIOR CREDIT APPLIED	.00	COPAY	.00		
NEW CREDIT BALANCE	.00	COINSURANCE	80.00		
NET DISBURSED	262.00				

STATUS CODES:
A - APPROVED   AJ - ADJUSTMENT   IP - IN PROCESS   R - REJECTED   V - VOID

Figure 1-7   Remittance advice.

- Provider identifier number
- Amount allowed by contract
- Amount paid provider
- Amount owed by patient

Usually, an RA is sent electronically to providers; patients receive a paper EOB. When the RA arrives at the provider's office, it is reviewed for accuracy. The medical insurance specialist compares each payment and explanation with the claim to check that:

- All procedures that were listed on the claim also appear on the payment transaction.
- Any unpaid charges are explained.
- The codes on the payment transactions match those on the claim.
- The payment listed for each procedure is as expected.

If any discrepancies are found when reviewing the RA, a request for a review of the claim is filed with the payer. In this process, the medical insurance specialist follows payers' or state rules to seek appropriate reimbursement for a claim. Occasionally, an overpayment may be received, and a refund check is issued by the medical practice.

Once the RA is reviewed, the amount of the payment (whether a paper check or an electronic payment) is recorded in the practice management program. Depending on the rules of the health plan, the patient may be billed for an outstanding balance. In other circumstances, an adjustment is made in the software and the patient is not billed.

STEP 9: GENERATE PATIENT STATEMENTS

If charges are billed to the patient, a statement is created in the practice management program and mailed to the patient. The **statement** lists all services performed, along with the charges for each service (see Figure 1-8). The statement lists the amount paid by the health plan and the remaining balance that is the responsibility of the patient.

statement a list of all services performed for a patient, along with the charges for each service.

Most medical practices have a regular schedule, referred to as a **billing cycle,** for sending statements to patients. For example, some practices bill half the patients on the fifteenth of the month and the other half on the thirtieth.

billing cycle regular schedule of sending statements to patients.

Family Care Center
285 Stephenson Boulevard
Stephenson, OH 60089
(614)555-0000

Statement Date	Chart Number	Page
09/30/2010	SMITHJA0	1

Make Checks Payable To:
Family Care Center
285 Stephenson Boulevard
Stephenson, OH 60089
(614)555-0000

James L. Smith
17 Blacks Lane
Stephenson, OH 60089

Date of Last Payment: 9/10/2010 Amount: -168.00 Previous Balance: 0.00

Patient: James L. Smith Chart Number: SMITHJA0 Case: Facial nerve paralysis

Dates	Procedure	Charge	Paid by Primary	Paid By Guarantor	Adjustments	Remainder
09/09/10	92516	210.00	-168.00		0.00	42.00

Amount Due
42.00

Figure 1-8 Patient statement.

STEP 10: FOLLOW UP PATIENT PAYMENTS AND HANDLE COLLECTIONS

accounting cycle the flow of financial transactions in a business.

accounts receivable (AR) monies that are flowing into a business.

The **accounting cycle** is the flow of financial transactions in a business—from making a sale to collecting payment for the goods or services delivered. In a medical practice, this is the cycle from treating the patient to receiving payments for services provided. Practice management software can be used to track **accounts receivable (AR)**—monies that are coming into the practice—and to produce financial reports.

At the end of each day, a report is generated that lists all charges, payments, and adjustments that occurred during that day (see Figure 1-9). To balance out a day, transactions listed on encounter forms (charges, payments, and adjustments) and totals from bank deposit entries are compared against the end-of-day report.

A monthly report summarizes the financial activity of the entire month. This report lists charges, payments, and adjustments and the total accounts receivable for the month. It is possible to balance out the month by totaling the daily charges, payments, and adjustments and then comparing the totals to the amounts listed on the monthly report.

Family Care Center
Patient Day Sheet
Ending 9/6/2010

Entry	Date	Document	POS	Description	Provider	Code	Modifier	Amount
ARLENSU0		**Susan Arlen**						
359	9/6/2010	1009060000	11		5	99212		54.00
361	9/6/2010	1009060000	11		5	EAPCPAY		-20.00
		Patient's Charges $54.00		Patient's Receipts -$20.00	Adjustments $0.00			Patient Balance $34.00
BELLHER0		**Herbert Bell**						
364	9/6/2010	1009060000	11		2	EAPCPAY		-20.00
362	9/6/2010	1009060000	11		2	99211		36.00
		Patient's Charges $36.00		Patient's Receipts -$20.00	Adjustments $0.00			Patient Balance $16.00
BELLJAN0		**Janine Bell**						
368	9/6/2010	1009060000	11		3	EAPCPAY		-20.00
365	9/6/2010	1009060000	11		3	99213		72.00
366	9/6/2010	1009060000	11		3	73510		124.00
		Patient's Charges $196.00		Patient's Receipts -$20.00	Adjustments $0.00			Patient Balance $176.00
BELLJON0		**Jonathan Bell**						
371	9/6/2010	1009060000	11		3	EAPCPAY		-20.00
369	9/6/2010	1009060000	11		3	99394		222.00
		Patient's Charges $222.00		Patient's Receipts -$20.00	Adjustments $0.00			Patient Balance $202.00
BELLSAM0		**Samuel Bell**						
372	9/6/2010	1009060000	11		2	99212		54.00
374	9/6/2010	1009060000	11		2	EAPCPAY		-20.00
		Patient's Charges $54.00		Patient's Receipts -$20.00	Adjustments $0.00			Patient Balance $34.00
BELLSAR0		**Sarina Bell**						
375	9/6/2010	1009060000	11		3	99213		72.00
377	9/6/2010	1009060000	11		3	EAPCPAY		-20.00
		Patient's Charges $72.00		Patient's Receipts -$20.00	Adjustments $0.00			Patient Balance $52.00

Figure 1-9   A sample page from a patient day sheet report.

It is also good practice to print reports that list the outstanding balances owed to the practice on a frequent basis. Regular review of these reports can alert the billing staff to accounts that require action to collect the amount due. A collection process is often started when patient payments are later than permitted under the practice's financial policy. Overdue accounts require diligent follow-up to maintain the practice's cash flow. Insurance claims that are not paid in a timely manner also require follow-up, to determine the reason for the non-payment and resubmit or appeal as appropriate.

CHAPTER REVIEW

USING TERMINOLOGY

Match the terms on the left with the definitions on the right.

_____ **1.** accounting cycle

_____ **2.** accounts receivable (AR)

_____ **3.** capitation

_____ **4.** coinsurance

_____ **5.** copayment

_____ **6.** diagnosis code

_____ **7.** encounter form

_____ **8.** explanation of benefits (EOB)

_____ **9.** fee-for-service

_____ **10.** health maintenance organization (HMO)

_____ **11.** health plan

_____ **12.** managed care

_____ **13.** patient information form

_____ **14.** payer

_____ **15.** policyholder

_____ **16.** preferred provider organization (PPO)

_____ **17.** premium

a. A paper document from a health plan that lists the amount of a benefit and explains how it was determined.

b. A document that contains personal, employment, and medical insurance information about a patient.

c. A form listing procedures relevant to the specialty of a medical office, used to record the procedures.

d. Private or government organization that insures or pays for health care.

e. An electronic document from a health plan that lists the amount of a benefit and explains how it was determined.

f. A small fixed fee paid by the patient at the time of an office visit.

g. An individual who has contracted with a health plan for coverage.

h. A payment made to a health plan by a policyholder for coverage.

i. A fixed amount that is paid to a provider in advance to provide medically necessary services to patients.

j. A type of insurance in which the carrier is responsible for the financing and delivery of health care.

k. A term used to describe money coming in to a business.

l. A type of managed care system in which providers are paid fixed rates at regular intervals.

m. An insurance plan in which policyholders are reimbursed for health care costs.

_____ **18.** procedure code

_____ **19.** remittance advice (RA)

n. Under an insurance plan, the portion or percentage of the charges that the patient is responsible for paying.

o. A network of health care providers who agree to provide services to plan members at a discounted fee.

p. A value that stands for a patient's illness, signs, or symptoms.

q. A number that represents medical procedures performed by a provider.

r. The flow of financial transactions in a business.

s. A plan, program, or organization that provides health benefits.

CHECKING YOUR UNDERSTANDING

Write "T" or "F" in the blank to indicate whether you think the statement is true or false.

20. Many patient information forms contain a place for the patient to sign to authorize the patient's health plan to send payments directly to a provider. _____

21. CPT-4 codes have eight digits. _____

22. *Coinsurance* refers to a small fixed fee that must be paid by the patient at the time of an office visit. _____

Answer the question below in the space provided.

23. List the ten steps in the billing and reimbursement cycle.

_____

_____

_____

Choose the best answer.

_____ 24. A patient information form contains information such as name, address, employer, and:

    a. procedure code

    b. insurance coverage information

    c. charges for procedures performed

_____ 25. A health maintenance organization (HMO) is one example of:

    a. a fee-for-service health plan

    b. a government plan

    c. a managed care health plan

_____ 26. In a managed care health plan, a _____ is usually collected from the patient at the office visit.

    a. deductible

    b. patient statement

    c. copayment

_____ 27. The most commonly used system of medical procedure codes is found in the:

    a. CPT

    b. ICD

    c. CMS-1500

_____ 28. Information about a patient's medical procedures that is needed to create an insurance claim is found on the:

    a. remittance advice

    b. encounter form

    c. patient information form

Information Technology and HIPAA

2

LEARNING OUTCOMES

When you finish this chapter, you will be able to:

◆ Discuss the role of information technology in medical offices.

◆ Describe the features of electronic medical record systems.

◆ Discuss the advantages of electronic prescribing.

◆ Explain the functions of a practice management program.

◆ Explain the role of a clearinghouse in processing electronic claims.

◆ Describe the purpose of the Health Insurance Portability and Accountability Act of 1996 (HIPAA).

◆ Explain how the HIPAA Electronic Transaction and Code Sets standards relate to insurance claims.

◆ Discuss how the HIPAA Privacy Rule protects patient health information.

◆ Describe the safeguards outlined in the HIPAA Security Rule.

KEY TERMS

administrative safeguards
audit/edit report
audit trail
autoposting
clearinghouse
CMS-1500 (08/05)
electronic data interchange (EDI)
electronic funds transfer (EFT)
electronic medical record (EMR)
electronic prescribing
HIPAA (Health Insurance Portability and Accountability Act of 1996)

HIPAA Electronic Transaction and Code Sets standards
HIPAA Privacy Rule
HIPAA Security Rule
information technology (IT)
National Provider Identifier (NPI)
physical safeguards
protected health information (PHI)
technical safeguards
walkout statement
X12-837 Health Care Claim (837P)

In the past, most administrative and financial tasks in medical offices were done on paper. Physicians' schedules were completed by hand in appointment books, and insurance claims were filled in by hand or typed on paper forms. Payments arrived in the mail from patients and insurance companies; bank deposit slips were prepared; and funds were deposited at the local bank.

Today, the health care industry is moving away from paper processes and relying instead on computers to accomplish daily tasks. The computer hardware and software that makes this automation possible is called **information technology (IT).**

information technology (IT) development, management, and support of computer-based hardware/software systems

MEDICAL OFFICE APPLICATIONS

The major applications of IT in medical practices are electronic medical records, electronic prescribing, and practice management. The following sections describe these uses of technology and highlight their advantages and disadvantages.

ELECTRONIC MEDICAL RECORDS

Information technology is increasingly used for storing, accessing, and sharing health information electronically. **Electronic medical record (EMR)** systems store physicians' reports of examinations, surgical procedures, tests, X-rays, and other clinical information. In addition to documenting patient care, EMR programs also provide access to data for research and quality improvement purposes. Some of the features and benefits of EMRs include:

electronic medical record (EMR) electronic collection and management of health data

◆ **Immediate access to health information** The EMR is accessible from workstations in the office as well as from remote sites such as hospitals, all at the same time. Retrieval of the information from an EMR is almost immediate, which is critical in emergency situations. Compared to sorting through papers in a paper folder, an EMR database can save seconds and even minutes when searching for vital patient information. Once information is updated in a patient record, the new information is immediately available to all who need access, whether across the hall or across town.

◆ **Computerized physician order management** Physicians can enter orders for medications, tests, and other services at any time. This information is then instantly transmitted to staff members for implementation.

◆ **Clinical decision support** An EMR system can provide access to the latest medical research to facilitate medical decision making.

◆ **Automated alerts and reminders** The system can provide medical alerts and reminders for office staff members to ensure that patients are scheduled for regular screenings and other preventive practices. Alerts can also be created to identify patient safety issues, such as possible drug interactions.

◆ **Electronic communication and connectivity** An EMR system can provide secure and easily accessible communication between physicians and staff members and, in some offices, between physicians and patients.

◆ **Patient support** Some EMR programs offer tools that allow patients to access their medical records and to request appointments electronically. The programs also offer patient education on health topics and instructions on preparing for common medical tests, such as an HDL cholesterol test.

◆ **Administrative and reporting** The EMR may include administrative tools including reporting systems that enable medical practices to comply with federal and state reporting requirements.

◆ **Error reduction** An EMR can decrease medical errors that are a result of illegible chart notes, since notes are no longer entered manually. The notes are entered electronically using a computer or a handheld device. However, the accuracy of the information in the EMR is only as good as the accuracy of the person entering the data into the computer device; it is still possible to click the wrong button or enter the wrong letter.

Despite these features and benefits, medical practices have been slow to change from paper to EMR systems. There are a number of reasons for this delay. A major obstacle to EMR implementation is the startup cost required to change to an electronic system. Electronic medical record systems. The cost of an EMR ranges from $3,621 to $32,000 per physician, according to a 2008 report from the AC Group, a research company, with more sophisticated programs at the higher end of the range.

Another disadvantage of EMRs is the learning curve required for staff members to become proficient users of the new technology. Practices may not have enough time available to train staff members on a new system.

Confidentiality and security concerns are also associated with EMR implementation. The storage of patient information on a computer and its transmission from one computer to another present significant risks. This topic is addressed later in this chapter in the section on the privacy and security of health information.

ELECTRONIC PRESCRIBING

Electronic prescribing refers to the use of computers and handheld devices to write and transmit prescriptions to a pharmacy in a secure digital format. Electronic prescribing systems range from simple

electronic prescribing the use of computers and handheld devices to write and transmit prescriptions to a pharmacy in a secure digital format.

solutions that record and send prescriptions to more complex programs that suggest the best drug for a patient based on the patient's medical history, the insurance coverage, and the overall effectiveness of the medication.

Electronic prescribing eliminates problems created by handwritten prescriptions. Illegible prescriptions not only slow down the prescribing process; they can also lead to dispensing and dosing errors at the pharmacy.

Most electronic systems include drug reference information, such as that found in the PDR (*Physician's Desk Reference*). Information about drug effectiveness, interactions, and standard dosing can assist the physician in selecting the best medication for a particular patient and condition.

Electronic prescribing can reduce problems resulting from inappropriate prescribing and drug interactions. Critical information about a patient's medical and medication history is available to the physician at the time the prescription is written. The patient's medical record is checked for known allergies and possible drug interactions. Used in this manner, electronic prescribing can prevent adverse drug interactions.

PRACTICE MANAGEMENT

Most offices use a practice management program (PMP) to complete routine office tasks, including patient scheduling, recording patient information, creating and transmitting electronic claims, receiving electronic payments, billing patients, creating financial reports, and collecting on overdue accounts. Some PMP's are capable of receiving data from electronic medical record programs. For example, an EMR can transmit information about patient visits to the PMP, including the patient's diagnosis and the services performed.

Practice management programs are critical to a medical office's survival, since accurate and timely records are required to determine whether the practice is profitable. These records are also important in meeting financial obligations and tax-reporting requirements.

Not all medical offices use the same PMP, but most programs operate in a similar manner. Initially, the program is prepared for use by entering basic facts about the practice itself. Often a computer consultant or an accountant helps set up these records. Information about many aspects of the business is recorded, including:

◆ Information about each patient, such as name, address, contact numbers, insurance coverage, and more

- Information about each provider, including facts about providers, referring providers, and outside providers such as labs

- Data about the health plans used by the practice's patients

- Codes used by the practice to note a diagnosis and the treatment provided, as well as the facility where the treatment was provided

Once all these data are in the program, the software can be used to perform many of the daily tasks of a medical practice. Medisoft, the practice management program used in *Computers in the Medical Office,* is one example of a PMP used in medical offices. The following sections provide additional information about the use of these programs.

Appointments

Practice management programs contain a computerized scheduling feature to keep track of patient appointments. (Chapter 11 covers this topic in depth.) When a patient telephones and requests an appointment, the program is used to search for an available time slot and to enter the appointment. Figure 2-1 shows an example of a computerized appointment schedule.

Each morning, the program prints a list of appointments for each provider in the practice. Appointments can easily be canceled or rescheduled, and the program also stores information about time reserved for hospital rounds, surgeries, seminars, lunches, vacations, and so on.

A major advantage of computerized scheduling is the ability to easily locate scheduled appointments. For example, if a patient calls to ask when her or his next appointment is scheduled, the medical

Family Care Center

Yan, Katherine   **Tuesday, September 7, 2010**

Time	Name	Phone	Length	Notes
Tuesday, September 07, 2010				
8:00a	Staff Meeting		60	
9:00a	Ramos, Maritza	(614)315-2233	30	
10:00a	Fitzwilliams, Sarah	(614)002-1111	15	
10:30a	Gardiner, John	(614)726-9898	15	
10:45a	Jones, Elizabeth	(614)123-5555	30	
12:00p	Lunch		60	

Figure 2-1 Sample computerized physician schedule.

office assistant enters the patient's name, and the program locates the appointment.

Computer scheduling also simplifies the entry of repeated appointments. Rather than looking through an appointment book for acceptable dates and times, the computer program performs the search and displays available dates and times.

Claims and Billing

The creation of accurate and timely insurance claims and patient statements is critical to a practice's financial survival. To generate claims and statements, a practice management program requires two basic types of information:

◆ **Patient data** Personal information about the patient, as well as information on the patient's medical insurance coverage

◆ **Transaction data** The date of the visit, the location of the treatment, the diagnosis and procedure codes, and the payments made at the time of the office visit

When patient and transaction information has been entered in the PMP and checked for accuracy, the software creates insurance claims. To transmit electronic claims, a medical office may send claims directly to a health plan or may employ a clearinghouse. A **clearinghouse** is a company that collects electronic insurance claims from medical practices and forwards the claims to the appropriate health plans (see Figure 2-2). Clearinghouses also translate claim data to fit the standard format required for physician claims.

clearinghouse a service company that receives electronic or paper claims from the provider, checks and prepares them for processing, and transmits them in HIPAA-compliant format to the correct carriers.

When a clearinghouse receives a claim, it performs an edit—a check to see that all necessary information is included in the claim file. It checks for missing data and obvious errors, such as procedures performed on a date that occurred before the patient's date of birth.

audit/edit report a report from a clearinghouse that lists errors to be corrected before a claim can be submitted to the payer.

After the basic edit is complete, an **audit/edit report** is sent from the clearinghouse to the practice. This report lists problems that need to be corrected before the claim can be sent to the health plan (see Figure 2-3). Ensuring "clean" claims before transmission greatly reduces the number of claim rejections and speeds payment.

Reimbursement

Physicians receive reimbursement for services from health plans and from patients. If a patient makes a payment at the time of an office visit, the amount is entered into the practice management program, and a **walkout statement** is given to the patient. A walkout statement lists the procedures performed, the charges for the procedures, and the amount paid by the patient (see Figure 2-4).

walkout statement a document listing charges and payments that is given to a patient after an office visit.

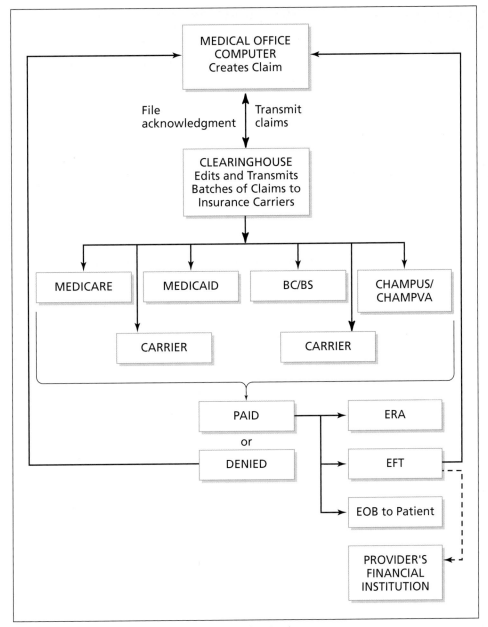

Figure 2-2 Example of claim flow using a clearinghouse.

A remittance advice (RA) with payment from a health plan usually pays for a number of patients and claims at once. The payments listed on the RA are entered in the practice management program (PMP) and applied to each patient's account. This process may be done manually as the medical office assistant matches payments with individual patient transactions in the PMP, and posts the payments in the program. Some practices use an automated process called **autoposting** to record this information in the program. In autoposting, the electronic data in the remittance advice is automatically posted to patient accounts in the PMP. While this approach saves the time that would be required to manually

autoposting an automated process for entering information on a remittance advice (RA) into a computer.

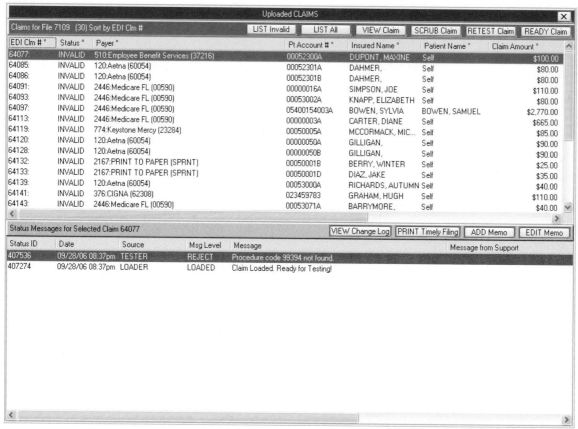

Figure 2-3 Sample audit/edit report.

enter the information, the application of payments still must be reviewed by a person to determine if any payments are not as expected.

ADVANTAGES OF COMPUTER USE

It is easy to understand why IT applications are so important in today's medical offices, since many tasks can be performed more efficiently using technology. As a result, computer literacy is now a requirement for employment in a medical office. In physician practices, there are a number of advantages to performing common tasks with computers:

◆ Information is stored in electronic files that can be used by more than one person at a time. The office's computers are linked together in a network that allows users to share files. Without a network, it is difficult for one person to review or update a document if another person is using it.

◆ Information is easy to find. Instead of looking in file cabinets and folders, staff members can retrieve patient information in a matter of seconds. Computerized databases also eliminate the problem of misplaced patient folders or charts.

Family Care Center
285 Stephenson Boulevard
Stephenson, OH 60089
(614)555-0000

Page: 1   9/6/2010

Patient:	Susan Arlen	**Instructions:**
	310 Oneida Lane	Complete the patient information portion of your insurance
	Stephenson, OH 60089	claim form. Attach this bill, signed and dated, and all other
		bills pertaining to the claim. If you have a deductible policy,
Chart #:	ARLENSU0	hold your claim forms until you have met your deductible.
Case #:	24	Mail directly to your insurance carrier.

Date	Description	Procedure	Modify	Dx 1	Dx 2	Dx 3	Dx 4	Units	Charge
9/6/2010	OF--established patient, low	99212		466.0				1	54.00
9/6/2010	East Ohio PPO Copayment	EAPCPAY						1	-20.00

Figure 2-4   Sample patient walkout statement.

◆ Less storage space is required for computer files, since data are stored on computer media such as CDs, not on paper. Storage space has been a major problem for medical offices, since they are required to keep patient records for a long time before discarding them.

◆ Computer databases are more efficient than manual filing systems; they save enormous amounts of time in a medical practice. For example, when medical records are stored electronically, a staff member does not have to pull patient charts at the start of each day and refile them at the end of the day. In addition, physicians can quickly access and update records as they see patients, using computer equipment in examining rooms.

◆ Computer use can reduce some types of errors. When using computers, information is entered once, checked for errors, and then used over and over again. For example, a patient's address and insurance policy number are entered once andaccessed when needed to create claims, bills, or correspondence.

A NOTE OF CAUTION: WHAT COMPUTERS CANNOT DO

While computers increase the efficiency of a practice and reduce errors, they are no more accurate than the individual entering the data. Many human errors occur during data entry, such as pressing the wrong key on the keyboard. Other errors are due to a lack of computer literacy—not knowing how to use a program to accomplish tasks. If people make mistakes while entering data, the information the computer produces will be incorrect.

Computers are very precise and also very unforgiving. While the human brain knows that *flu* is short for *influenza*, the computer does not know this, and it regards flu and influenza as two distinct conditions. If a computer user accidentally enters a name as *ORourke* instead of *O'Rourke*, a person might know what is meant; the computer does not. It would probably respond with a message such as "No such patient exists in the database." For this reason, proper training in the use of computer programs is essential for medical office personnel.

HIPAA AND ELECTRONIC EXCHANGE OF INFORMATION

The increasing reliance on computers to store and exchange information continues to present a number of technical and security challenges. In the early 1990s, health care industry leaders, the Department of Health and Human Services (DHHS), and the U.S. Congress became increasingly concerned about the lack of standardization in the business of health care. At that time, it was estimated that more than four hundred different formats existed for the electronic processing of health claims. In addition, at least twenty-six cents of each health care dollar was going toward administrative costs, such as:

◆ Enrolling an individual in a health plan

◆ Paying health insurance premiums

◆ Checking eligibility

◆ Obtaining authorization to refer a patient to a specialist

◆ Processing claims

◆ Notifying a provider about the payment of a claim

HIPAA (Health Insurance Portability and Accountability Act of 1996) federal act that set forth guidelines for standardizing the electronic data interchange of administrative and financial transactions, exposing fraud and abuse in government programs, and protecting the security and privacy of health information.

In 1996, as a result of ongoing work, Congress passed the **Health Insurance Portability and Accountability Act of 1996 (HIPAA).** The act is the most significant legislation affecting the health care field since the Medicare and Medicaid programs were introduced in 1965. The legislation was designed to:

◆ Ensure the portability of insurance coverage as employees moved from job to job

◆ Increase accountability and decrease fraud and abuse in healthcare

- Improve the efficiency of health care transactions and mandate standards for health information

- Ensure the security and privacy of health information

One section of the legislation, known as HIPAA Administrative Simplification legislation, focuses on mandating nationwide standards for health information and protecting the security and privacy of health information. This legislation contains a number of rules, including:

1. HIPAA Electronic Transaction and Code Sets standards

2. HIPAA Privacy Rule

3. HIPAA Security Rule

4. Final Enforcement Rule

HIPAA ELECTRONIC TRANSACTION AND CODE SETS STANDARDS

HIPAA legislation seeks to reduce administrative costs and to minimize complexities in the health care industry by requiring the use of standardized electronic formats for the transmission of administrative and financial data. The **HIPAA Electronic Transaction and Code Sets standards** describe a particular electronic format that providers and health plans must use to send and receive health care transactions. The Centers for Medicare and Medicaid (CMS) is responsible for enforcing the Electronic Transaction and Code Sets Standards.

HIPAA Electronic Transaction and Code Sets standards regulations requiring electronic transactions such as claim transmission to use standardized formats.

The electronic transmission of data—called **electronic data interchange (EDI)**—involves sending information from computer to computer. Many different EDI systems have been used in health care, causing a confusing array of software programs required to decipher messages.

electronic data interchange (EDI) the exchange of routine business transactions from one computer to another using publicly available communications protocols.

To address this situation, the HIPAA legislation standardized EDI formats. HIPAA states that any practice working with electronic transactions must send and receive data in a standard format. The electronic formats are based on EDI standards called ASC X12, after the initials of the national committee that developed them, and a number has been assigned to each standard transaction.

The HIPAA standards cover electronic transactions that are frequently exchanged between medical offices and health plans and that contain patient-identifiable health-related administrative information, including health claims, health plan eligibility, enrollment and disenrollment, payments for care and health plan premiums, claim status, first injury reports, coordination of benefits, and others. The electronic formats are referred to as:

- **X12-270/271 Health Care Eligibility Benefit Inquiry and Response** Questions and answers about whether patients' health plans cover planned treatments and procedures

- **X12-276/277 Health Care Claim Status Request and Response** Questions and answers between providers—such as medical offices and hospitals—and payers about claims that are due to be paid

- **X12-278 Health Care Services Review—Request for Review and Response** Questions and answers between patients, or providers on their behalf, and managed care organizations for approval to see medical specialists

- **X12-835 Claims Payment and Remittance Advice** The payment and RA are sent from the payer to the provider; the payment may be via **electronic funds transfer (EFT)** from the payer directly to the provider's bank, similar to an ATM transaction

- **X12-837 Health Care Claim or Encounter** Data about the billing provider who requests payment, the patient, and the diagnoses/procedures that a provider sends to a payer

In most physician practices, the claim format is the HIPAA-standard **X12-837 Health Care Claim,** or **837P.** This claim is called the professional claim because it is used to bill for a physician's services. A hospital's claim is called an institutional claim, and there are also HIPAA dental claims and drug claims. Some small medical offices are exempt from the HIPAA requirement to send electronic claims. These practices use the **CMS-1500 (08/05)** paper claim, which is the currently mandated paper claim form.

Practices that use clearinghouses to transmit 837P claims are required by HIPAA to have a contract that has procedures that the business associate must follow to ensure compliance with HIPAA rules on privacy, security, and transactions.

In addition to standards for electronic transactions for claims, the Administrative Simplification legislation establishes standard medical code sets for use in health care transactions. For example, ICD-9-CM codes are required for diagnoses, and CPT-4 codes are mandated for procedures.

HIPAA legislation also requires the use of a national standard identifier for all health care providers. In the past, each health plan assigned a unique identification number to a provider. It was common for a provider to have a different identification number for each health plan; Medicare used a Unique Physician Identification Number (UPIN), Blue Cross and Blue Shield assigned provider numbers, and

electronic funds transfer (EFT) a system that transfers money electronically.

X12-837 Health Care Claim (837P) HIPAA standard format for electronic transmission of a professional claim from a provider to a health plan.

CMA-1500 (08/05) The mandated paper claim form that can be used in some practices of less than 10 fulltime employees.

other plans also had unique provider identifiers. The **National Provider Identifier (NPI)** is a ten-position numerical identifier consisting of all numbers. The numbers do not contain any information about health care providers, such as the state in which they practice or their provider type or specialization. Under HIPAA legislation, any individual or organization that provides health care services must obtain an NPI. *Individual* refers to physicians, dentists, nurses, chiropractors, pharmacists, physical therapists, and others; *organization* includes hospitals, home health agencies, clinics, nursing homes, laboratories, and others. The NPI replaces all previous identification numbers.

National Provider Identifier (NPI) a standard identifier for all health care providers consisting of ten numbers.

PRIVACY REQUIREMENTS

As part of the Administrative Simplification provisions, the **HIPAA Privacy Rule** protects individually identifiable health information. Health information is information about a patient's past, present, or future physical or mental health or payment for health care. If this information can be used to find out the person's identification, it is referred to as **protected health information (PHI).** Except for treatment, payment, and health care operations, the Privacy Rule limits the release of protected health information without the patient's consent. The Final Enforcement Rule mandates that the Privacy Rule is enforced by the Office for Civil Rights.

HIPAA Privacy Rule regulations for protecting individually identifiable information about a patient's past, present, or future physical and mental health and payment for health care that is created or received by a health care provider.

protected health information (PHI) information about a patient's past, present, or future physical or mental health or payment for health care that can be used to identify the person.

The privacy rule must be followed by all covered entities—health plans, health care clearinghouses, and health care providers—and their business associates. The rules mandate that a covered entity must:

◆ Adopt a set of privacy practices that are appropriate for its health care services

◆ Notify patients about their privacy rights and how their information can be used or disclosed

◆ Train employees so that they understand the privacy practices

◆ Appoint a staff member to be the privacy official responsible for seeing that the privacy practices are adopted and followed

◆ Secure patient records containing individually identifiable health information so that they are not readily available to those who do not need them

Under the HIPAA Privacy Rule, medical practices must have a written Notice of Privacy Practices (see Figure 2-5). This document describes the medical office's practices regarding the use and disclosure of PHI. It also establishes the office's privacy complaint procedures, explains that disclosure is limited to the minimum necessary information, and discusses how consent for other types of information release is obtained. Medical practices are required to display the Notice of Privacy Practices in a prominent place in the office. The office must make a good-faith effort to obtain a patient's written

NOTICE OF PRIVACY PRACTICES

OUR COMMITMENT TO YOUR PRIVACY

Our practice is dedicated to maintaining the privacy of your protected health information (PHI). In conducting our business, we will create records regarding you and the treatment and services we provide to you. We are required by law to maintain the confidentiality of health information that identifies you. We also are required by law to provide you with this notice of our legal duties and the privacy practices that we maintain in our practice concerning your PHI. By federal and state law, we must follow the terms of the notice of privacy practices that we have in effect at the time.

We realize that these laws are complicated, but we must provide you with the following important information:

- How we may use and disclose your PHI
- Your privacy rights in your PHI
- Our obligations concerning the use and disclosure of your PHI

The terms of this notice apply to all records containing your PHI that are created or retained by our practice. We reserve the right to revise or amend this Notice of Privacy Practices. Any revision or amendment to this notice will be effective for all of your records that our practice has created or maintained in the past, and for any of your records that we may create or maintain in the future. Our practice will post a copy of our current Notice in our offices in a visible location at all times, and you may request a copy of our most current Notice at any time.

WE MAY USE AND DISCLOSE YOUR PROTECTED HEALTH INFORMATION (PHI) IN THE FOLLOWING WAYS:

The following categories describe the different ways in which we may use and disclose your PHI.

1. Treatment. Our practice may use your PHI to treat you. For example, we may ask you to have laboratory tests (such as blood or urine tests), and we may use the results to help us reach a diagnosis. We might use your PHI in order to write a prescription for you, or we might disclose your PHI to a pharmacy when we order a prescription for you. Many of the people who work for our practice — including, but not limited to, our doctors and nurses — may use or disclose your PHI in order to treat you or to assist others in your treatment. Additionally, we may disclose your PHI to others who may assist in your care, such as your spouse, children or parents. Finally, we may also disclose your PHI to other health care providers for purposes related to your treatment.

2. Payment. Our practice may use and disclose your PHI in order to bill and collect payment for the services and items you may receive from us. For example, we may contact your health insurer to certify that you are eligible for benefits (and for what range of benefits), and we may provide your insurer with details regarding your treatment to determine if your insurer will cover, or pay for, your treatment. We also may use and disclose your PHI to obtain payment from third parties that may be responsible for such costs, such as family members. Also, we may use your PHI to bill you directly for services and items. We may disclose your PHI to other health care providers and entities to assist in their billing and collection efforts.

Figure 2-5 Exceprt from a Notice of Privacy Practices.

Acknowledgment of Receipt of Privacy Practices Notice

PART A: The Patient.

Name: _____

Address: _____

Telephone: _____ E-mail: _____

Patient Number: _____ Social Security Number: _____

PART B: Acknowledgment of Receipt of Privacy Practices Notice.

I, _____ , acknowledge that I have received a Notice of Privacy Practices.

Signature: _____ Date: _____
If a personal representative signs this authorization on behalf of the individual, complete the following:

Personal Representative's Name: _____

Relationship to Individual: _____

PART C: Good-Faith Effort to Obtain Acknowledgment of Receipt.

Describe your good-faith effort to obtain the individual's signature on this form: _____

_____

_____

Describe the reason why the indvidual would not sign this form. _____

_____

_____

SIGNATURE.
I attest that the above information is correct.

Signature: _____ Date: _____

Print Name: _____ Title: _____
Include this acknowledgment of receipt in the individual's records.

Figure 2-6 Acknowledgement of Receipt of Privacy Practices form.

acknowledgment of having received and read the Notice of Privacy Practices in the form of a signed Acknowledgment of Receipt of Notice of Privacy Practices (see Figure 2-6).

SECURITY REQUIREMENTS

The **HIPAA Security Rule** outlines safeguards to protect the confidentiality, integrity, and availability of health information that is stored on a computer system or transmitted across computer

HIPAA Security Rule regulations outlining the minimum administrative, technical, and physical safeguards required to prevent unauthorized access to protected health care information.

networks, including the Internet. While the HIPAA Privacy Rule applies to all forms of protected health information, whether electronic, paper, or oral, the Security Rule covers only PHI that is created, received, maintained, or transmitted in electronic form. The Final Enforcement Rule specifies that the Security Rule is enforced by the Centers for Medicare and Medicaid Services (CMS).

The security standards are divided into three categories: administrative, physical, and technical safeguards.

administrative safeguards administrative policies and procedures designed to protect electronic health information outlined by the HIPAA Security Rule.

Administrative safeguards are administrative policies and procedures designed to protect electronic health information. The management of security is assigned to one individual, who conducts an assessment of the current level of data security. Once that assessment is complete, security policies and procedures are developed or modified to meet current needs. Security training is provided to educate staff members on the policies and to raise awareness of security and privacy issues.

physical safeguards mechanisms required to protect electronic systems, equipment, and data from threats, environmental hazards, and unauthorized intrusion.

Physical safeguards are the mechanisms required to protect electronic systems, equipment, and data from threats, environmental hazards, and unauthorized intrusion. Threats include computer hackers, disgruntled employees, or angry patients. Health information stored on computers is also at risk from physical threats, such as unplanned system outages or storage media failures.

Electronic information is also at risk from environmental hazards, such as fire, flood, or earthquake. For this reason, medical practices create regular backups of computerized information. Many practices back up their files at the end of each day. The backup files are stored at a remote physical location to minimize the likelihood of data loss in a large-scale disaster. In the event of major disaster, data from the remote site can easily be recovered.

Unauthorized intrusion refers to access by individuals who do not have a "need to know." For example, individuals who are not working with confidential patient information should not be able to view this type of information on an office computer monitor. To prevent intrusion, offices limit physical access to computers. Security measures can be as simple as a lock on the door or as advanced as an electronic device that requires fingerprint authentication to gain access.

technical safeguards automated processes used to protect data and control access to data.

Technical safeguards are the automated processes used to protect data and control access to data. Access to information is granted on an as-needed basis. For example, the individual responsible for scheduling may not need access to billing data. Examples of technical safeguards include computer passwords, antivirus and firewall software, and secure transmission systems for sending patient data from one computer to another.

As an additional security measure, computer programs can keep track of data entry and create an **audit trail**—a report that shows who has accessed information and when. When new data are entered or existing data are changed, a log records the time and date of the entry as well as the name of the computer operator. The practice manager reviews the log on a regular basis to detect irregularities. If an error has been made, the program lists the name of the person and the date the information was entered.

audit trail a report that traces who has accessed electronic information, when information was accessed, and whether any information was changed.

CHAPTER REVIEW

USING TERMINOLOGY

Match the terms on the left with the definitions on the right.

_____ **1.** audit/edit report

_____ **2.** protected health information (PHI)

_____ **3.** clearinghouse

_____ **4.** electronic prescribing

_____ **5.** national provider identifier (NPI)

_____ **6.** electronic data interchange (EDI)

_____ **7.** practice management program (PMP)

_____ **8.** electronic medical records (EMR)

_____ **9.** HIPAA Security Rule

_____ **10.** HIPAA Electronic Transaction and Code Sets standards

_____ **11.** information technology (IT)

_____ **12.** walkout statement

_____ **13.** X12-837 Health Care Claim (837P)

a. Regulations that require electronic transactions to use standardized formats.

b. A software program that automates many of the administrative and financial tasks required to run a medical practice.

c. A document listing charges and payments that is given to a patient after an office visit.

d. A national standard identifier for all health care providers consisting of ten numbers.

e. Computer hardware and software systems.

f. The electronic format of the claim used by physicians' offices to bill for services.

g. The use of computers and handheld devices to write and transmit prescriptions to a pharmacy in a secure digital format.

h. The electronic collection and management of health information.

i. A report that lists errors in a claim.

j. An organization that receives claims from a provider, checks and prepares them for processing, and transmits them to insurance carriers in a standardized format.

k. The transfer of business transactions from one computer to another using communications protocols.

l. Information about a patient's past, present, or future physical or mental health or payment for health care that can be used to identify the person.

m. Regulations outlining the minimum safeguards required to prevent unauthorized access to electronic health care information.

CHECKING YOUR UNDERSTANDING

Write "T" or "F" in the blank to indicate whether you think the statement is true or false.

14. The HIPAA Electronic Transaction and Code Sets standards specify standard medical code sets, such as ICD-9-CM and CPT-4. _____

15. Computer programs use audit trails to help ensure the privacy and confidentiality of patient health care information. _____

16. All medical offices, regardless of size, must use the HIPAA-standard X12-837claim. _____

17. The HIPAA standards require a practice that uses a clearinghouse to have a contract that states the procedures that must be followed to ensure HIPAA compliance. _____

18. Computerized databases are more efficient than manual filing systems. _____

Answer the question below in the space provided.

19. List five advantages of using computers in a medical practice.

_____

_____

_____

Choose the best answer.

_____ 20. The HIPAA Security Rule specifies the _____ , technical, and physical safeguards required to prevent unauthorized access to health care information.

    a. administrative

    b. clinical

    c. legal

_____ 21. Electronic medical records are used to record data such as physicians' reports of examinations, surgical procedures, tests results, and:

    a. billing codes

    b. X-rays

    c. insurance claims

_____ **22.** Many medical offices assign _____ to individuals who have access to computer data as a security measure.

    a. identification numbers

    b. private offices

    c. passwords

_____ **23.** The HIPAA standard electronic format for the exchange of payment and remittance advice is the:

    a. X12-835

    b. X12-278

    c. X12-271

_____ **24.** _____ reports are designed to provide payers with "clean" claims, thus reducing the number of claim rejections due to missing or incorrect data.

    a. Clearinghouse

    b. Electronic data interchange

    c. Audit/edit

MEDISOFT ADVANCED TRAINING

Chapter 3
Introduction to Medisoft

Chapter 4
Entering Patient Information

Chapter 5
Entering Insurance, Account, and Condition Information

Chapter 6
Entering Charge Transactions and Patient Payments

Chapter 7
Creating Claims

Chapter 8
Posting Insurance Payments and Creating Patient Statements

Chapter 9
Printing Reports

Chapter 10
Collections in the Medical Office

Chapter 11
Scheduling

Introduction to Medisoft

3

WHAT YOU NEED TO KNOW

To use this chapter, you need to know how to:

- Start your computer and Microsoft Windows.
- Use the keyboard and mouse.

LEARNING OUTCOMES

In this chapter, you will learn how to:

- Start Medisoft.
- Select options on the Medisoft menus.
- Use the icons on the Medisoft toolbar.
- Enter, edit, and delete data.
- Back up and restore data.
- Use Medisoft's Help features.
- Exit Medisoft.
- Use Medisoft's file maintenance features.

KEY TERMS

backup data
database
knowledge base
MMDDCCYY format
packing data
purging data
rebuilding indexes
recalculating balances
restoring data

WHAT IS MEDISOFT?

Medisoft is a practice management program. Information on patients, providers, insurance carriers, and patient and insurance billing is stored and processed by the system. Medisoft is widely used by medical practices throughout the United States. It is typically used to accomplish the following daily work in a medical practice:

◆ Enter information on new patients and change information on established patients as needed

◆ Enter transactions, such as charges, to patients' accounts

◆ Submit insurance claims to payers

◆ Record payments and adjustments from patients and insurance companies

◆ Print walkout statements and remainder statements for patients

◆ Monitor collections activities

◆ Print standard reports and create custom reports

◆ Schedule appointments

Many of the general working concepts used in operating Medisoft are similar to those in other software programs. Thus, you should be able to transfer many skills taught in this book to other practice management programs.

HOW MEDISOFT DATA ARE ORGANIZED AND STORED

database a collection of related bits of information

Information entered into Medisoft is stored in databases. A **database** is a collection of related pieces of information.

MEDISOFT DATABASES

Medisoft stores these major types of data:

◆ **Provider data** The provider database has information about the physician(s) as well as the practice, such as name, address, phone number, and tax and medical identifier numbers.

◆ **Patient data** Each patient information form is stored in the patient database. The patient's unique chart number and personal information—name, address, phone number, birth date, Social Security number, gender, marital status, and employer—are examples of information stored in this database.

◆ **Insurance carriers** The insurance carrier database contains the name, address, and other data about each insurance carrier used by patients, such as the type of plan. Usually, this database also contains information on each carrier's electronic media claim (EMC) submission.

◆ **Diagnosis codes** The diagnosis code database contains the International Classification of Diseases, Ninth Revision, Clinical Modification (ICD-9-CM) codes that indicate the reason a service is provided. The codes entered in this database are those most frequently used by the practice. The practice's encounter form or superbill often serves as a source document when the Medisoft system is first set up.

◆ **Procedure codes** The procedure code database contains the data needed to create charges. The Current Procedural Terminology (CPT-4) codes most often used by the practice are selected for this database. The practice's encounter form is often a good source document for the codes. Other claim data elements, such as place of service (POS) and the charge for each procedure, are also stored in the procedure code database.

◆ **Transactions** The transaction database stores information about each patient's visits, diagnoses, and procedures, as well as received and outstanding payments. Transactions in the form of charges, payments, and adjustments are also stored in the transaction database.

Within Medisoft, each database is linked, or related, to each of the others by having at least one fact in common. For example, information entered in the patient database is shared with the transaction database, linking the two. Information is entered only once; Medisoft selects the data from each database as needed.

THE STUDENT DATA TEMPLATE

Before a medical office begins using Medisoft, basic information about the practice and its patients must be entered in the computer. The author has created a database—the Student Data Template—that you will use to complete the exercises in this book. Check with your instructor to determine whether the Student Data Template has already been loaded on your computer. If your instructor has not already loaded the data, go to the Online Learning Center at www.mhhe.com/cimo6e, and download the Student Data Template file. You will need to load the database before you do the exercises in this chapter.

THE MEDISOFT MENU BAR

Medisoft offers choices of actions through a series of menus. Commands are issued by clicking options on the menu bar or by clicking shortcut buttons on the toolbar. The menu bar lists the names of the menus in Medisoft: File, Edit, Activities, Lists, Reports,

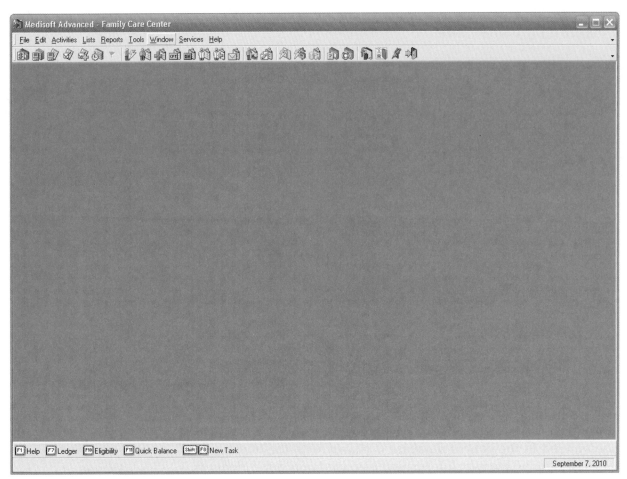

Figure 3-1   Main Medisoft window

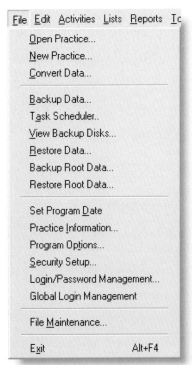

Figure 3-2   File menu

Tools, Window, Services, and Help (see Figure 3-1). Beneath each menu name is a pull-down menu of one or more options.

File Menu   The File menu is used to enter information about the medical office practice when first setting up Medisoft. It is also used to back up data, restore data, set program security options, perform file maintenance activities, and change the program date (see Figure 3-2).

Edit Menu   The Edit menu contains the basic commands needed to move, change, or delete information (see Figure 3-3). These commands are Cut, Copy, Paste, and Delete.

Activities Menu   Most medical office data collected on a day-to-day basis are entered through options on the Activities menu (see Figure 3-4). This menu is used to perform most billing tasks in a medical practice, including:

◆   Entering financial transactions

◆   Creating insurance claims

◆   Entering deposits

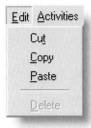

Figure 3-3 Edit menu

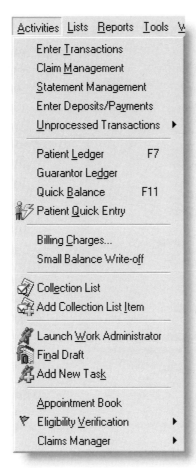

Figure 3-4 Activities menu

Lists Reports Tools Window Services Hel

Patients/Guarantors and Cases
Patient Recall
Patient Treatment Plans
Patient Entry Template

Procedure/Payment/Adjustment Codes
MultiLink Codes
Diagnosis Codes

Insurance ▶
Addresses
EDI Receivers
Referring Providers
Provider ▶

Billing Codes
Contact List

Claim Rejection Messages
Patient Payment Plan

Figure 3-5 Lists menu

◆ Creating patient statements

◆ Viewing summaries of patient account information

◆ Calculating billing charges

◆ Writing off small account balances

◆ Performing collections activities

◆ Launching the appointment scheduler

Patient insurance eligibility is also verified by selecting the Eligibility Verification option on the Activities menu.

Lists Menu   Information on new patients, such as name, address, and employer, is entered through the Lists menu (see Figure 3-5). If information needs to be changed on an established patient, it is also updated through this menu. The Lists menu also provides access to lists of codes, insurance carriers, providers, billing codes, contacts, and payment plans. These lists may be updated and printed when necessary.

Reports Menu   The Reports menu is used to print reports about patients' accounts and other reports about the practice (see Figure 3-6). Medisoft comes with a number of standard report formats, such as

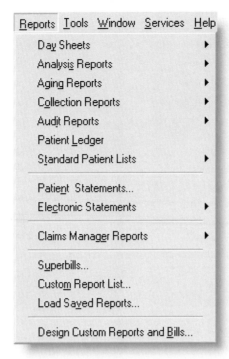

Figure 3-6   Reports menu

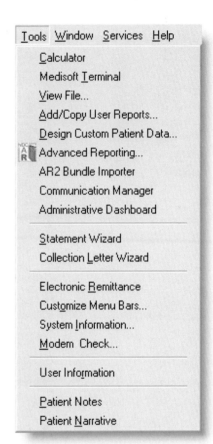

Figure 3-7   Tools menu

day sheets, aging reports, and patient ledgers. Practices may create their own report formats using the Design Custom Reports and Bills option.

Tools Menu   The Tools menu provides access to Medisoft's built-in calculator and other options. The Tools menu is also used to view the contents of a file as well as a profile of the computer system (see Figure 3-7). Custom collection letters and patient statements can be easily created by using several wizards that are available. The new Communications Manager and Administrative Dashboard features are also found on the Tools menu.

Window Menu   Using the Window menu, it is possible to switch back and forth between several open windows. For example, if the Patient List dialog box and the Transaction Entry dialog box were both open, the Window menu would look like the menu in Figure 3-8. The Window menu also has an option to close all windows.

Services Menu   The Services menu is used by practices to manage enrollment in electronic services such as claims manager, eligibility verification, and electronic prescribing (see Figure 3-9).

Help Menu   The Help menu, shown in Figure 3-10, is used to access Medisoft's built-in Help feature and also provides a link to Medisoft support on the World Wide Web. The Help menu also contains options for registering the program.

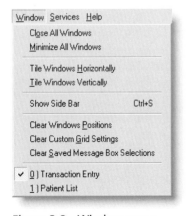

Figure 3-8   Window menu

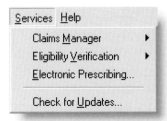

Figure 3-9   Services menu

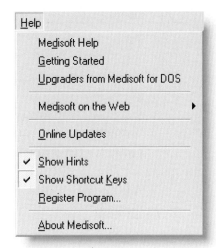

Figure 3-10   Help menu

EXERCISE 3-1

Practice using the Medisoft menus.

1. Start Medisoft.

2. Click the Lists menu on the menu bar.

3. Click Patients/Guarantors and Cases. The Patient List dialog box is displayed.

4. Click the Close button at the bottom of the dialog box.

5. Click the Activities menu.

6. Click Enter Transactions. The Transaction Entry dialog box appears.

7. Click the Close button in the upper-right corner of the window.

THE MEDISOFT TOOLBAR

Located below the menu bar, the toolbar contains a series of buttons with icons that represent the most common activities performed in Medisoft. These buttons are shortcuts for frequently used menu commands. When you click on a button, the corresponding Medisoft dialog box opens. For example, clicking the Claim Management button opens the same dialog box as selecting the Claim Management option on the Activities menu. Throughout this book, the buttons can be used instead of the pull-down menus to perform common tasks. The toolbar contains twenty-six buttons (see Figure 3-11 and Table 3-1).

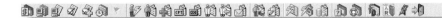

Figure 3-11   Medisoft toolbar

Table 3-1   Medisoft Toolbar Buttons

Button	Button Name	Opens	Activity
	Transaction Entry	Transaction Entry dialog box	Enter, edit, or delete transactions
	Claim Management	Claim Management dialog box	Create and transmit insurance claims
	Statement Management	Statement Management dialog box	Create statements
	Collection List	Collection List dialog box	View, add, edit, or delete items on collection list
	Add Collection List Item	Add Collection List Items dialog box	Add items to the collection list
	Appointment Book	Office Hours	Schedule appointments
	View Eligibility Verification Results (F10)	Eligibility Verification Results dialog box	Review results of eligibility verification inquiries
	Patient Quick Entry	Patient Quick Entry dialog box	Use predefined template to enter new patients
	Patient List	Patient List dialog box	Enter patient information
	Insurance Carrier List	Insurance Carrier List dialog box	Enter insurance carriers
	Procedure Code List	Procedure/Payment/Adjustment Code List dialog box	Enter procedure codes
	Diagnosis Code List	Diagnosis List dialog box	Enter diagnosis codes
	Provider List	Provider List dialog box	Enter providers
	Referring Provider List	Referring Provider List dialog box	Enter referring providers
	Address List	Address List dialog box	Enter addresses
	Patient Recall Entry	Patient Recall dialog box	Enter Patient Recall data
	Custom Report List	Open Report dialog box	Open a custom report
	Quick Ledger	Quick Ledger dialog box	View a patient's ledger
	Quick Balance	Quick Balance dialog box	View a patient's balance
	Enter Deposits and Apply Payments	Deposit List dialog box	Enter deposits and payments
	Show/Hide Hints	Show or Hide Hints	Turn the Hints feature on and off
	Medisoft Help	Medisoft Help	Access Medisoft's built-in help feature
	Edit Patient Notes in Final Draft	Final Draft untitled document	Use built-in word processor to create and edit patient notes
	Launch Advanced Reporting	Advanced Reporting dialog box	Provides enhanced reporting capabilities
	Launch Work Administrator	Assignment List	Assign tasks to practice staff
	Exit Program	Exit Program	Exit the Medisoft program

EXERCISE 3-2

Practice using buttons on the toolbar.

1. Click the Provider List button. The Provider List dialog box opens.

2. Close the dialog box by clicking the X in the upper-right corner of the window.

3. Click the Procedure Code List button. The Procedure/Payment/ Adjustment List dialog box is displayed.

4. Close the dialog box by clicking the Close button in the lower-right section of the window.

ENTERING AND EDITING DATA

All data, whether patients' addresses or treatment procedures, are entered into Medisoft through the menus on the menu bar or through the buttons on the toolbar. Selecting an option from the menus or toolbar opens a dialog box. The Tab key is used to move between text boxes within a dialog box. Some information, such as a patient's name, is entered by keying data into a text box. At other times, selections are made from a list of choices already present, such as when making a selection from the drop-down list of providers already in the database.

CHANGING THE MEDISOFT PROGRAM DATE

Medisoft is a date-sensitive program. When transactions are entered in the program, the dates must be accurate, or the data entered will be of little value to the practice. Many times, date-sensitive information is not entered into Medisoft on the same day that the event or transaction occurred. For example, Friday afternoon's office visits may not be entered into the program until Monday. If the Medisoft Program Date is not changed to Friday's date before entering the data, all the information entered on Monday will be stored as Monday's transactions. For this reason, it is important to know how to change the Medisoft Program Date.

For the exercises in this book, you will need to change the Medisoft Program Date to the date specified at the beginning of the each exercise. Most of the exercises in this text/workbook take place in the year 2010. When a date is entered that is in the future (relative to the actual date on which the entry is made), the program displays one of

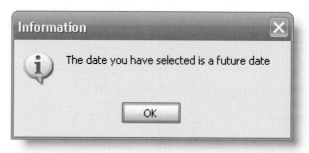

Figure 3-12a   Dialog box that appears when a future date is entered

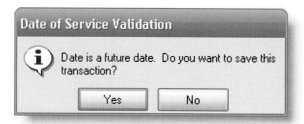

Figure 3-12b   Dialog box that appears when a future date is entered while entering patient visit transactions

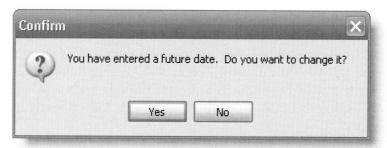

Figure 3-12c   Dialog box that appears when a future date is entered while entering deposits

several dialog boxes (see Figures 3-12a, b, and c). For example, if the exercise date is September 10, 2010, but the data are actually being entered on February 9, 2009, the program recognizes that a future date has been entered.

Depending on where in the program the date is entered, the dialog box will vary. If a change is made to the pop-up calendar, the dialog box in Figure 3-12a appears as a notification that the date selected is in the future. To keep the future date, click the OK button.

When entering patient office visit transactions, the Date of Service Validation window appears and asks whether the transaction should be saved (see Figure 3-12b). To keep the future date and save the transaction, it is necessary to click the Yes button.

When entering deposits, a Confirm dialog box appears and asks whether the date should be changed (see Figure 3-12c). To keep the future date, the No button must be clicked.

Slightly different procedures for changing the program date are used in Windows XP and Windows Vista. Please follow the instructions for your computer's operating system.

Windows XP   The following steps are used to change the Medisoft Program Date in Windows XP:

1. Click Set Program Date on the File menu. A pop-up calendar is displayed (see Figure 3-13). *Note:* You can also click directly on the date that is displayed in the lower-right corner of the window.

2. To change the month, click the word displayed for the current month, and a pop-up list of months appears. Click the desired month on the pop-up list (see Figure 3-14). If the month is in the future, a pop-up message appears to remind you that you have selected a future date. To continue with the date change, click the OK button. This will also happen if you select a day or a year in the future.

3. To change the year, follow the same procedure. Click the current year, and select the desired year from the pop-up list (see Figure 3-15). Note that the year pop-up list includes 1990 through 2009 only. To change the calendar to 2010, click 2009 and then click the right arrow button to advance one month at a time until 2010 is reached.

4. Select the desired day of the month by clicking on that date in the calendar. If the month is in the future, a pop-up message appears to remind you that you have selected a future date. To continue with the date change, click the OK button. This will also happen if you select a day or a year in the future. The calendar closes, and the desired date is displayed on the status bar.

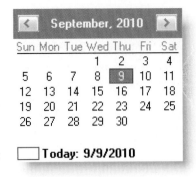

Figure 3-13   Medisoft pop-up calendar

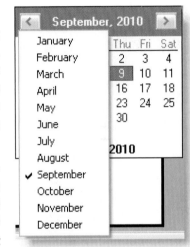

Figure 3-14   Calendar month pop-up list

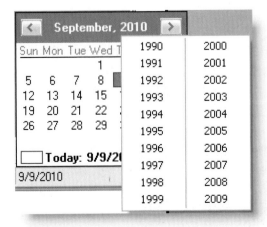

Figure 3-15   Calendar year pop-up list

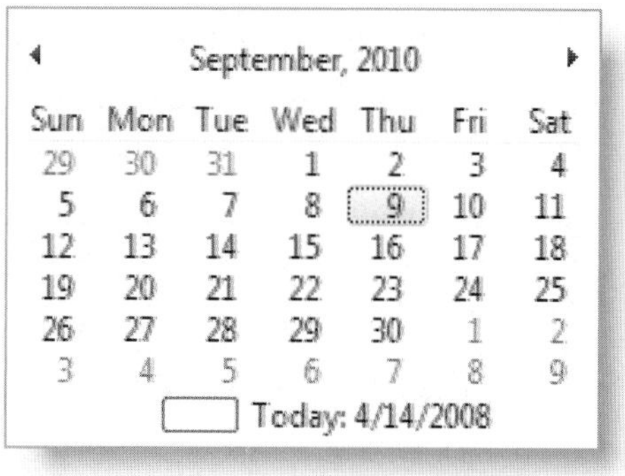

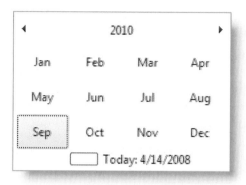

Figure 3-16 Medisoft pop-up calendar

Figure 3-17 Calendar month window

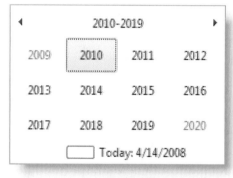

Figure 3-18 Calendar year window

Windows Vista The following steps are used to change the Medisoft Program Date in Windows Vista:

1. Click Set Program Date on the File menu. A pop-up calendar is displayed in the lower-right corner of the window(see Figure 3-16). *Note:* You can also click directly on the date that is displayed in the lower-right corner of the window.

2. To change the month, click the word displayed for the current month, and the abbreviations for the months appear in the calendar window. Click the desired month (see Figure 3-17).

3. To change the year, follow the same procedure. Click the current year, and select the desired year from the years that appear in the window (see Figure 3-18).

4. Select the desired day of the month by clicking on that date in the calendar. If the month is in the future, a pop-up message appears to remind you that you have selected a future date. To continue with the date change, click the OK button. This will also happen if you select a day or a year in the future. The calendar closes, and the desired date is displayed on the status bar.

MMDDCCYY format a specific way in which dates must be keyed, in which *MM* stands for the month, *DD* stands for the day, *CC* represents the century, and *YY* stands for the year

In most Medisoft dialog boxes, dates must be entered in the MMDDCCYY format. In the **MMDDCCYY format,** *MM* stands for the month, *DD* stands for the day, *CC* represents century, and *YY* stands for the year. Each day, month, century, and year entry must contain two digits, and no punctuation can be used. For example, February 1, 2010, would be keyed *02012010.*

> **WARNING!** Dates are very important! If incorrect dates are used when entering data, the information in reports will be inaccurate. Be sure to change the Medisoft Program Date as specified at the beginning of each exercise.

EXERCISE 3-3

Practice entering information and correcting errors.

1. Click the Activities menu.

2. Click Enter Transactions.

3. Click the triangle button in the Chart box. The Chart drop-down list is opened (see Figure 3-19).

4. To select James Smith, key the first two letters of his chart number (SMITHJAØ): **SM.** Notice that when "SM" is keyed, the system goes to the entry for the first patient whose chart number begins with *SM*, in this case James Smith.

5. Press the Tab key.

6. To edit a transaction, click in the field that needs to be changed. Click in the Procedure field. Notice that the entry in the field becomes highlighted.

7. Click again in the Procedure field. A pop-up list of procedure codes is displayed.

8. Select a new code from the list by clicking on it. Scroll down the pop-up list of codes, and click 99396. Notice that the new code is displayed in the Procedure field, but the entry in the Amount field has not changed. This does not happen until the Tab key is pressed. Press the Tab key now, and watch the entry in the Amount field change.

9. Press the Tab key repeatedly, and watch as the cursor moves from box to box.

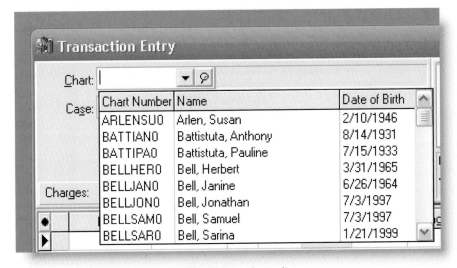

Figure 3-19 Transaction Entry Chart drop-down list

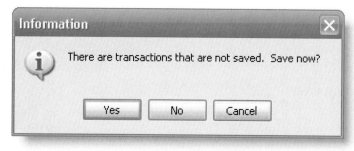

Figure 3-20 Transaction Entry save warning dialog box

10. Exit the Transaction Entry dialog box by clicking the Close button or by clicking the close icon in the upper-right corner of the dialog box. An Information box is displayed, asking whether the changes should be saved (see Figure 3-20). In this case, click the No button. The changes are not saved, and the Transaction Entry window closes.

SAVING DATA

Information entered into Medisoft is saved by clicking the Save button that appears in most dialog boxes. In most medical practices, data are saved to a hard disk. For the purposes of this book, your instructor will tell you where to save your data. This may be a hard disk, a directory on a network drive, a flash drive, a CD-RW, or some other type of storage medium. The letter identifying the drive may be C:\, but it could also be another letter, such as F:\, G:\, H:\, or S:\.

DELETING DATA

In some Medisoft dialog boxes, there are buttons for the purpose of deleting data. For example, to delete an insurance carrier, the entry for the carrier is clicked in the Insurance Carrier List dialog box. Then, the Delete button is clicked (see Figure 3-21).

Insurance Carrier List

Search for: [　　　　　　　　] Field: Name

Code	Name	Type	Street 1
14	AARP Medigap	Other	342 Center St.
4	Blue Cross/Blue Shield	Blue Cross/Shield	340 Boulevard
5	ChampVA	ChampsVA	240 Center Street
13	East Ohio PPO	PPO	10 Central Avenue
2	Medicaid	Medicaid	248 West Main Street
1	Medicare	Medicare	246 West Main Street
15	OhioCare HMO	HMO	147 Central Avenue
3	Tricare	Champus	249 Center Street

Edit　New　Delete　Print Grid　Close

Figure 3-21 Insurance Carrier List dialog box with Delete button highlighted

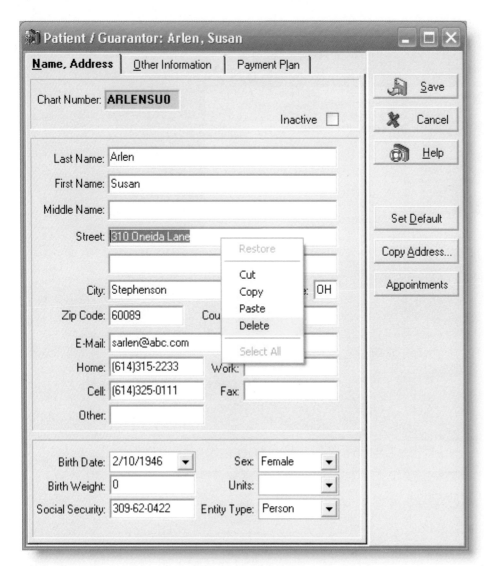

Figure 3-22 Shortcut menu with Delete option available

Medisoft will ask for a confirmation before deleting the data. In other dialog boxes, there is no button for deleting data. In this situation, select the text that is to be deleted, and either click the Delete key on the keyboard or click the right mouse button. A shortcut menu is displayed that contains an option to delete the entry (see Figure 3-22).

USING MEDISOFT HELP

Medisoft offers users three different types of help.

Hints   As the cursor moves over certain fields, hints appears on the status bar at the bottom of the screen. For example, when the cursor is over the New Patient button, a related hint is displayed (see Figure 3-23). The Hint feature can be turned on or off by clicking Show Hints on the Help menu.

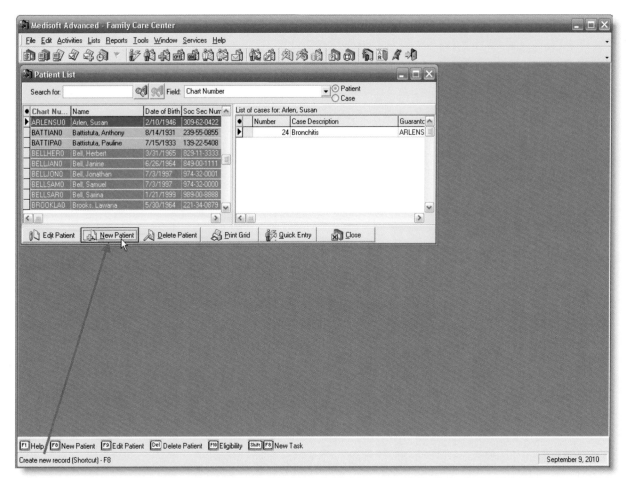

Figure 3-23 Hint displayed on status bar

Built-in For more detailed help, Medisoft has an extensive help feature built into the program itself, which is accessed by selecting Medisoft Help on the Help menu (see Figure 3-24).

Online The Help menu also provides access to Medisoft help available on the Medisoft corporate website at http://www.Medisoft.com (see Figure 3-25). The website contains a searchable **knowledge base,** which is a collection of up-to-date technical information about Medisoft products.

knowledge base a collection of up-to-date technical information

EXERCISE 3-4

Practice using Medisoft's built-in help feature.

1. Click the Help menu.

2. Click Medisoft Help. Medisoft displays a list of topics for which help is available.

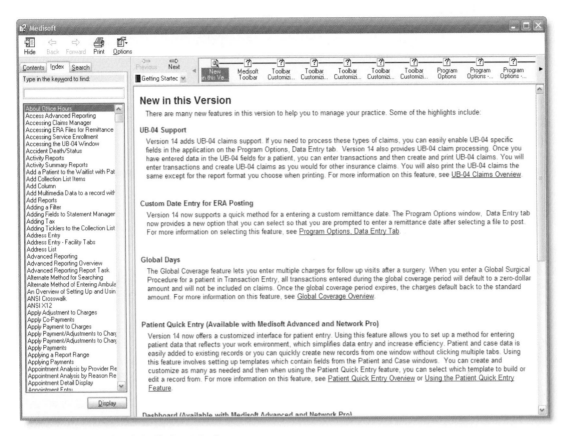

Figure 3-24 Medisoft built-in Help feature

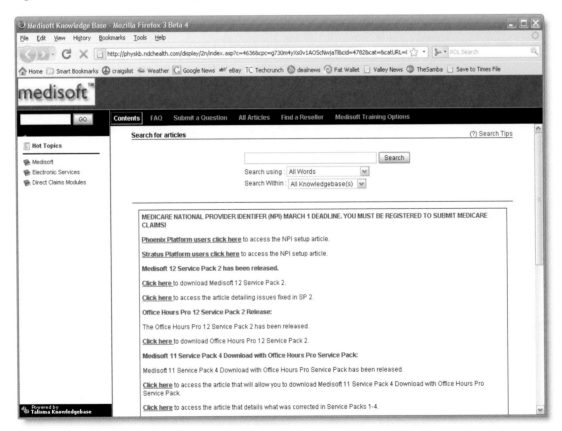

Figure 3-25 Medisoft online Knowledge Base

3. Locate Diagnosis Entry in the left column. Double-click Diagnosis Entry. Information on entering diagnosis codes is displayed on the right side of the window.

4. Click the Close box to close the Help window.

EXERCISE 3-5

Practice using Medisoft's online help.

1. Access the Internet. Click Medisoft on the Web > Knowledge Base option on the Help menu (see Figure 3-26). The Knowledge Base area of the website is displayed.

2. Enter *transactions* in the search box.

3. Select Medisoft on the Search Within drop-down list.

4. Accept the All Categories entry.

5. Click the Search button.

6. FAQs, or Frequently Asked Questions, appear at the top of the list of articles.

7. Select an article, and click on the title to read it.

8. Click the Close box to exit the Medisoft Knowledge Base. Terminate your Internet connection, if appropriate.

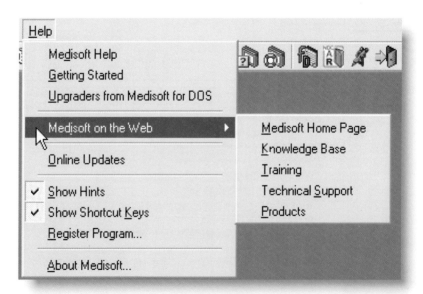

Figure 3-26 Medisoft on the Web submenu

EXITING MEDISOFT

Medisoft is exited by clicking Exit on the File menu or by clicking the Close box. To avoid the inconvenience of exiting and restarting Medisoft many times during a day when the computer is needed for a different program, Medisoft can be made temporarily inactive by using the Minimize button, the first of the three small buttons displayed in the upper-right corner of the window. Medisoft can be reactivated at any time by clicking the Medisoft button on the Windows taskbar.

MAKING A BACKUP FILE WHILE EXITING MEDISOFT

Data are periodically saved on removable media, such as CD-RWs or flash drives, through a process known as backing up. The extra copy of data files made at a specific point in time is known as **backup data.** Backup data can be used to restore data to the system in the event the data in the system are accidentally lost or destroyed. Backups are performed on a regular schedule, determined by the practice. Many practices back up data at the end of each day. A copy of backup data is usually stored at a location other than the office, in case of a natural or man-made disaster at the office facility.

backup data   a copy of data files made at a specific point in time that can be used to restore data to the system

In a school setting, files are also backed up regularly to store each student's work securely and separately. If you are a student using this book in a school environment, it is important to make a backup copy of your work after each Medisoft session. This ensures that you can restore your work during the next session and be able to use your own data even if another student uses the computer after you or if, for any reason, the data on the school computer are changed or corrupted.

In Medisoft, the Backup Data option on the File menu can be used to make a backup copy of the active database at any time. By default, Medisoft also displays a Backup Reminder dialog box every time the program is exited. The Backup Reminder dialog box gives you the opportunity to back up your work every time you exit Medisoft (see Figure 3-27). To perform the backup, click the Back Up Data Now. A Backup Warning dialog box may appear, indicating that if others are using the same practice data, they should exit Medisoft before the backup is made (see Figure 3-28). To continue to exit the program without making a backup, click the Exit Program button. The following exercise provides practice.

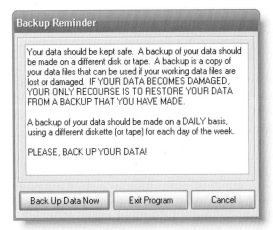

Figure 3-27   Backup Reminder dialog box

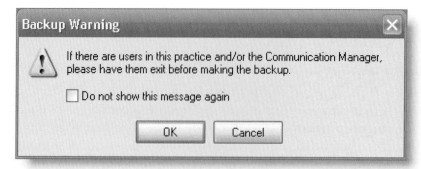

Figure 3-28   Backup Warning dialog box

EXERCISE 3-6

Practice backing up your work on exiting Medisoft.

1. To exit Medisoft, click Exit on the File menu, or click the Exit button on the toolbar.

2. The Backup Reminder dialog box appears, displaying three options: Backup Data Now, Exit Program, or Cancel. For the purposes of this text, it is recommended that you back up your work each time you exit the program. Your instructor will tell you where to save your backup.

3. Click the Back Up Data Now button. If a Backup Warning dialog box appears, click the OK button.

4. The Medisoft Backup dialog box is displayed (see Figure 3-29). Depending on the last time the dialog box was accessed, the Destination File Path and Name box may already contain an entry. Your instructor will tell you what to enter in this field.

5. Medisoft automatically displays the location of the database files to be backed up in the Source Path box in the lower half of the dialog box.

6. Click the Start Backup button.

7. The program backs up the latest database files and displays an Information dialog box indicating that the backup is complete. Click OK to continue.

8. The Medisoft Backup dialog box disappears, and the Medisoft program closes.

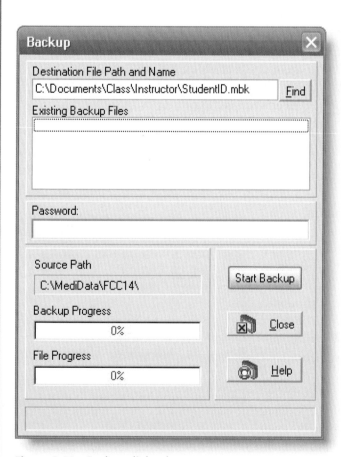

Figure 3-29   Backup dialog box

RESTORING THE BACKUP FILE

The process of retrieving data from backup storage devices is referred to as **restoring data.** Whenever a new Medisoft session begins, the following steps can be used to restore the backup file, if required. If you share a computer in an instructional environment, it is recommended that you perform a restore before each new session to be sure you are working with your own data.

restoring data the process of retrieving data from backup storage devices

In this example, backups are stored on the H drive, and the Medisoft program files are located on the C drive.

To restore H:\StudentID.mbk to the Medisoft directory on the C: drive (C:\MediData\FCC14):

1. Start Medisoft.

2. Check the program's title bar at the top of the screen to make sure the Family Care Center data set is the active data set. (If it is not, use the Open Practice option on the File menu to select it.)

3. Open the File menu, and click Restore Data.

4. When the Warning box in Figure 3-30 appears, click OK.

5. The Restore dialog box appears (see Figure 3-31). In the Backup File Path and Name box at the top of the dialog box, key *H:\StudentID.mbk* if this name is not already displayed.

6. The Destination Path at the bottom of the box should already say C:\Medisoft\FCC14. Leave this as it is.

7. Click the Start Restore button.

8. When the Confirm box appears, click OK.

9. An Information dialog box appears indicating that the restore is complete. Click OK to continue.

10. The Restore dialog box disappears. You are ready to begin the next session.

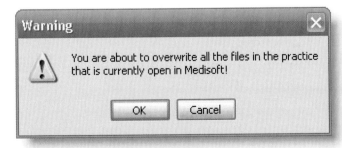

Figure 3-30 Restore warning box

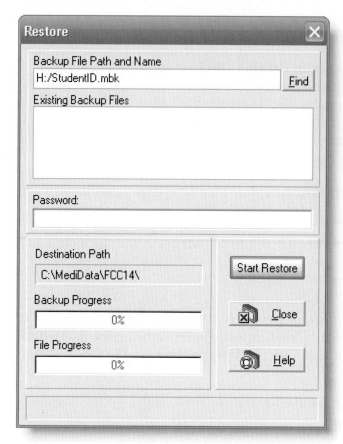

Figure 3-31 Restore dialog box

FILE MAINTENANCE UTILITIES

In addition to the backup and restore features, Medisoft provides four features to assist in maintaining data files stored in a system. These four features are found on tabs in the File Maintenance dialog box (see Figure 3-32).

1. Rebuild Indexes

2. Pack Data

3. Purge Data

4. Recalculate Balances

The dialog box is accessed by clicking File Maintenance on the File menu. If the medical office's database is large, Medisoft's utilities may take a long time to finish. For this reason, it is usually a good idea to use the utility functions at the end of the day or when the system will not be needed for a while.

WARNING! Do not attempt to perform the utility functions listed in this chapter unless told to do so by your instructor. Loss of data could occur.

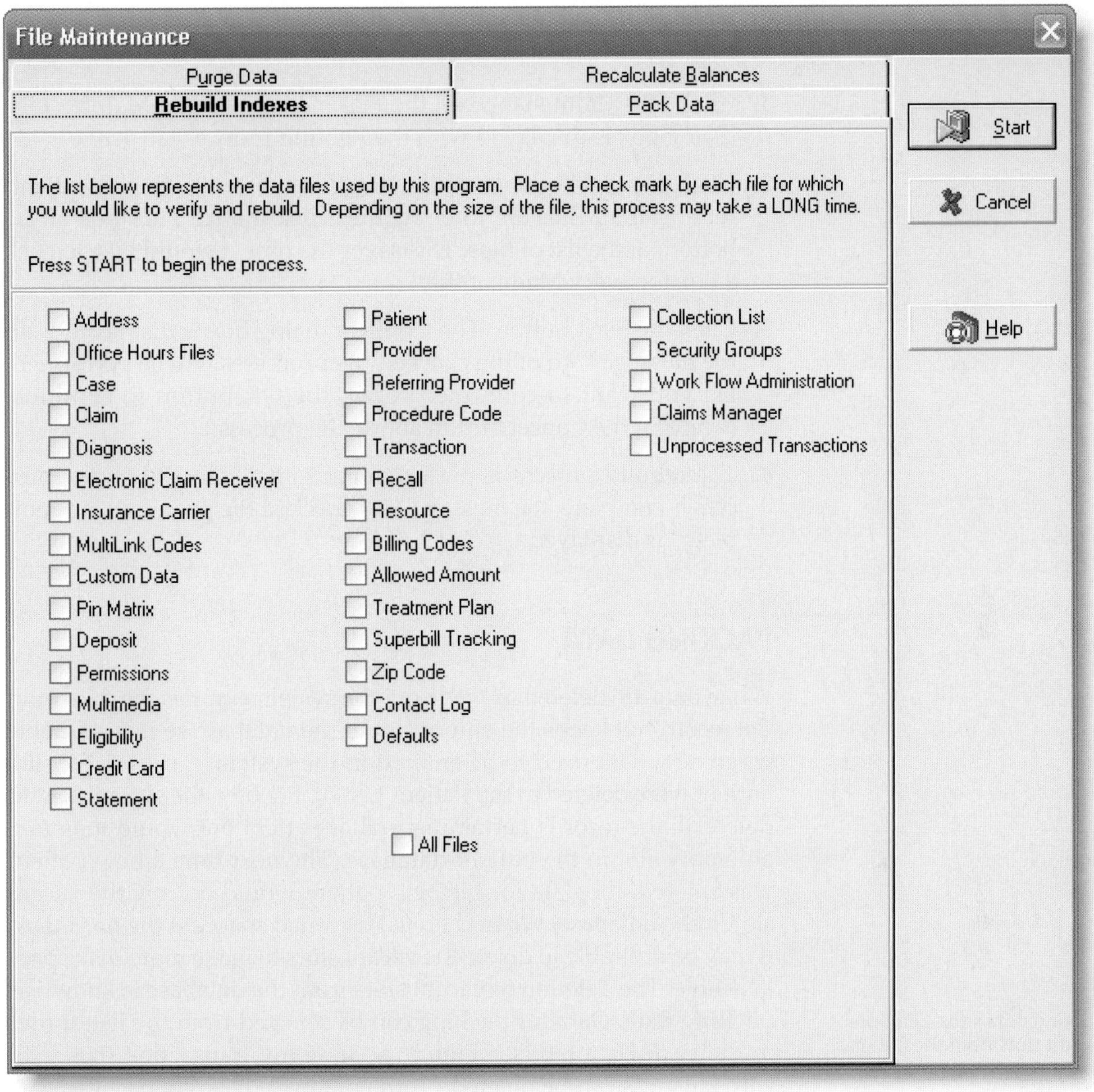

File Maintenance

Purge Data	Recalculate Balances
Rebuild Indexes	Pack Data

Start

Cancel

Help

The list below represents the data files used by this program. Place a check mark by each file for which you would like to verify and rebuild. Depending on the size of the file, this process may take a LONG time.

Press START to begin the process.

- Address
- Office Hours Files
- Case
- Claim
- Diagnosis
- Electronic Claim Receiver
- Insurance Carrier
- MultiLink Codes
- Custom Data
- Pin Matrix
- Deposit
- Permissions
- Multimedia
- Eligibility
- Credit Card
- Statement

- Patient
- Provider
- Referring Provider
- Procedure Code
- Transaction
- Recall
- Resource
- Billing Codes
- Allowed Amount
- Treatment Plan
- Superbill Tracking
- Zip Code
- Contact Log
- Defaults

- Collection List
- Security Groups
- Work Flow Administration
- Claims Manager
- Unprocessed Transactions

- All Files

Figure 3-32 File Maintenance dialog box

REBUILDING INDEXES

Rebuilding indexes is a process that checks and verifies data and corrects any internal problems with the data. The rebuild does not check or verify the content of the data. For example, the system will not check whether John Fitzwilliams paid $50 on his last visit. Rebuilding does not change the content of any data files. To keep files working efficiently, files should be rebuilt about once a month. Files to be rebuilt are selected from the list of files in the Rebuild Indexes tab (refer back to Figure 3-32). If the database is large, rebuilding indexes can take a long time.

rebuilding indexes a process that checks and verifies data and corrects any internal problems with the data

To rebuild files in Medisoft in an office, you would complete the following steps:

1. Click File Maintenance on the File menu. The File Maintenance dialog box is displayed with the Rebuild Indexes tab active.

2. Click in each check box next to the files that are to be verified and rebuilt. If all files are to be rebuilt, click the All Files box at the bottom of the list of files. This saves the time it would take to click a box for every Medisoft file.

3. Click the Start button. The Confirm dialog box is displayed with the message "All of the checked file processes will be performed. Do you want to continue?" Click the OK button to continue. (Clicking the Cancel button aborts the process.)

4. The rebuild process is performed automatically. When the process is complete, the message "All checked file processes are complete" is displayed.

PACKING DATA

When data are deleted in Medisoft, the system empties the data from the record but keeps the empty slot in the database so it is available when new data need to be entered in the system. For example, if a patient were deleted in the Patient List dialog box, the system would delete all the records pertaining to that patient but would maintain an empty slot in the patient database. The next time a new patient was entered, the data for the new patient would occupy the vacant slot in the database. When there is not much space on the hard disk, it may be desirable to delete the vacant slots to make more disk space available. The deletion of vacant slots from the database is known as **packing data.** Data for packing can be selected from the list of files in the Pack Data tab (see Figure 3-33). (Only transaction files with zero balances can be deleted.) If the database is large, packing data can take a long time.

packing data the deletion of vacant slots from the database

To pack files in an office situation, you would complete the following steps:

1. Click File Maintenance on the File menu. The File Maintenance dialog box is displayed with the Rebuild Indexes tab active. Make the Pack Data tab active.

2. Click in each check box next to the files that are to be packed.

3. If all files are to be packed, click the All Files box at the bottom of the list of files.

4. Click the Start button. The Confirm dialog box is displayed with the message "All of the checked file processes will be performed.

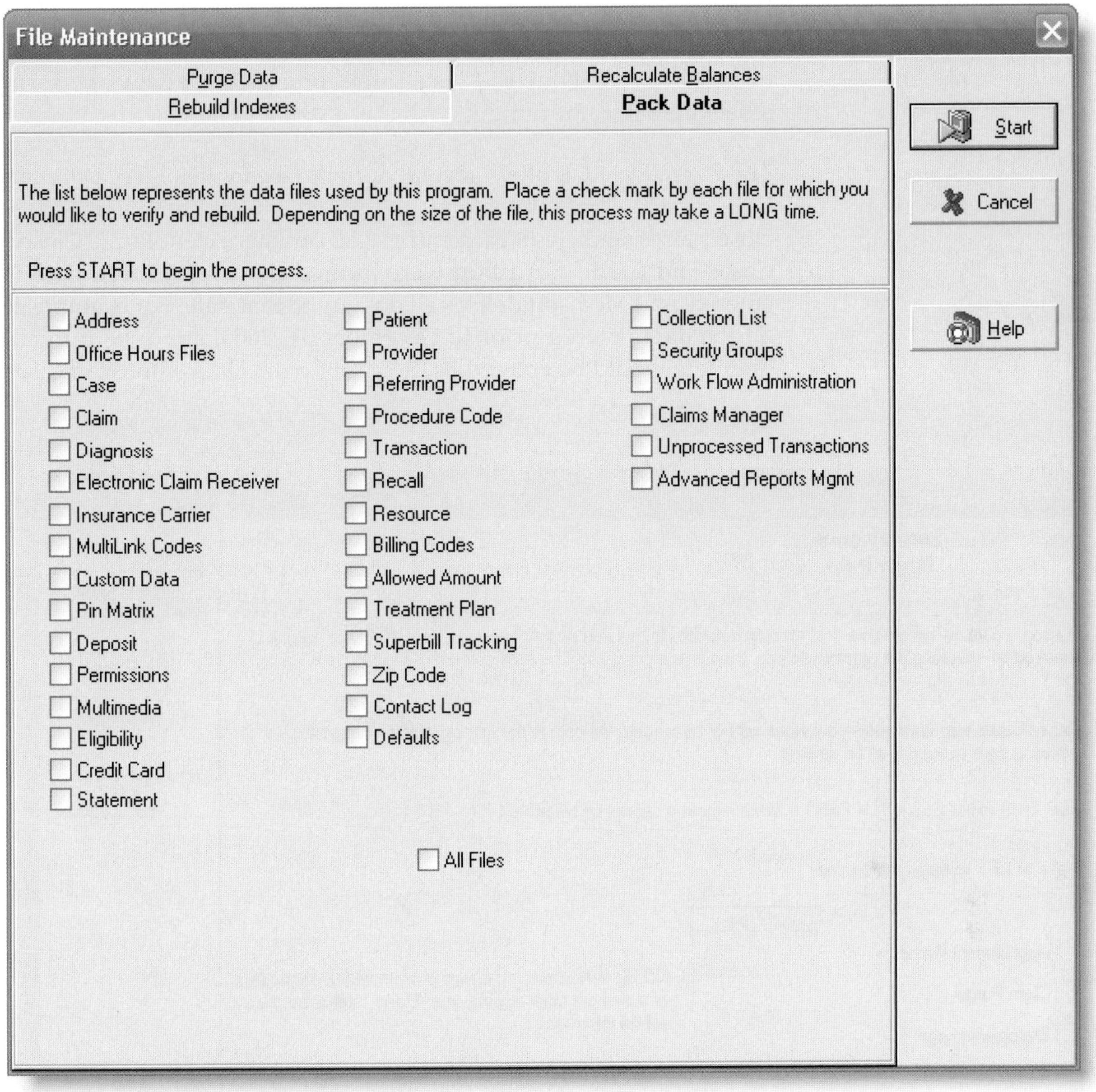

Figure 3-33 Pack Data tab

Do you want to continue?" Click the OK button to continue. (Clicking the Cancel button aborts the process.)

5. The pack process is performed automatically. When the process is complete, the message "All checked file processes are complete" is displayed.

PURGING DATA

The process of deleting files of patients who are no longer seen by a provider in a practice is called **purging data.** Purging data frees space on the computer and permits the system to run more

purging data the process of deleting files of patients who are no longer seen by a provider in a practice

efficiently. However, purging should be done with great caution. Once data are purged from the system, they cannot be retrieved, except from a backup file. As a safety precaution, always perform a backup before purging.

The Purge Data tab offers several options (see Figure 3-34). Data can be purged for appointments, claims, statements, appointment recalls, closed cases, and credit card entries. All options except Purge Closed Cases and Credit Card Purge are purged by date. A cutoff date is entered, and Medisoft deletes all data up to that date. For example, if all the data entered prior to December 31, 2000, are to be purged, that date would be entered as the cutoff date. Data entered in cases

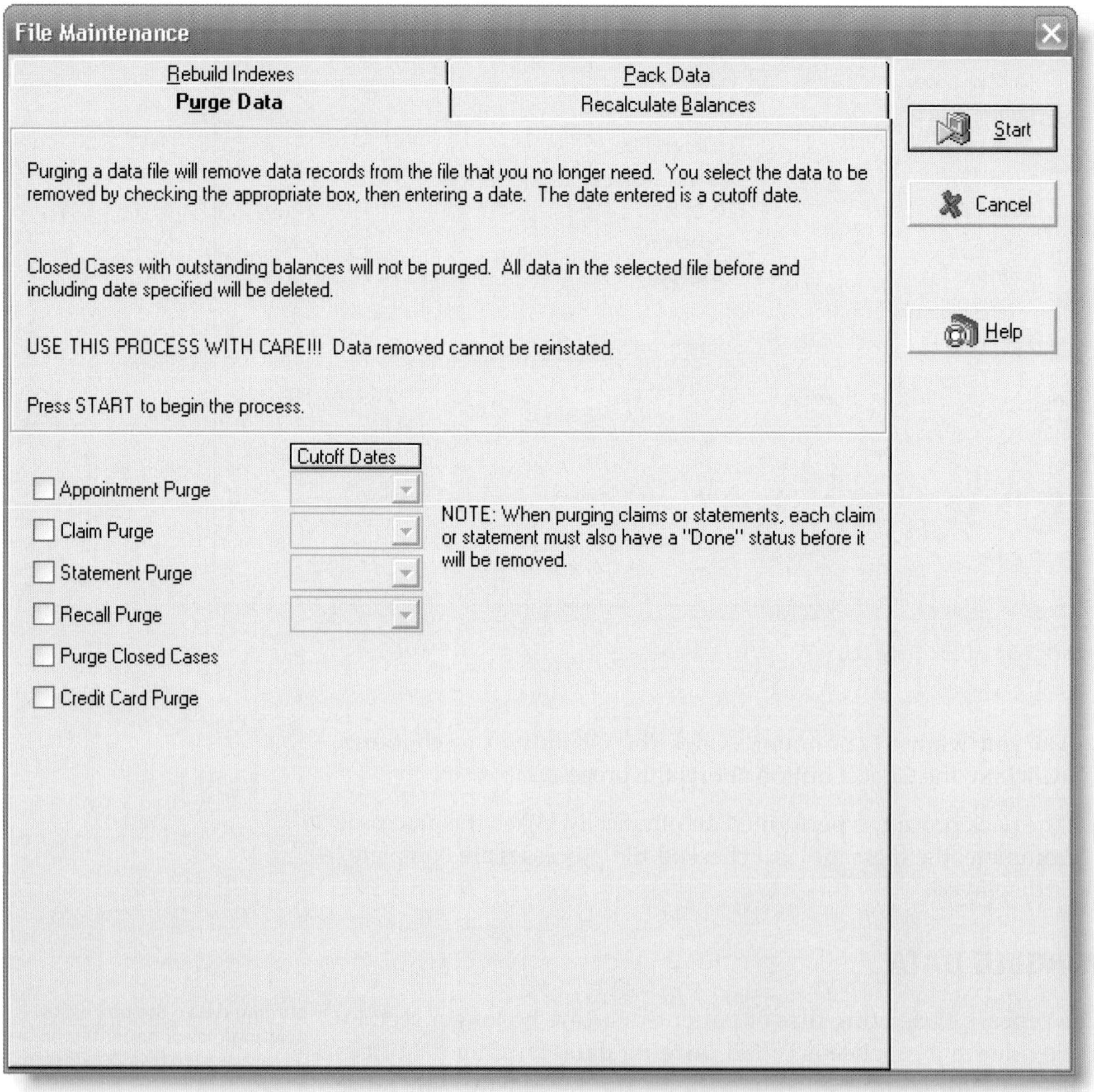

Figure 3-34   Purge Data tab

that have been closed are purged by clicking the check box labeled Purge Closed Cases.

To purge data in an office situation, you would complete the following steps:

1. Click File Maintenance on the File menu. The File Maintenance dialog box is displayed with the Rebuild Indexes tab active. Make the Purge Data tab active.

2. Click in each check box next to the files that are to be purged. Enter a cutoff date in the Cutoff Dates box.

3. Click the Start button. The Confirm dialog box is displayed with the message "All of the checked file processes will be performed. Do you want to continue?" Click the OK button to continue. (Clicking the Cancel button aborts the process.)

4. The purge process is performed automatically. When the process is complete, the message "All checked file processes are complete" is displayed.

RECALCULATING PATIENT BALANCES

As transaction entries are changed or deleted, there are times when the balance listed on the screen is not accurate. **Recalculating balances** refers to the process of updating balances to reflect the most recent changes made to the data. This feature is accessed through the Recalculate Balances tab on the File Maintenance dialog box (see Figure 3-35).

recalculating balances the process of updating balances to reflect the most recent changes made to the data

When balances are recalculated, the system reviews every patient's data and recalculates the balances. The process can be time-consuming. Individual patient balances can be recalculated in the Transaction Entry dialog box by clicking the Account Total column.

To recalculate balances in an office situation, you would complete the following steps:

1. Click File Maintenance on the File menu. The File Maintenance dialog box is displayed with the Rebuild Indexes tab active. Make the Recalculate Balances tab active.

2. Click to place a check mark in the appropriate box(es).

3. Click the Start button. The Confirm dialog box is displayed with the message "All of the checked file processes will be performed. Do you want to continue?" Click the OK button to continue. (Clicking the Cancel button aborts the process.)

4. The recalculate process is performed automatically. When the process is complete, the message "All checked file processes are complete" is displayed.

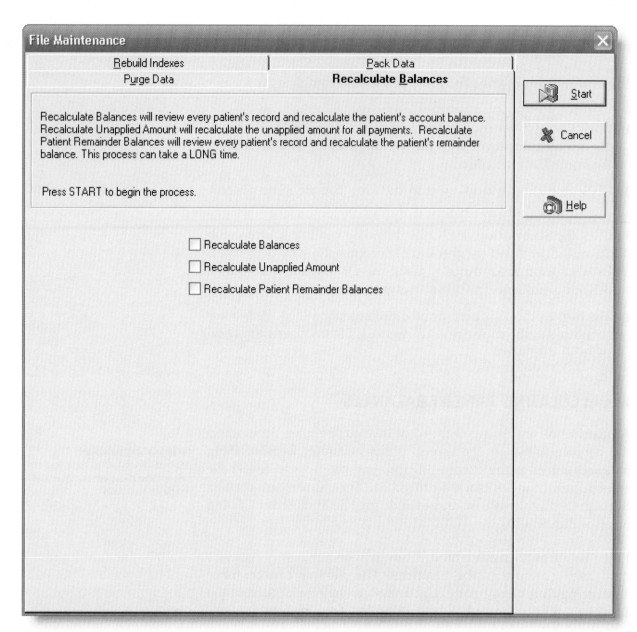

Figure 3-35   Recalculate Balances tab

CHAPTER REVIEW

USING TERMINOLOGY

Match the terms on the left with the definitions on the right.

_____ **1.** backup data

_____ **2.** knowledge base

_____ **3.** MMDDCCYY format

_____ **4.** packing data

_____ **5.** database

_____ **6.** purging data

_____ **7.** rebuilding indexes

_____ **8.** recalculating balances

_____ **9.** restoring data

a. The process of retrieving data from backup storage devices.

b. A searchable collection of up-to-date technical information.

c. A collection of related pieces of information.

d. The process of updating balances to reflect the most recent changes made to the data.

e. The process of deleting files of patients who are no longer seen by a provider in a practice.

f. A way in which dates must be keyed.

g. A copy of data files made at a specific point in time that can be used to restore data to the system.

h. A process that checks and verifies data and corrects any internal problems with the data.

i. The deletion of vacant slots from the database.

CHECKING YOUR UNDERSTANDING

Answer the questions below in the space provided.

10. Describe two ways of issuing a command in Medisoft.

_____

_____

11. What are two ways data are entered in a box?

_____

_____

12. What three types of Medisoft help are available?

_____

_____

_____

13. Which menu provides access to Office Hours, Medisoft's scheduling feature?

_____

14. What is the purpose of the buttons on the toolbar?

_____

_____

15. What is the format for entering dates in Medisoft?

_____

16. Describe two ways of exiting Medisoft.

_____

_____

17. Why is it important to back up data regularly?

_____

_____

18. Why is extra caution required when purging data?

_____

_____

19. When is a data restore performed?

_____

_____

20. In Medisoft, where are the two places a patient's balance can be recalculated?

_____

_____

APPLYING KNOWLEDGE

Answer the questions below in the space provided.

21. Use Medisoft's built-in Help to look up information on the following topics:

   a. How to enter diagnosis codes.

   b. How to print procedure code lists from the Medisoft database.

22. You come to work on a Monday morning and find that the office computer is not working. The system manager informs everyone that the computer's hard disk crashed and that all data that were not backed up are lost. What do you do?

_____

_____

AT THE COMPUTER

Answer the following questions at the computer:

23. How many options are there in the Reports menu?

_____

24. What is the first choice on the Lists menu?

_____

25. List the options on the Activities menu.

_____

_____

26. Set the Medisoft Program Date to December 1, 2010, and then exit Medisoft.

_____

Entering Patient Information

4

WHAT YOU NEED TO KNOW

To use this chapter, you need to know how to:

◆ Start Medisoft.

◆ Move around the Medisoft menus.

◆ Use the Medisoft toolbar.

◆ Enter and edit data in Medisoft.

◆ Exit Medisoft.

LEARNING OUTCOMES

In this chapter, you will learn how to:

◆ Use the Medisoft Search feature.

◆ Assign a chart number for a new patient.

◆ Enter personal and employer information for a new patient.

◆ Locate and change information for a patient.

KEY TERMS

chart number
established patient
guarantor
new patient

HOW PATIENT INFORMATION IS ORGANIZED IN MEDISOFT

Figure 4-1
Patient List
shortcut button

Patient information is accessed through the Patient List dialog box. The Patient List dialog box is displayed when Patients/Guarantors and Cases is clicked on the Lists menu or when the corresponding shortcut button is clicked on the toolbar (see Figure 4-1).

The Patient List dialog box (see Figure 4-2) is divided into two primary sections. The left side of the window displays information about patients, and the right side of the window contains information about cases. Cases are covered in Chapter 5.

SHORT CUT The quickest way to open a patient or case is to double-click on the line associated with a patient or case.

On the upper-right side of the Patient List dialog box, there are two radio buttons: Patient and Case. When the Patient radio button is clicked, the left side of the window becomes active. Correspondingly, when the Case radio button is clicked, the right side of the window becomes active. The command buttons at the bottom of the dialog box vary, depending on which side of the window is active. When the Patient window is active, the command buttons at the bottom of the screen include Edit Patient, New Patient, Delete Patient, Print Grid, Quick Entry, and Close.

The Patient window contains the following data: Chart Number, Name, Date of Birth, Social Security Number, Patient ID #2, Patient Type, Phone 1, Provider, Last Name, Billing Code, and Patient Indicator. There is not enough room in the Patient window to display all this information, so only a portion is visible at one time. The additional patient information can be viewed by using the scroll bar,

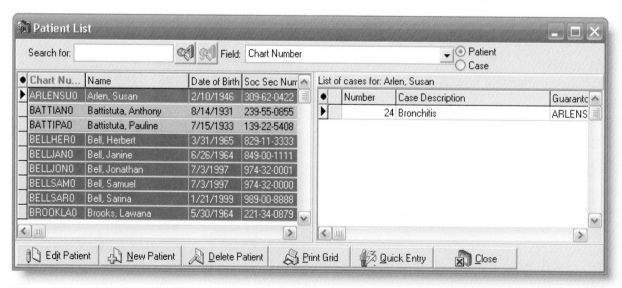

Figure 4-2 Patient List dialog box

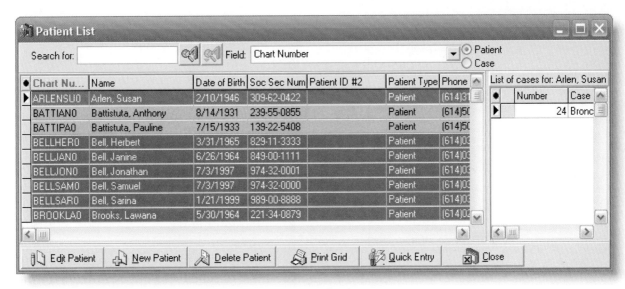

Figure 4-3   Patient window expanded to show additional columns

maximizing the dialog box, or resizing the Patient area of the dialog box (see Figure 4-3).

Information in the Patient window is color-coded. In the exercises in this text/workbook, these patient identification color codes are assigned to represent the patient's insurance carrier (see Figure 4-4).

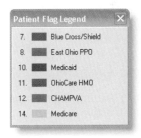

Figure 4-4   Color legend for Patient List window

ENTERING NEW PATIENT INFORMATION

A **new patient** is a patient who has not received services from the same provider or a provider of the same specialty within the same practice for a period of three years. An **established patient** is a patient who has been seen by a provider in the practice in the same specialty within three years.

Information on a new patient is entered in Medisoft by clicking the New Patient button at the bottom of the Patient List dialog box (see Figure 4-5). This action opens the Patient/Guarantor dialog box (see Figure 4-6). The Patient/Guarantor dialog box contains three tabs: the Name, Address tab, the Other Information tab, and the Payment Plan tab.

There are several buttons located on the right side of the Patient/ Guarantor dialog box. These buttons include:

Save   Saves the information entered in the dialog box.

Cancel   Closes the dialog box and discards any information entered.

new patient   a patient who has not received services from the same provider or a provider of the same specialty within the same practice for a period of three years

established patient   a patient who has been seen by a provider in the practice in the same specialty within three years

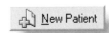

Figure 4-5   New Patient button

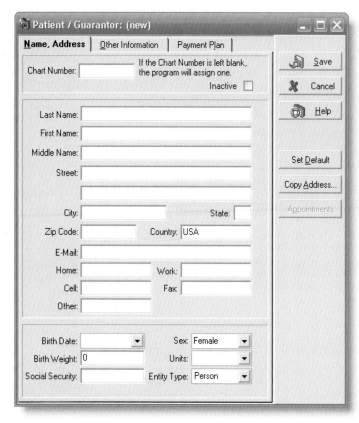

Figure 4-6 Patient/Guarantor dialog box with Name, Address tab active

Help Displays the Medisoft help window for Patient/Guarantor Entry.

Set Default Sets the information in this window as the default for all new patients. (To undo, hold the CTRL key down, and this button changes to Remove Default.)

Copy Address Copies demographic information from another patient or guarantor entry.

Appointments Opens a window with a list of scheduled appointments for the patient. (The Appointments button is grayed and cannot be selected if a patient has no appointments scheduled.)

NAME, ADDRESS TAB

The Name, Address tab is where basic patient information is entered (see Figure 4-6).

Chart Number

chart number a unique number that identifies a patient

The **chart number** is a unique number that identifies a patient. In Medisoft, a chart number links together all the information about a patient that is stored in the different databases, such as name, address, charges, and insurance claims. Each patient is assigned an eight-character chart number. If the chart number box for a patient is left blank, the system will assign a number.

Medical practices may use different methods for assigning chart numbers, although these general guidelines must be followed:

◆ No special characters, such as hyphens, periods, or spaces, are allowed.

◆ No two chart numbers can be the same.

For the purposes of this book, the following method will be used for assigning chart numbers:

◆ The first five characters of the chart number are the first five letters of a patient's last name. If the patient's last name has fewer than five characters, add the beginning letters of the patient's first name.

◆ The next two characters are the first two letters of a patient's first name. (If the first two letters of the first name were used to complete the first five letters, the next two letters of the patient's first name are used.)

◆ The last character is always a zero, displayed in this book with the symbol "Ø."

For example, the chart number for John Fitzwilliams would begin with the first five letters of his last name (FITZW), followed by the first two characters of his first name (JO), followed by a zero (Ø). John's complete chart number would be FITZWJOØ. Following the same rules, John's daughter Sarah would have a chart number of FITZWSAØ.

EXERCISE 4-1

Create a chart number for each of these patients, and write it in the space provided.

Albert Wong _____

Jessica Sypkowski _____

John James _____

Personal Data

In addition to the chart number, personal information about a patient is entered in the Name, Address tab.

Name, Address, Phone Numbers, E-Mail   Medisoft provides fields for name and address as well as a number of fields for contact methods. There are boxes for e-mail address, home phone, work phone, cell phone, fax, and other. Phone and fax numbers must be entered without parentheses or hyphens.

Birth Date   The patient's birth date is entered in the Birth Date box using the MMDDCCYY format.

Sex   This drop-down list contains choices for the patient's gender: male or female.

Birth Weight   If the patient is a newborn, the birth weight is entered in this field.

Units   This field indicates whether the birth weight is listed in pounds or grams.

Social Security   The nine-digit Social Security number is entered without hyphens; Medisoft automatically adds hyphens.

SHORT CUT   The Copy Address button saves time when entering patients with the same address, such as family members. Clicking on the Copy Address button provides an option to copy demographic information from a patient already in the database.

Entity Type This field is used for the direct transmission of electronic claims to an insurance carrier. The options in this field are person or non-person.

OTHER INFORMATION TAB

The Other Information tab within the Patient/Guarantor dialog box contains facts about a patient's employment and other miscellaneous information (see Figure 4-7).

Type The Type drop-down list is used for billing purposes to designate whether an individual is a patient or guarantor.

guarantor an individual who is not a patient of the practice, but who is the insurance policyholder for a patient of the practice

In the Medisoft Patient/Guarantor dialog box, individuals are classified into two categories: patient and guarantor. A patient is an individual who is a patient of the practice, whether or not he or she is also the insurance policyholder. The term **guarantor** refers to an individual who is not a patient of the practice but who is the insurance policyholder for a patient of the practice. For example, if the

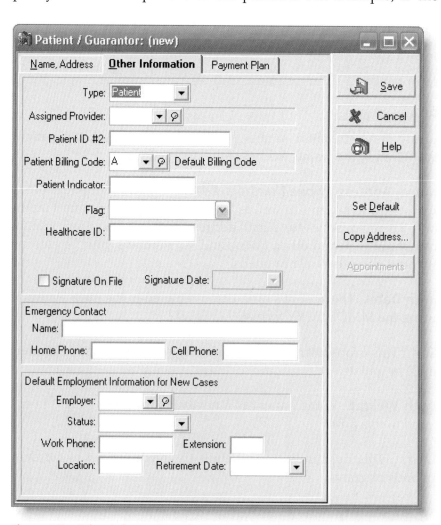

Figure 4-7 Other Information tab

insurance policy of a parent who is not a patient provides coverage for a child who is a patient, the parent is the guarantor.

Information about the patient is always entered in Medisoft in the Name/Address tab. When the patient is not the policyholder, information about the guarantor must also be entered in the Medisoft database for insurance claims to be processed. This information is collected from the patient information or patient update form.

Assigned Provider   The Assigned Provider drop-down list contains codes assigned to the doctors in the practice (see Figure 4-8). The code for the specific doctor who provides care to this patient is selected.

Patient ID #2   The Patient ID #2 box is used by some medical practices as a second identification system in addition to chart numbers.

Patient Billing Code   The Patient Billing Code is an optional field used to categorize patients according to the billing codes that the practice has set up in Medisoft. For example, Billing Code A might be for patients with insurance coverage, B for cash patients, and so on. Some practices use billing codes to classify patients according to a billing cycle—patients with Billing Code A are billed on the first of the month, and those with Billing Code B on the fifteenth of the month. The Billing Code field is not used in the exercises in this book.

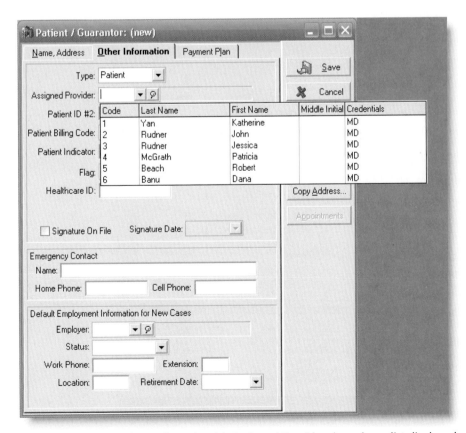

Figure 4-8   Other Information tab with Assigned Provider drop-down list displayed

Patient Indicator   The Patient Indicator is an optional field that practices can use to classify types of patients, such as workers' compensation patients, cash patients, and diabetic patients.

Flag   This field can be used to organize patients into groups and assign a color code to each group. In this text/workbook, the flag is assigned to patients' insurance plans.

Healthcare ID   The Healthcare ID is not used at present; it is included for future implementation of the HIPAA legislation.

Signature on File   A check mark in the Signature on File check box means that the patient's signature is on file for the purpose of submitting insurance claims. This box must be completed. If it is not, the insurance carrier will not accept and process insurance claims.

Signature Date   The date keyed in the Signature Date box is the date the patient signed the insurance release form.

Emergency Contact   Information about how to contact someone in case of a patient emergency is entered in these fields.

Employer   The code for the patient's employer is selected from the drop-down list of employers in the database (see Figure 4-9). If the patient's employer is not in the database, this information must

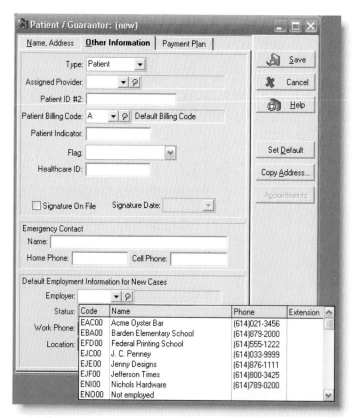

Figure 4-9   Other Information tab with Employer drop-down list displayed

be entered before the code can be selected. (This process is described later in the chapter.)

Status   The Status drop-down list displays the following choices for the patient's employment status: Not employed, Full time, Part time, Retired, and Unknown.

Work Phone and Extension   Work phone numbers should be entered without parentheses or hyphens.

Location   Some companies have multiple locations. If the patient supplies information on the specific company location, it is entered in this box.

Retirement Date   The Retirement Date box is filled in only if the patient is already retired. Retirement dates should be entered in the MMDDCCYY format.

When all the fields in the Name, Address tab and the Other Information tab have been filled in, entries should be checked for accuracy. If any information needs to be corrected, it can easily be changed. Once the information has been checked and necessary corrections made, data are saved by clicking the Save button.

PAYMENT PLAN TAB

The Payment Plan tab is used when a patient's account is overdue and a payment plan has been created to pay down the remaining balance (see Figure 4-10).

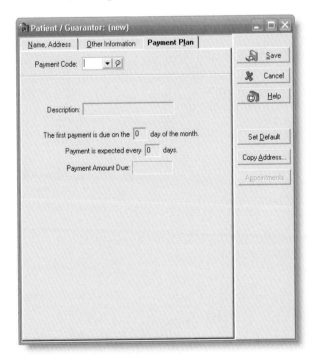

Figure 4-10   Payment Plan tab

EXERCISE 4-2

Using Source Document 1 (located in Part 4 of this book), complete the Patient/Guarantor dialog box for Hiro Tanaka, a new patient of Dr. Yan.

1. Start Medisoft by clicking the Start button and selecting All Programs, Medisoft, Medisoft Advanced Patient Accounting.

2. On the Lists menu, click Patients/Guarantors and Cases, or click the corresponding shortcut button on the toolbar.

3. Scroll down the list of patients to make sure Hiro Tanaka is not already in the patient database.

4. Click the New Patient button.

5. Create a chart number for this patient. Remember, in this text/workbook the chart number should be the first five letters of the patient's last name, followed by the first two letters of the patient's first name, followed by a Ø. Click the Chart Number box, and enter the chart number.

6. Click the Last Name box, and fill in the patient information. Fill in the rest of the boxes (for which you have data) on the Name, Address tab, pressing the Tab key to move from box to box.

7. Click the Other Information tab, and fill in the appropriate boxes. Be sure to select an Assigned Provider (Dr. Yan is Tanaka's assigned provider) so the exercises in this chapter will work.

8. Select Tanaka's insurance carrier in the Flag field.

9. Make no entries in the following boxes: Patient ID #2, Patient Indicator, Healthcare ID, and Emergency Contact boxes. Accept the default entry in the Patient Billing Code box. Click the Signature on File box and enter *10/04/2010* as the Signature Date. A Confirm box appears, stating that you have entered a future date and asking whether you want to change it. Click No. A Warning box is displayed, stating that the date entered is in the future. Click OK.

10. Since Tanaka's employer is not in the database, leave the employer boxes blank for now.

11. Check your entries for accuracy, and make corrections if necessary.

12. Click the Save button to save the data on Tanaka.

13. Verify that Tanaka has been added to the list in the Patient List dialog box.

14. Close the Patient List dialog box.

ADDING AN EMPLOYER TO THE ADDRESS LIST

If the patient's employer does not appear on the Employer drop-down list in the Other Information tab, it must be entered using the Address

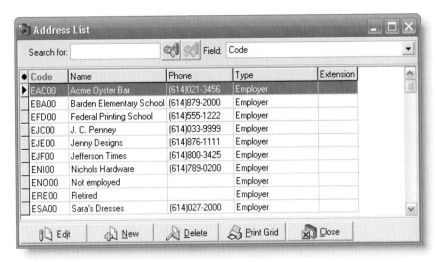

Figure 4-11 Address List dialog box

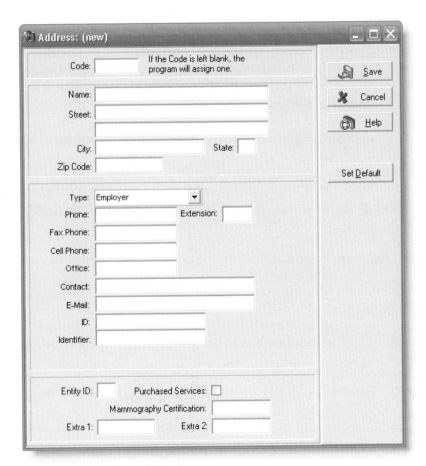

Figure 4-12 Address dialog box

feature. Addresses are entered by clicking the Addresses command on the Lists menu, which displays the Address List dialog box (see Figure 4-11). Addresses are entered by clicking the New button.

Clicking the New button at the bottom of the Address List dialog box displays the Address dialog box (see Figure 4-12).

The Address dialog box contains the following boxes:

Code   The code for an employer should begin with the letter *E* to indicate that this is an employer. Codes can be a combination of letters and numbers up to a maximum of five characters. If a code is not assigned, the system will assign one.

Name and Address   The employer's name is entered in the Name box. This field allows up to thirty characters. The employer's street, city, state (two characters only), and ZIP code are entered in the boxes provided.

Type   The Type drop-down list displays a list of kinds of addresses: Attorney, Employer, Facility, Laboratory, Miscellaneous, and Referral Source. For example, when the address being entered is that of an employer, "Employer" would be selected.

Phone, Extension, Fax Phone, Cell Phone   In the Phone box, the employer's phone number is entered, without parentheses or hyphens. If there is an extension, it is entered in the Extension box. If there is a cell phone, it is entered in the Cell Phone box. The employer's fax number is entered in the Fax Phone box.

Office   This field can be used to note a particular office within an organization.

Contact   The Contact box is used to enter the name of an individual at the place of employment. If there is no contact person, the box is left blank.

E-Mail   This box provides a field for the employer's e-mail address.

ID   If there is an identification number for the employer, it is entered in the ID box.

Identifier   The Identifier field is in place for future implementation of HIPAA legislation.

Entity ID   Enter a two-digit code that indicates the type of entity:

FA	Facility
LI	Independent lab
TL	Testing lab
77	Service location

Purchased Services   Click this check box if the practice purchases services from this facility or laboratory.

Mammography Certification   If this entity is certified to perform mammography procedures, enter the certification number.

SHORT CUT

Throughout Medisoft, the F8 function key serves as a shortcut for entering data. For example, clicking once in the Employer box on the Other Information tab and then pressing F8 brings up the Address dialog box, in which a new employer can be entered. The F8 key shortcut enables users to enter data in Medisoft in another part of the program without leaving the current dialog box. Once the F8 key is pressed, the dialog box used to enter new addresses is opened, with the Patient List and Patient/Guarantor dialog box still open in the background (see Figure 4-13).

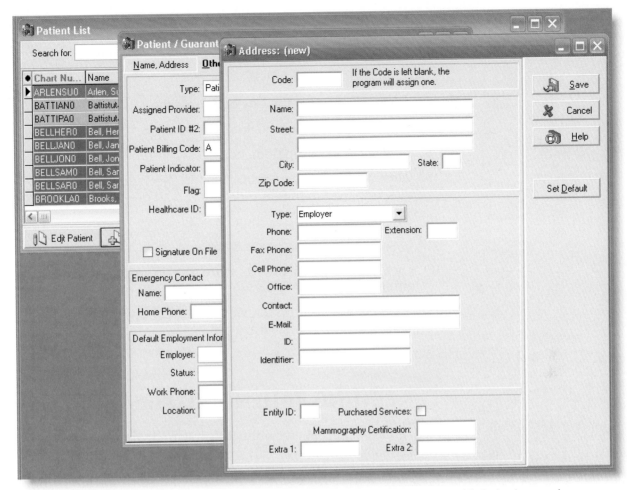

Figure 4-13   Address dialog box with Patient List and Patient/Guarantor boxes visible in background

Extra 1, Extra 2   The Extra 1 and Extra 2 boxes are available to keep track of additional information that needs to be recorded and stored for future reference.

When all the information on the employer has been entered, it is saved by clicking the Save button.

EXERCISE 4-3

Practice entering information about an employer.

1. Click Addresses on the Lists menu. The Address List dialog box is displayed.

2. Click the New button at the bottom of the dialog box. The Address dialog box is displayed.

3. In the Code box, key **EMCØØ** for McCray Manufacturing, Inc. (*E* for employer, followed by the first two letters of the employer's name, followed by two zeros). Press the Tab key.

4. Key *McCray Manufacturing Inc.* in the Name box. Press the Tab key.

5. In the Street box, key *1311 Kings Highway.* Press the Tab key twice.

6. Key *Stephenson* in the City box. Press the Tab key.

7. Key *OH* in the State box. Press the Tab key.

8. Key *60089* in the Zip Code box. Press the Tab key.

9. Verify that Employer is displayed in the Type box. If it is not, click Employer in the drop-down list, and press the Tab key.

10. Key *6145550000* in the Phone box. Press the Tab key.

11. Leave the remaining boxes blank.

12. Click the Save button to store the information you have entered.

13. Click the Close button to exit the Address List dialog box.

EDITING PATIENT INFORMATION

From time to time, patients notify the practice that they have moved, changed jobs or insurance carriers, and so on. When this happens, information needs to be updated in Medisoft's patient/guarantor database.

The process of changing information about a patient is similar to that of entering information for a new patient. The Patients/Guarantors and Cases command is selected from the Lists menu. A search is usually performed to locate the chart number of the patient whose record needs to be updated. Clicking the Edit button displays the Patient/Guarantor dialog box, where changes can be made. Clicking the Save button stores the changes.

SEARCHING FOR PATIENT INFORMATION

A patient who comes to a medical practice for the first time fills out a patient information form. The information on this form needs to be entered into the Medisoft patient/guarantor database before insurance claims can be submitted. However, before information on a patient is entered into the system, it is important to search the database to be certain that the patient does not already exist there.

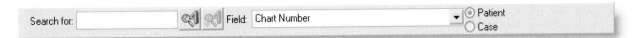

Figure 4-14   Search for and Field boxes

Medisoft provides two options for conducting searches: Search for and Field boxes, and Locate buttons.

SEARCH FOR AND FIELD OPTION

The Search for and Field boxes at the top of many dialog boxes provide a quick way to search for information in Medisoft (see Figure 4-14).

The Search for box contains the text that is to be searched on. The entry in the Field box controls how the list is sorted. Figure 4-15 displays the Field options in the Patient List dialog box.

When a selection is made in the Field box, the information is resorted by the selected criteria. For example, if Social Security Number is selected in the Field box, the entries in the List window are listed in numerical order by Social Security number, from lowest to highest (see Figure 4-16).

The Search for and Field feature is used in the following Medisoft dialog boxes: Patient List, Insurance Carrier List, Procedure/Payment/Adjustment List, Diagnosis Code List, Address List, Provider List, and Referring Provider List. Table 4-1 displays the Field box options for each of these Medisoft dialog boxes.

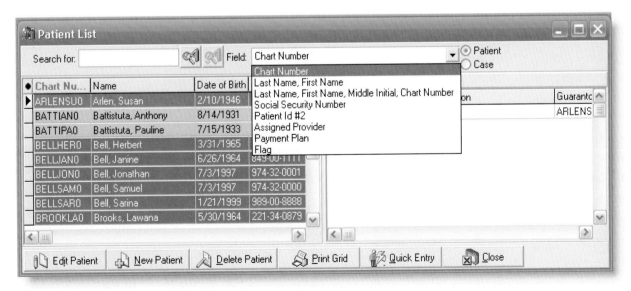

Figure 4-15   Field options in the Patient List dialog box

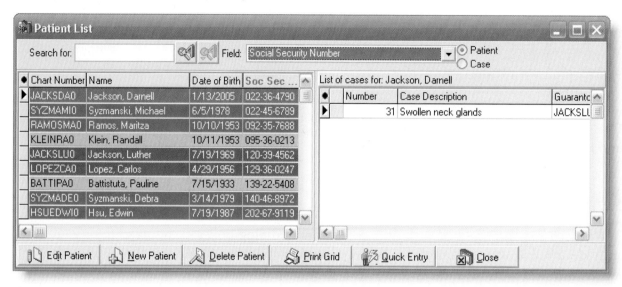

Figure 4-16 List window sorted by Social Security number

Table 4-1	Field Options for Medisoft Searches

List Window	Field Options
Patient List	Flag; Payment Plan; Patient ID #2; Assigned Provider; Social Security Number; Last Name, First Name, Middle Initial, Chart Number; Last Name, First Name; Chart Number
Insurance Carrier List	Code, Name
Procedure/Payment/Adjustment List	Type, Code 1, Description
Diagnosis Code List	Code 1, Description
Address List	Type, Name, Code,
Provider List	Code; Last Name, First Name
Referring Provider List	Code; Last Name, First Name

After an entry is made in the Field box, the search criteria are entered in the Search field. As each letter or number is entered, the list automatically filters out records that do not match. For example, if the Field box is set to Last Name, First Name in the Patient List dialog box and *S* is entered in the Search field, the program eliminates all data from the list except patients whose last names begin with *S* (see Figure 4-17).

To restore the Patient list to its default setting (all patients listed), delete the entry in the Search for box.

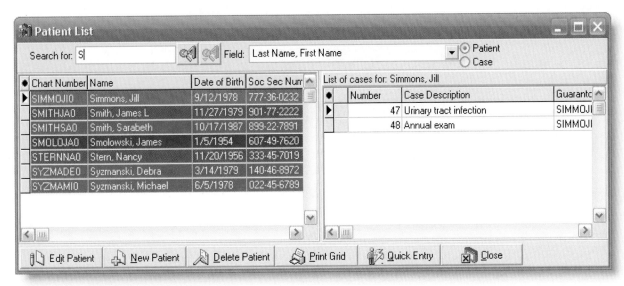

Figure 4-17   Patient List dialog box with search for patients whose last names begin with *S*

EXERCISE 4-4

Use the Search feature to locate information on James Smolowski.

1. On the Lists menu, click Patients/Guarantors and Cases, or click the corresponding shortcut button. The Patient List dialog box is displayed, and the cursor is blinking in the Search for box. Confirm that the entry in the Field box is Last Name, First Name.

2. Enter the first letter of the patient's last name. Notice that when you keyed *S*, the list window filtered the data so that only patients whose last names begin with *S* are listed. Now enter the second letter of his last name, *m.* The list now displays only those patients whose last names begin with the letters *Sm*. Now enter the third letter, *o.* Smolowski is the only patient whose name begins with the letters *Smo*, so he is the only patient listed.

3. To restore the Patient window so that all patients are listed, delete the letters entered in the Search for box.

4. Click the Close button to exit the Patient List dialog box.

LOCATE BUTTONS OPTION

Another option for finding information in Medisoft is to use the Locate buttons (see Figure 4-18).

When a Locate button is clicked, a Locate dialog box is displayed. Figure 4-19 shows the Locate Patient dialog box.

Field Value

The information entered in the Field Value box at the top of the window can be part of a name, birth date, payment date or amount, or assigned provider. Any combination of numbers and letters can be used.

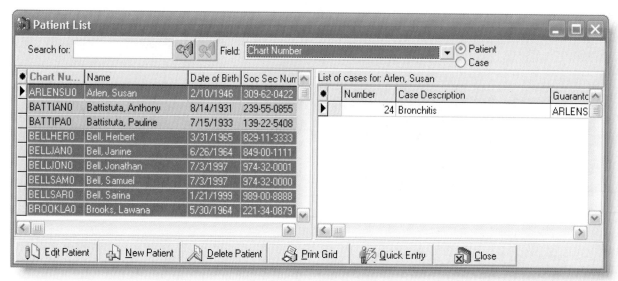

Figure 4-18   Locate buttons highlighted in yellow

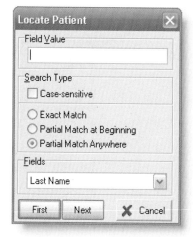

Figure 4-19   Locate Patient
dialog box

SHORT CUT   To make
searching easier, right-
click a column heading
in a window that con-
tains several columns.
From the shortcut
menu that appears,
select Locate, or press
ALT + L. This opens a
Locate window that
defaults the Fields se-
lection to the column
you selected.

Search Type

Case Sensitive   Use to make the search sensitive to uppercase or lowercase letters.

Exact Match   Use when an entry in the Field Value box is exactly as entered in the program.

Partial Match at Beginning   Use when unsure of the correct spelling or entry at the end of the word.

Partial Match Anywhere   Use when unsure of the correct spelling or entry.

Fields

The Fields box provides a drop-down list from which to choose the field that contains the information that is being matched. For example, if searching for a patient by last name, select the Last Name field. The available fields are determined by the type of information you are working with. For example, if you are looking for a particular Chart Number, you have nineteen fields from which to choose as the basis of your search. Searching for cases gives access to up to ninety-one fields.

Once the criteria are selected, clicking the First button starts a search for the first match to the criteria. If a match is found, the Locate window is closed, and the search result is highlighted in the Search window. If a match is not found, a message is displayed. Clicking the Next button begins a search for the next criteria match, and so on. When the program reaches the end of the list, a message is displayed indicating that the search is complete.

EXERCISE 4-5

Practice searching for and editing information on Hiro Tanaka.

1. Open the Patient List dialog box. Confirm that the Field box entry is Last Name, First Name.

2. Search for Hiro Tanaka by keying the first few letters of her last name in the Search for box. Notice that as soon as the *T* is entered, all patients except Tanaka disappear from the Patient List window, because Tanaka is the only patient whose last name begins with *T*.

3. Click the Edit Patient button.

4. Click the Other Information tab.

5. Click the triangle button in the Employer box. Click McCray Manufacturing Inc. on the drop-down list. Notice that the program automatically enters the phone number in the Work Phone box.

6. Select Full time from the Status drop-down list.

7. Click the Save button to store the information you have entered.

8. Close the Patient List dialog box.

ON YOUR OWN EXERCISES

At the end of each chapter, you will apply what you have learned in an On Your Own exercise. This exercise is similar to the exercises you completed throughout the chapter, with one important difference: step-by-step instructions are not provided. You must rely on what you learned and practiced in the chapter to complete the On Your Own exercise.

ON YOUR OWN EXERCISE 1 Entering a New Patient

Lisa Wright is a new patient who has just arrived for her office visit with Dr. Jessica Rudner. Using Source Document 2, complete the Patient/Guarantor dialog box. (*Note:* Not all text boxes will have entries.)

Remember to create a backup of your work before exiting Medisoft! To help you keep track of your work, name the backup file after the chapter you are working on, for example, StudentID-c4.mbk.

Electronic Medical Record Exchange

Transferring Patient Information

Some practice management programs and electronic medical record programs are able to exchange patient information. This saves time and reduces errors, since patient information is entered in one program and then transferred to the other, eliminating the need to enter the information twice.

Patient information in Medisoft, such as displayed in the illustration below, is transferred to an electronic medical record program.

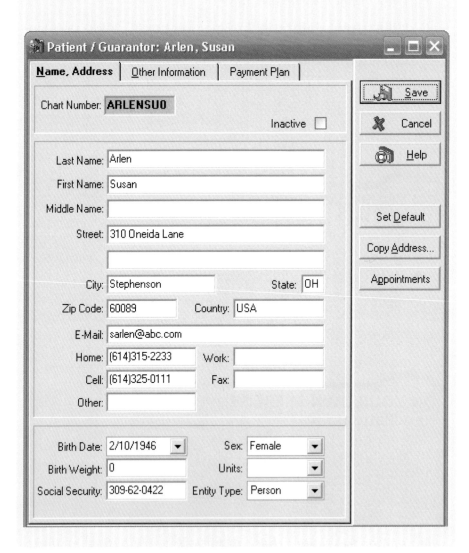

The next screen capture shows a list of patient information that has been received by Medisoft from an electronic medical record program. As you can see, the list includes information on new patients as well as updated information about established patients.

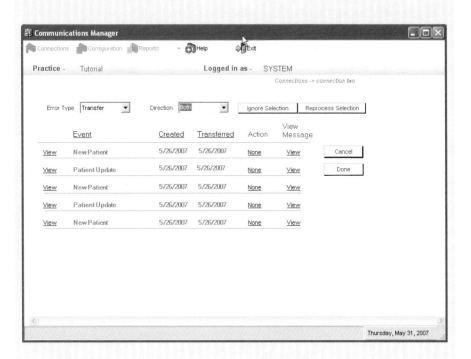

Name: _____   Date: _____

CHAPTER 4 WORKSHEET

After completing all the exercises in the chapter, answer the following questions in the spaces provided.

1. What is entered in the Chart Number field for Hiro Tanaka (Name, Address tab)?

   _____

2. Which patient is found as a result of the search in Exercise 4-4?

   _____

3. Which patient is found as a result of the search in Exercise 4-5?

   _____

4. What is the entry in the Employer field for Hiro Tanaka (Other Information tab)?

   _____

5. What is the entry in the Signature Date box for Hiro Tanaka (Other Information tab)?

   _____

6. What is entered in the Chart Number field for Lisa Wright (Name, Address tab)?

   _____

7. What is entered in the Flag field for Lisa Wright (Other Information tab)?

   _____

8. What is entered in the Work Phone field for Hiro Tanaka (Other Information tab)?

   _____

9. What is entered in the Status field for Lisa Wright (Other Information tab)?

   _____

10. What is entered in the Birth Date field for Lisa Wright (Name, Address tab)?

   _____

CHAPTER REVIEW

USING TERMINOLOGY

Define the terms in the space provided.

1. chart number

_____

_____

2. established patient

_____

_____

3. guarantor

_____

_____

4. new patient

_____

_____

CHECKING YOUR UNDERSTANDING

Answer the questions below in the space provided.

5. To search for Paul Ramos, can you key either "Paul" or "Ramos"? Explain.

_____

_____

6. Create a chart number for a patient named William Burroughs.

_____

_____

7. Sam Wu has no insurance of his own but is covered by his wife's insurance policy. How would you indicate this in the Patient/Guarantor dialog box?

_____

_____

8. A patient's address is 11 West Main Street, Anytown, WI 55555. What would you enter in the City box located in the Patient/Guarantor dialog box?

_____

_____

9. How would you enter the Social Security number 123-45-6789?

_____

_____

APPLYING KNOWLEDGE

Answer the following question in the space provided.

10. Jane Taylor-Burke comes to the office. She thinks she saw Dr. Yan a few years ago for a flu shot, but she is not sure. You need to decide whether to enter Ms. Taylor-Burke as a new patient in the Medisoft database. What should you do?

_____

_____

AT THE COMPUTER

Answer the following questions at the computer.

11. How many patients in the database have the last name of Smith?

_____

_____

12. List the name of the patient who is found when you search for the letters *JO*.

_____

_____

13. What is Li Y. Wong's chart number?

_____

_____

14. In the Patient List dialog box, search for information on Leila Patterson. What steps did you take to find the information?

_____

_____

Entering Insurance, Account, and Condition Information

5

WHAT YOU NEED TO KNOW

To use this chapter you need to know how to:

◆ Use the Medisoft Search feature.

◆ Enter patient information in Medisoft.

◆ Locate and change information about an established patient.

LEARNING OUTCOMES

When you finish this chapter, you will be able to:

◆ Determine when to create a new case.

◆ Set up a new case.

◆ Enter information on a patient's insurance policy.

◆ Enter information about an accident or illness.

◆ Enter information on a patient's diagnosis.

◆ Edit information in an existing case.

◆ Close a case.

◆ Delete a case.

KEY TERMS

capitated plan
case
chart
primary insurance carrier

record of treatment and
   progress
referring provider
sponsor

WORKING WITH CASES

case a grouping of transactions for visits to a physician's office, organized around a condition

A **case** is a grouping of transactions for visits to a physician's office organized around a condition. When a patient comes for treatment, a case is created.

A case is set up to contain the transactions that relate to a particular condition. For example, all treatments and procedures for a patient's bronchial asthma would be stored in a case called "bronchial asthma." Services performed and charges for those services would be entered in the system and linked to the bronchial asthma case.

WHEN TO SET UP A NEW CASE

A new case should be set up each time a patient comes to see the physician for a new condition or when there is a change in the provider or insurance carrier. For example, suppose that a patient has been seeing a physician regularly for treatment of bronchial asthma. All the transactions for this treatment would be contained in one case. Then suppose that the patient has an accident and comes in for treatment of a sprained ankle. The sprained ankle is a new condition. A new case would be set up in Medisoft for the sprained ankle treatments.

When a patient changes insurance carriers, a new case should be set up, even if the same condition is being treated under the new carrier. This makes it easier to submit insurance claims to the appropriate carrier. Transactions that took place while the previous policy was in effect must be submitted under that policy. Transactions that occur after the change in policies must be submitted to the new carrier. By opening a new case, transactions for the two insurance carriers can be kept separate. The information needed to submit claims to the previous carrier is still intact, while information for claims under the new policy is current.

A patient may require more than one case per office visit if treatment is provided for two or more unrelated conditions. For example, a patient who visits the physician complaining of migraine headaches may also ask for an influenza vaccination. Since the two conditions are unrelated, two cases would need to be created: one for the migraine headaches, and one for the vaccination. In contrast, a patient who is treated for shortness of breath and chest pain during exertion would require one case if the physician determines that the two complaints are related to the same diagnosis.

It is common for patients to have more than one case open at any one time. In the example mentioned earlier, the patient's bronchial asthma case and sprained ankle case would be open at the same time. While the patient is being treated for the ankle injury, the bronchial asthma treatment is continuing. Some cases are for chronic conditions and remain open a long time. Other cases, such as for treatment of influenza, may be of short duration. Cases are closed when the patient is no longer being treated for the condition, when the insurance policy in the case is no longer in effect, or when the patient leaves the practice.

CASE COMMAND BUTTONS

In Medisoft, cases are created, edited, and deleted from within the Patient List dialog box. The Patient List dialog box is accessed by choosing Patients/Guarantors and Cases from the Lists menu. When the Case radio button in the Patient List dialog box is clicked, the following command buttons appear at the bottom of the Patient List dialog box: Edit Case, New Case, Delete Case, Copy Case, Print Grid, Quick Entry, and Close (see Figure 5-1).

Edit Case   The Edit Case button is used to add, delete, or change information in an existing case. When the Edit Case button is clicked, the Case dialog box is displayed. Case information to be updated is contained in eleven different tabs. For example, if a patient changes insurance carriers, information needs to be updated in the Policy 1, 2, or 3 tab. The only item in the Case dialog box that cannot be changed is the Case Number. All other boxes are edited by moving the cursor to the box and making the change, whether this involves rekeying, selecting and deselecting check boxes, or clicking a different option on a drop-down list.

> **SHORT CUT** Cases can also be opened for editing by double-clicking on the case number/description in the Case window within the Patient List dialog box.

New Case   The New Case button creates a new case.

Delete Case   The Delete Case button deletes a case from the system if the case has no open transactions. Open transactions are charges

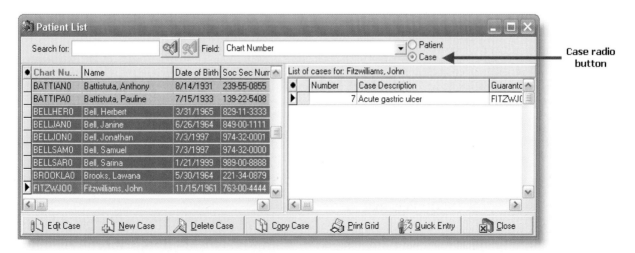

Figure 5-1   Patient List dialog box with Case radio button selected

that have not been fully paid by the insurance carrier or the policy-holder. The Delete Case button should be used with caution; once deleted, information cannot be retrieved. Cases should be deleted only when it is definite that the patient's records will never be needed again. Medical offices usually have policies about when a patient's records are deleted, such as five years after the patient's last visit to the practice. In most instances, it is more appropriate to close a case than to delete it. Cases are closed by clicking the Case Closed box in the Personal tab of the Case dialog box.

Cases are deleted in the Patient List dialog box. With the Case radio button clicked, the specific case to be deleted is selected by clicking the line that displays the case number and description. The case is then deleted by clicking the Delete Case button at the bottom of the dialog box. The system will ask, "Are you sure you want to delete this case?" Clicking the Yes button deletes the case from the system.

Copy Case   The Copy Case button copies all the information from an existing case into a new case. This feature is useful when creating a new case for a patient who already has a case in the system. Copy Case makes it unnecessary to reenter the information in all ten tabs; instead, the information in the existing case is copied into a new case. Then the information that needs to be changed can be edited to reflect the new case. Sometimes the new case requires few changes; other times data must be changed in all the tabs of the Case folder. For this reason, when copying a case it is important to check each tab to make sure the copied information is accurate for the new case. The information that remains the same from the previous case can be left as is.

Print Grid   The Print Grid button is used to select or deselect columns of information for printing purposes.

Quick Entry   The Quick Entry button is used in practices that customize the way patient data are entered.

Close   The Close button closes the Patient List dialog box.

> **SHORT CUT** When creating a new case for an established patient, it is faster to use the Copy Case button than to create a new case using the New Case button.

CREATING A NEW CASE FOR A NEW PATIENT

Clicking the New Case button brings up the Case dialog box (see Figure 5-2). Information about a patient is entered in eleven different tabs in the Case dialog box:

1. Personal

2. Account

3. Diagnosis

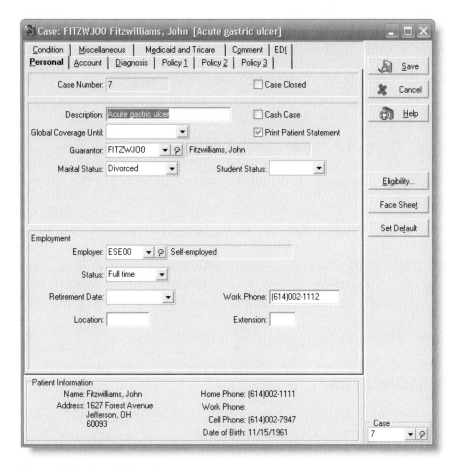

Figure 5-2 Case dialog box

4. Policy 1

5. Policy 2

6. Policy 3

7. Condition

8. Miscellaneous

9. Medicaid and Tricare

10. Comment

11. EDI

The information required to complete the eleven tabs comes from documents found in a patient's chart. The **chart** is a folder that contains all records pertaining to a patient. The new patient information form supplies basic information, such as name and address, as well as information about insurance coverage, allergies, whether the condition is related to an accident, and the referral source. The **record of treatment and progress** contains the physician's notes about a patient's condition and diagnosis. The encounter form is a list of services performed and the charges for them.

chart a folder that contains all records pertaining to a patient

record of treatment and progress a physician's notes about a patient's condition and diagnosis

There are several buttons located on the right side of the Case folder. These buttons include:

Save   Saves the information entered in the dialog box.

Cancel   Closes the dialog box and discards any information entered.

Help   Displays the Medisoft help window for the Case folder.

Eligibility   Displays an option to verify eligibility for the patient and case.

Face Sheet   Prints a sheet of information about the patient and case.

Set Default   Sets the information in the case as the default for new cases for this patient. To remove the default, hold down the CTRL key and this button changes to a Remove Default button.

Case   Displays a list of the patient's cases.

PERSONAL TAB

The Personal tab contains basic information about a patient and his or her employment (see Figure 5-3).

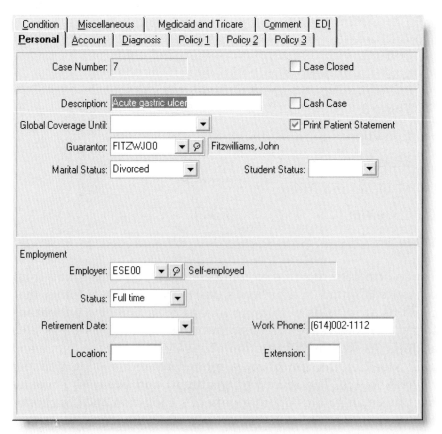

Figure 5-3   Personal tab

Case Number   The case number is a sequential number assigned by Medisoft. To avoid confusion, case numbers are unique; no two patients ever have the same case number.

Case Closed   A case is marked as closed by placing a check mark in the Case Closed box. At times it is appropriate to close a case. Closing a case indicates that no more data will be entered into the case. When is it appropriate to close a case? Policies vary from practice to practice, but generally cases are closed when a patient changes insurance carriers, has recovered completely from a condition (such as the flu), or is no longer a patient at the practice.

Description   Information entered in the Description box indicates a patient's complaint, or reason for seeing a physician. For example, if a patient comes to see a physician for an annual physical examination, the Description box would read "annual physical." Other examples of entries are sore throat, stomach pains, dog bite, and accident at work. A patient's complaint can be found in his or her chart.

Global Coverage Until   Certain services are paid for under what are known as "global fees." These fees include reimbursement for services performed at different times by the same provider (or group) when performed in conjunction with one medical procedure or episode of care. For example, in a global surgical package, preoperative, intraoperative, and postoperative services are included in the single payment for a surgical procedure. The entry in this field indicates the date on which charges are no longer considered part of the global fee.

Cash Case   If the Cash Case box is checked, the patient is paying cash and has no insurance coverage.

Guarantor   The Guarantor box lists the name of the person responsible for paying the bill. The drop-down list contains the chart numbers and names of all potential guarantors in the database.

Print Patient Statement   If this box is checked, a statement for the patient is automatically printed when statements for the practice are printed.

Marital Status   The drop-down list provides the following choices to indicate a patient's marital status: Divorced, Legally separated, Married, Single, Unknown, or Widowed.

Student Status   The Student Status drop-down list is used to indicate whether a patient is a full-time student, a part-time student, or a nonstudent. If a patient's status is not known, the box should be left blank.

Employer   The Employer box contains the default employer information that has been entered in the Patient/Guarantor dialog box.

If it is necessary to change the employer, the default can be overridden by clicking another employer code on the drop-down list.

Status The Status box lists a patient's employment status as recorded in the Patient/Guarantor dialog box. To change the selection that appears in the Status box, another selection is clicked on the drop-down list. The options are Full-time, Not employed, Part-time, Retired, and Unknown.

Retirement Date The Retirement Date box should be filled in only when a patient is already retired. There are two ways of entering the retirement date. The date can be entered in the Retirement Date box, or it can be selected from the pop-up calendar that appears when the triangle button to the right of the box is clicked.

Work Phone The Work Phone box contains a patient's work phone number.

Location If a patient has supplied a specific work location, such as "Fifth Avenue Branch," it is entered in the Location box.

Extension The Extension box lists a patient's work phone extension.

Saving Cases

After the information in the tab has been checked for accuracy and edited as necessary, the case must be saved. Data recorded in the Case dialog box are stored by clicking the Save button on the right side of the Case dialog box. Clicking the Cancel button exits the Case dialog box without saving the newly entered information.

EXERCISE 5-1

Create a new case for patient Hiro Tanaka, and enter information in the Personal tab. The information needed to complete this exercise is found on Source Document 1.

Date: October 4, 2010

1. Start Medisoft and restore the data from your last work session.

2. Change the Medisoft Program Date to the date listed above, October 4, 2010.

3. On the Lists menu, click Patients/Guarantors and Cases. The Patient List dialog box is displayed.

4. Search for Hiro Tanaka by keying *T* in the Search for box. The arrow should point to the entry line for Hiro Tanaka.

5. Click the Case radio button to activate the case portion of the Patient List dialog box.

6. Click the New Case button. The dialog box labeled Case: TANAKHI0 Tanaka, Hiro (new) is displayed. The Personal tab is the current active tab. Notice that some information is already filled in.

7. Enter Tanaka's reason for seeing the doctor in the Description box.

8. Choose the correct entry for Tanaka's marital status from the drop-down list in the Marital Status box. The Student Status box can be left blank.

9. Notice that the information on Tanaka's employment is already filled in. The system copies the information entered in the Patient/Guarantor dialog box to the case file for you.

10. Check your entries for accuracy.

11. Click the Save button to save the case information you just entered. The Patient List dialog box redisplays. Notice that the case you just created is listed in the area of the dialog box labeled List of cases for: Tanaka, Hiro.

12. Do not close the Patient List dialog box.

ACCOUNT TAB

The Account tab includes information on a patient's assigned provider, referring provider, and referral source, as well as other information that may be used in some medical practices but not others (see Figure 5-4).

Assigned Provider   The Assigned Provider box is automatically filled in with the code number and name of the assigned provider listed in the Patient/Guarantor dialog box. The drop-down list provides a complete list of providers in the practice. If necessary, the Assigned Provider selection can be changed by clicking another provider on the list.

Referring Provider   A **referring provider** is a physician who recommends that a patient see a specific other physician. The Referring Provider box contains the name of the physician who referred the patient to the practice. The referring provider's name and code are selected from the drop-down list. If the referring provider is not listed on the drop-down list, he or she will need to be added to the Referring Provider list, which is found on the Lists menu. It is not necessary to close the Case dialog box to add a referring provider to the database. To add a new referring provider, click in the Referring Provider box and press the F8 key, or click Referring Providers on the Lists menu. The Referring Provider List dialog box opens in front of the other dialog boxes displayed on the screen, and a new provider can be entered.

referring provider   a physician who recommends that a patient see a specific other physician

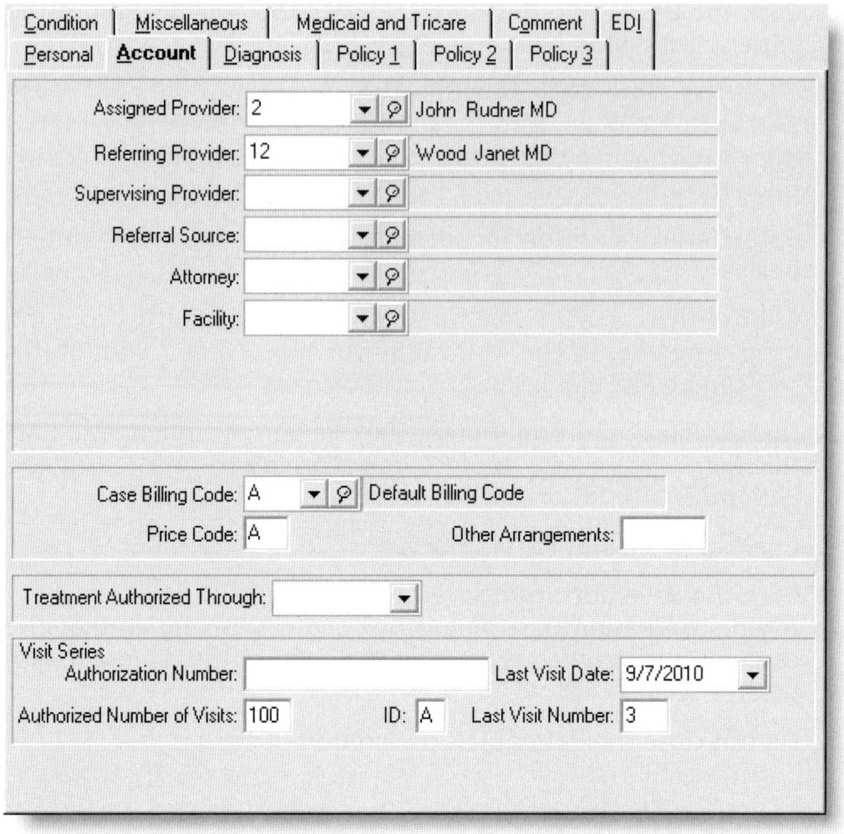

Figure 5-4   Account tab

Supervising Provider   When the provider rendering services is being supervised by a physician, the supervising physician's information is included on the claim.

Referral Source   If known, the source of a patient's referral is selected from the drop-down list of choices.

Attorney   The Attorney box is used for accident cases. If a patient has an attorney, the name of the attorney should be selected from the drop-down list. If the attorney is not listed, he or she will need to be added to the system by clicking Addresses on the Lists menu and entering information about the attorney.

Facility   The Facility box lists the place where a patient is receiving treatment. A facility is selected from the drop-down list. When necessary, facilities can be added to the database by clicking Addresses on the Lists menu and entering the necessary information.

Case Billing Code   The Case Billing Code box is a one- or two-character box used by some practices to classify and sort patients by insurance carrier, diagnosis, billing cycle, or other kinds of information.

Price Code   The Price Code box determines which set of fees is used when entering transactions for this case. The Price Code fees are entered and stored in the Amounts tab of the Procedure/Payment/Adjustment List dialog box, accessed through the Lists menu.

Other Arrangements   If a special arrangement is made for billing, it is indicated in the Other Arrangements box.

Treatment Authorized Through   A date can be entered in this box if the insurance carrier has authorized treatment only through a certain date.

Visit Series   Information in the Visit Series section of the Account tab is used primarily by psychotherapy practices and chiropractors.

ID   A pre-authorized visit series is assigned an ID value, which is entered in the ID field. An entry may be one letter (A-Z) or number (1-9). When one series of pre-authorized visits is completed, the program automatically changes to the next series.

EXERCISE 5-2

Complete the Account tab for Hiro Tanaka. The information needed to complete this exercise is found on Source Document 1.

Date: October 4, 2010

1. Confirm that Hiro Tanaka is still listed in the Patient List dialog box and that the Case radio button is selected.

2. Click the Edit Case button to add information to Tanaka's case file. The Case dialog is displayed, with the Personal tab active.

3. Make the Account tab active. The word *Account* should now be displayed in boldface type, and the boxes on the Account tab should be visible.

4. Notice that the Assigned Provider box is already filled in with the name of Tanaka's assigned provider, Katherine Yan. The system copies this information from data stored in the Patient/Guarantor dialog box.

5. Click the name of Tanaka's referring provider on the Referring Provider drop-down list. Press Tab.

6. Accept the default entry of "A" in the Price Code box.

7. Check your work for accuracy.

8. Save the changes. The Patient List dialog box is redisplayed.

9. Do not close the Patient List dialog box.

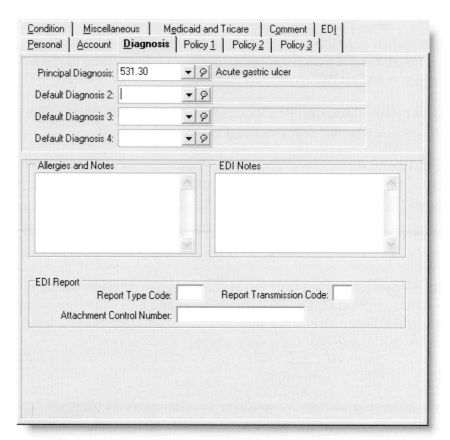

Figure 5-5 Diagnosis tab

DIAGNOSIS TAB

The Diagnosis tab contains a patient's diagnosis, information about allergies, and electronic media claim (EDI) notes (see Figure 5-5).

Principal Diagnosis and Default Diagnosis 2, 3, and 4   A patient's diagnosis is selected from the drop-down list of diagnoses. If a patient has more than one diagnosis for the same condition, the primary diagnosis is entered in the Principal Diagnosis field. Additional diagnoses are entered in the Default Diagnosis 2, 3, and 4 fields. The program can be changed to display up to eight diagnoses if required.

Allergies and Notes   If a patient has allergies or other special conditions that need to be recorded, they are entered in the Allergies and Notes box.

EDI Notes   If a patient's claims require special handling when submitted electronically, notes about the procedure, such as an explanation about the charges for supplies, are listed in this box.

EDI Report   The Report Type Code is a two-character code that indicates the title or contents of a document, report, or supporting item sent with electronic claims. The Report Transmission Code is a two-character code that defines the timing, transmission method, or format by which reports are sent with electronic claims. The value entered in the Attachment Control Number field is a unique reference number up to seven digits long.

EXERCISE 5-3

Complete the Diagnosis tab for Hiro Tanaka. The information needed to complete this exercise is found on Source Documents 1 and 3.

Date: October 4, 2010

1. Edit the case for Hiro Tanaka.

2. Make the Diagnosis tab active.

3. From the list of choices in the drop-down list, select Tanaka's diagnosis.

4. In the Allergies and Notes box, enter information on Tanaka's allergies.

5. Check your work for accuracy.

6. Save the changes. The Patient List dialog box is redisplayed.

7. Do not close the Patient List dialog box.

POLICY 1 TAB

The Policy 1 tab is where information about a patient's primary insurance carrier and coverage is recorded (see Figure 5-6).

The **primary insurance carrier** is the first carrier to whom claims are submitted. There may also be a secondary carrier (Policy 2 tab) or a tertiary carrier (Policy 3 tab).

primary insurance carrier the first carrier to whom claims are submitted

Insurance 1 The Insurance 1 box lists the code number and name of the insurance carrier. The drop-down list shows the carriers already in the system. If the carrier is not listed, it must be added to the database. It is not necessary to close the Case dialog box to add an insurance carrier to the database. When Insurance Carriers is clicked on the Lists menu, the Insurance Carrier List dialog box is displayed in front of the other dialog boxes on the screen.

Policy Holder 1 The Policy Holder box lists the person who is the insured under a particular policy. For example, if the patient is a child covered under his or her parent's insurance plan, the parent's chart number would be entered in this box. The insured's chart number is selected from the choices on the drop-down list. (If the insured is not a patient of the practice, he or she must be entered as a guarantor in Medisoft, and a chart number must be established.)

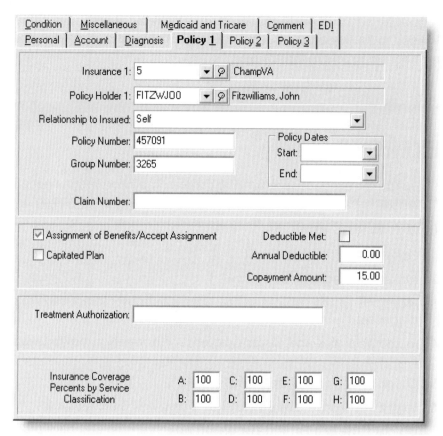

Figure 5-6   Policy 1 tab

Relationship to Insured   This box describes a patient's relationship to the individual listed in the Policy Holder 1 box.

Policy Number   A patient's policy number is entered in the Policy Number box.

Group Number   The group number for a patient's policy is entered in the Group Number box.

Claim Number   This field is used on property, casualty, and auto claims. The number is assigned by the property and casualty payer, usually during eligibility determinations.

Policy Dates—Start/End   The date a patient's insurance policy went into effect is entered in the Policy Dates—Start box. If the date is not known, the date the patient first came to the practice for treatment can be entered. If the policy has ended, such as because the carrier changed or the coverage expired, the date on which coverage terminated is entered in the Policy Dates—End box.

Assignment of Benefits/Accept Assignment   For physicians who are participating in an insurance plan, a check mark in the Accept Assignment box indicates that the provider accepts payment directly from the insurance carrier.

Capitated Plan   In a **capitated plan,** payments are made to the physician from a managed care company for patients who select the physician as their primary care provider, regardless of whether the patients visit the physician or not. A check mark in this box indicates that this insurance plan is capitated.

Deductible Met   This box is checked if the patient has met the deductible for the current year.

Annual Deductible   The dollar amount of the insured's insurance plan deductible is entered in this box.

Copayment Amount   The dollar amount of a patient's copayment per visit is entered in the Copayment Amount box.

Treatment Authorization   This field is used to record the treatment authorization code from an insurance company, usually for UB-04 hospital claims. The UB-04 is the standard uniform bill (UB) that is used for institutional health care providers. The UB-04 replaced the UB-92 in 2007.

Insurance Coverage Percents by Service Classification   The percentage of fees that an insurance carrier covers is entered in the Insurance Coverage Percents by Service Classification box. Some insurance plans pay different percentages of charges based on the type of service provided. For example, a plan may pay 80 percent of necessary medical procedures, 100 percent of lab work, and 50 percent of outpatient mental health charges.

capitated plan   an insurance plan in which payments are made to a physician by a managed care company for a patient who selects the physician as his or her primary care provider, regardless of whether the patient visits the physician

EXERCISE 5-4

Complete the Policy 1 tab for Hiro Tanaka. The information needed to complete this exercise is found on Source Document 1.

Date: October 4, 2010

1. Edit the case for Hiro Tanaka.

2. Make the Policy 1 tab active.

3. Select Tanaka's primary insurance carrier from the drop-down list in the Insurance 1 box. Press Tab.

4. The program completes the Policy Holder 1 field with the name of the patient. Since Tanaka is the policyholder, accept this entry.

5. Notice that the Relationship to Insured box already has "Self" entered. Since this is correct, do not make any changes.

6. Enter Tanaka's insurance policy number in the Policy Number box. Press Tab.

7. Enter Tanaka's group number in the Group Number box. Press Tab.

8. In the Policy Dates—Start box, key **01012010** (January 1, 2010) as the start date of the policy. Press Tab. The program displays a Confirm message stating that the date entered is in the future and asking whether you want to change it. Click No.

9. Dr. Yan accepts assignment for this carrier, so click the Assignment of Benefits/Accept Assignment box.

10. The insurance plan is capitated, so check the Capitated Plan box.

11. Key **20** in the Copayment box if it does not already appear. Press Tab.

12. Key **100** in each of the Insurance Coverage Percents by Service Classification boxes.

13. Check your work for accuracy.

14. Save the changes.

15. Do not close the Patient List dialog box.

POLICY 2 TAB

Claims are usually not submitted to a secondary carrier until the primary carrier has paid. The secondary carrier must have access to the remittance advice of the primary carrier to see what has already been paid on the claim. Delayed secondary billing may be set up so a claim is not created for the secondary carrier until a response has been received from the primary carrier.

The boxes in the Policy 2 tab are the same as those in the Policy 1 tab, with a few exceptions. The Copayment Amount, Capitated Plan, and Annual Deductible boxes are only in the Policy 1 tab. Only the Policy 2 tab has a Crossover Claim box (see Figure 5-7).

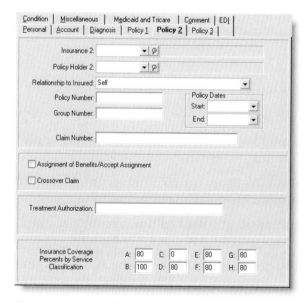

Figure 5-7 Policy 2 tab

Crossover Claim   The Crossover Claim box is used when a patient has Medicare as the primary carrier and Medicaid as the secondary carrier. Because Medicare is the primary carrier, it pays first on a claim and then submits the claim directly to the Medicaid carrier for you.

POLICY 3 TAB

The Policy 3 tab does not contain the Copayment Amount, Capitated Plan, Annual Deductible, and Crossover Claim boxes. Otherwise, the boxes are the same as those in the Policy 1 and Policy 2 tabs (see Figure 5-8).

CONDITION TAB

The Condition tab stores data about a patient's illness, accident, disability, and hospitalization (see Figure 5-9). This information is used by insurance carriers to process claims.

Injury/Illness/LMP Date   The date of a patient's injury, illness, or last menstrual period (LMP) is entered in the Injury/Illness/LMP Date box. (For an illness, the date when the symptoms first appeared is entered.)

Illness Indicator   The Illness Indicator box specifies whether a patient's condition is an illness, a last menstrual period in the case of a pregnancy, or an injury.

First Consultation Date   The date of a patient's first visit for a particular condition is entered in the First Consultation Date box. The actual date can be entered, or the pop-up calendar can be activated and dates selected.

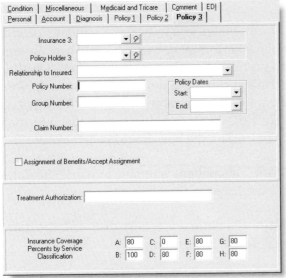

Figure 5-8   Policy 3 tab

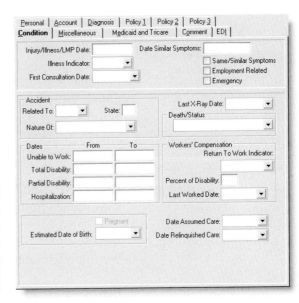

Figure 5-9   Condition tab

Date Similar Symptoms   If a patient has had similar symptoms in the past, enter the date of those symptoms in the Date Similar Symptoms box.

Same/Similar Symptoms   A check mark in the Same/Similar Symptoms box indicates that a patient has had the same or similar symptoms in the past.

Employment Related   If the Employment Related box is checked, it means that the illness or accident is in some way related to a patient's employment.

Emergency   If a patient sees the provider on an emergency visit, a check mark is entered in the Emergency box.

Accident—Related To   The Accident—Related To box indicates whether a patient's condition is related to an accident. The drop-down list offers three choices: Auto, if an automobile accident is involved; No, if it is not accident-related; and Yes, if it is accident-related but not related to an auto accident. If a patient's condition is accident-related, the State and Nature Of boxes should also be completed.

Accident—State   The abbreviation for the state in which the accident occurred is entered in this box.

Accident—Nature Of   This box provides additional information about the type of accident. The following choices can be selected from the drop-down list: Injured at home, Injured at school, Injured during recreation, Work injury/Self employed, Work injury/Non-collision, Work injury/Collision, and Motorcycle injury.

Last X-ray Date   The date of the last X-rays for the current condition are entered in this box.

Death/Status   The Death/Status box indicates a patient's condition according to the Karnofsky Performance Status Scale. There are eleven options: Able to carry on normal activity, Cares for self, Dead, Disabled, Moribund (a terminal condition near death), Normal, Normal activity with effort, Requires considerable assistance, Requires occasional assistance, Severely disabled, and Very sick. If this information is not provided by the physician, the box should be left blank.

Dates—Unable to Work   If a patient is unable to work, the dates of the absence from work are listed in these boxes.

Dates—Total Disability   If a patient is totally disabled, the dates of the total disability are entered in these boxes.

Dates—Partial Disability   If a patient is partially disabled, the dates of the partial disability are listed in these boxes.

Dates—Hospitalization If a patient is hospitalized, the dates of the hospitalization are entered in these boxes.

Workers' Compensation—Return to Work Indicator If a patient has been out of work on workers' compensation, the patient's return to work status is selected from the drop-down list of choices: Conditional, Limited, or Normal. If the status is Conditional or Limited, the Percent of Disability box should also be completed.

Workers' Compensation—Percent of Disability This box indicates a patient's percentage of disability upon returning to work.

Last Worked Date The last day the patient worked is listed in this box.

Pregnant This box is checked if a woman is pregnant.

Estimated Date of Birth If the patient is pregnant, enter the date the baby is due.

Date Assumed Care This field is used when providers share postoperative care. Enter the date the provider assumed care for this patient.

Date Relinquished Care This field is used when providers share postoperative care. Enter the date the provider relinquished care of the patient.

EXERCISE 5-5

Complete the Condition tab for Hiro Tanaka. The information needed to complete this exercise is found on Source Documents 1, 3, and 4.

Date: October 4, 2010

1. Edit the case for Hiro Tanaka.

2. Make the Condition tab active.

3. Enter the date of the injury in the Injury/Illness/LMP Date box.

4. Leave the Illness Indicator box blank.

5. In the First Consultation Date box, enter the date Tanaka first saw Dr. Yan for this condition. Press Tab. The program displays a Confirm message stating that the date entered is in the future, and asking whether you want to change it. Click No.

6. Since this visit resulted from a non-work-related accident, leave the Date Similar Symptoms box, the Same/Similar Symptoms box, and the Employment Related box blank.

7. Since this was an emergency visit, place a check mark in the Emergency box by clicking it.

8. Choose Auto in the Accident—Related To box.

9. In the Accident—State box, enter the two-letter abbreviation for the state in which the accident occurred.

10. Tanaka was injured while driving home from a softball game. Complete the Accident—Nature Of box regarding the type of accident with Injured during recreation.

11. Enter the dates Tanaka was unable to work in the Dates—Unable to Work boxes.

12. Enter the dates Tanaka was totally disabled in the Dates—Total Disability boxes.

13. Enter the dates Tanaka was partially disabled in the Dates—Partial Disability boxes.

14. Enter the dates Tanaka was hospitalized in the Dates—Hospitalization boxes.

15. Leave the remaining fields blank.

16. Check your work for accuracy.

17. Save the changes.

18. Do not close the Patient List dialog box.

MISCELLANEOUS TAB

The Miscellaneous tab records a variety of miscellaneous information about the patient and his or her treatment (see Figure 5-10).

Outside Lab Work If the Outside Lab Work box is checked, the lab work was performed by a lab other than the physician's office. If the

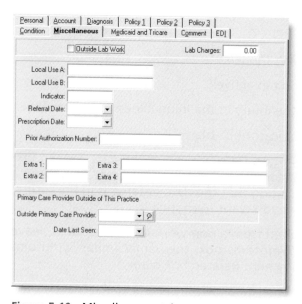

Figure 5-10 Miscellaneous tab

lab bills the provider rather than the patient, then the provider bills the patient for the lab work even though it was performed by an outside lab.

Lab Charges The charges for lab work, whether performed inside or outside the practice, are entered in the Lab Charges box.

Local Use A and B These boxes may be used by some medical practices to record information specific to the local office.

Indicator If an indicator code is used to categorize patients or services, it is entered in the Indicator box. For example, patients might be categorized according to the primary diagnosis. Services might be divided into such categories as lab work, consultations, and hospital visits.

Referral Date If the patient was referred to the provider, enter the date of the referral.

Prescription Date This field is required for hearing and vision claims.

Prior Authorization Number Before some services are performed, prior authorization must be obtained from the appropriate insurance carrier. If an insurance carrier has issued an authorization number for treatment that has not yet occurred, the number is entered in the Prior Authorization Number box.

Extra 1, 2, 3, and 4 The Extra 1, 2, 3, and 4 boxes are used for different purposes depending on the medical practice.

Outside Primary Care Provider If a patient is covered by a managed care plan and the patient's primary care provider is outside the medical practice, the name of the provider is selected from the drop-down list in this box.

Date Last Seen The Date Last Seen box lists the date a patient was last seen by the outside primary care provider.

MEDICAID AND TRICARE TAB

For patients covered by Medicaid or TRICARE, the Medicaid and Tricare tab is used to enter additional information about the government programs (see Figure 5-11).

Medicaid

EPSDT EPSDT stands for Early and Periodic Screening, Diagnosis, and Treatment. This is a Medicaid program for patients under the age of twenty-one who need screening and diagnostic services to

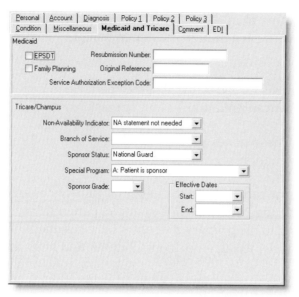

Figure 5-11 Medicaid and Tricare tab

determine physical or mental problems as well as treatment for conditions discovered. It also includes well-baby checkup examinations. A check mark in the EPSDT box indicates that a patient's visit is part of the EPSDT program.

Family Planning   A check mark in the Family Planning box specifies that a patient's condition is related to Medicaid family planning services.

Resubmission Number   For claims being resubmitted to Medicaid, the resubmission number is entered in this box.

Original Reference   For claims being resubmitted to Medicaid, the original reference number is recorded in the Original Reference box.

Service Authorization Exception Code   This code is required on some Medicaid claims. If a service authorization code was not obtained before seeing the patient, select one of the following codes:

1   Immediate/Urgent Care

2   Services Rendered in a Retroactive Period

3   Emergency Care

4   Client as Temporary Medicaid

5   Request from County for Second Opinion to Recipient Can Work

6   Request for Override Pending

7   Special Handling

TRICARE

TRICARE is the government insurance program that serves spouses and children of active-duty service members, military retirees and their families, some former spouses, and survivors of deceased military members (Army, Navy, Air Force, Marine Corps, Coast Guard, Public Health Service, and NOAA, the National Oceanic and Atmospheric Administration).

Non-Availability Indicator The Non-Availability Indicator box specifies whether a nonavailability (NA) statement is required. The choices on the drop-down list are NA statement not needed, NA statement obtained, and Other carrier paid at least 75%.

Branch of Service The Branch of Service box indicates the particular branch of service: Army, Air Force, Marines, Navy, Coast Guard, Public Health Service, NOAA, and ChampVA.

Sponsor Status The **sponsor** is the active-duty service member. The sponsor's family members are covered by the TRICARE insurance plan. The drop-down list in the Sponsor Status box provides choices to indicate the sponsor's status in the service, such as Active, Medal of Honor, or Reserves.

sponsor in TRICARE, the active-duty service member

Special Program The Special Program drop-down list contains codes for special TRICARE programs.

Sponsor Grade The two-character sponsor grade is entered in the Sponsor Grade box.

Effective Dates The start date of the TRICARE policy is entered in the Effective Dates—Start box. If there is an end date, it is entered in the Effective Dates—End box. Specific dates can be entered, or a selection can be made from the pop-up calendar.

COMMENT TAB

The Comment tab is used to enter case notes (see Figure 5-12). Notes entered in this box will print on statements if statements are formatted to include case comments.

EDI TAB

The EDI tab is used to enter information for electronic claims specific to this case (see Figure 5-13). Only fields that are relevant for the particular case need to be completed.

Care Plan Oversight # If a physician is billing for home health and hospice care plan oversight (CPO), enter the care plan oversight number.

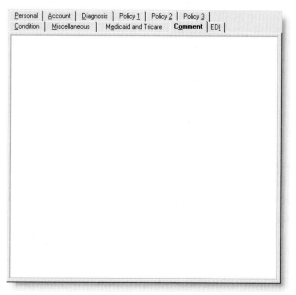

Figure 5-12   Comment tab

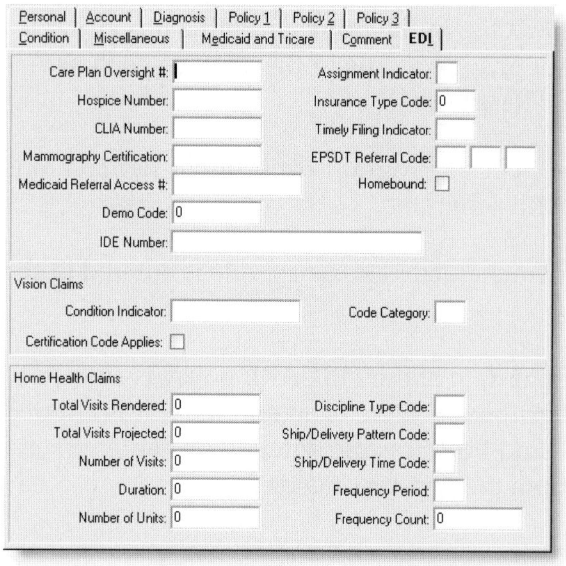

Figure 5-13   EDI tab

Hospice Number   If a physician is billing for hospice care, enter the hospice number.

CLIA Number   When laboratory claims are billed electronically, the Clinical Laboratory Improvement Act (CLIA) number must be included in the claim. This number is assigned to labs and required on all laboratory claims billed to Medicare.

Mammography Certification   This box lists the provider's or facility's mammography certification number.

Medicaid Referral Access #   The referring physician's Medicaid referral access number for the patient is entered in this field.

Demo Code   This field is used when filing claims for this patient under demonstration projects.

IDE Number   The IDE number is required when there is an investigational device exemption on the claim. This is usually for vision claims but can also be assigned for other types of claims.

Assignment Indicator   The entry in this field is the assignment indicator for this case. Valid codes are:

A   Assigned

B   Assignment accepted on clinical lab services only

C   Not assigned

P   Patient refuses to assign benefits

Insurance Type Code   The type of insurance that the patient has is selected in the Insurance Type Code field. This is required when sending Medicare secondary claims. Valid codes are:

12   Medicare secondary working-aged beneficiary or spouse with employer group health plan

13   Medicare secondary end-stage renal disease beneficiary in the 12-month coordination period with an employer's group health plan

14   Medicare secondary, no-fault insurance including auto is primary

15   Medicare secondary workers' compensation

16   Medicare secondary public health service (PHS) or other federal agency

41   Medicare secondary black lung

42   Medicare secondary Veteran's Administration

43   Medicare secondary disabled beneficiary under age 65 with large-group health plan (LGHP)

47   Medicare secondary, other liability insurance is primary

Timely Filing Indicator   If a response to a request for information from an insurance carrier was delayed, the reason for the delay is entered. Valid entries are:

1   Proof of eligibility unknown or unavailable

2   Litigation

3   Authorization delays

4   Delay in certifying provider

5	Delay in supplying billing forms
6	Delay in delivery of custom-made appliances
7	Third-party processing delay
8	Delay in eligibility determination
9	Original claim rejected or denied due to a reason unrelated to the billing limitation rules
10	Administration delay in the prior approval process
11	Other

EPSDT Referral Code   The patient's referral code for the EPSDT program is entered in this field.

Homebound   If the patient is under homebound care, this box should be checked.

Vision Claims

If a provider submits vision claims, entries are made in these fields.

Condition Indicator   The code indicator is entered in this field.

Certification Code Applies   This box is checked if a certification code is applicable.

Code Category   The code category for the vision device is entered in this field.

Home Health Claims

If a provider submits home health claims, these fields are filled in.

Total Visits Rendered   This field indicates the total number of visits.

Total Visits Projected   This field lists the total number of visits projected.

Number of Visits   The total number of visits is entered in this field.

Duration   The duration of the home health visits is recorded in this field.

Number of Units   This field contains the number of units for the home visits.

Discipline Type Code   The provider's discipline type code is entered.

Ship/Delivery Pattern Code   Enter the pattern code for the home visits.

Ship/Delivery Time Code   This field records the time code for the home visits.

Frequency Period   The frequency period for the home visits is listed.

Frequency Count   The frequency count for the home visits is entered.

EDITING CASE INFORMATION ON AN ESTABLISHED PATIENT

Information in an existing case is modified by selecting the case to be edited and clicking the Edit Case button at the bottom of the Patient List dialog box. (The Case radio button must be clicked for the Edit Case button to be displayed.) Alternatively, a case can be opened for editing by double-clicking directly on the case line in the right half of the dialog box.

EXERCISE 5-6

John Fitzwilliams, an established patient, has just remarried. Edit the information in his Case dialog box to reflect this change.

Date: October 4, 2010

1. Click in the Search For field and press the backspace key to delete the *T* that was entered to search for Hiro Tanaka. The Patient List once again displays the complete list of patients.

2. Enter *F* in the Search For field. All patients who have last names beginning with the letter *F* are displayed. Click anywhere in the listing for John Fitzwilliams to select his entry.

3. Click the Case radio button. Verify that Acute Gastric Ulcer is listed in the Case area of the dialog box.

4. Click the Edit Case button.

5. In the Personal tab, change the entry in the Marital Status box from Divorced to Married.

6. Check your work for accuracy.

7. Save the changes.

8. Close the Patient List dialog box.

Electronic Medical Record Exchange

Creating Cases for Imported Transactions

Transactions received from an electronic medical record will not always be related to an existing case in Medisoft. As illustrated below, the Unprocessed Transactions Edit dialog box contains a blank Case field and a message, "Case number does not exist. (Error)."

To process the transaction, a new case must be created. This can be done from the Unprocssed Transactions Edit dialog box, simply by pressing the F8 shortcut key, which opens a new case dialog box in Medisoft.

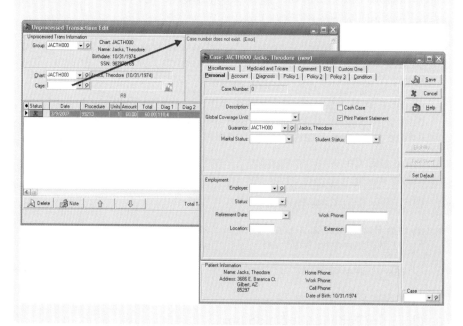

Name: _____   **Date:** _____

CHAPTER 5 WORKSHEET

After completing all the exercises in the chapter, answer the following questions in the spaces provided.

1. What is the entry in the Referring Provider box for Hiro Tanaka (Account tab)?

_____

2. What is the entry in the Allergies and Notes box for Hiro Tanaka (Diagnosis tab)?

_____

3. What is the code for John Fitzwilliams's employer (Personal tab)?

_____

4. What is listed in the Principal Diagnosis field for Hiro Tanaka (Diagnosis tab)?

_____

5. Is Hiro Tanaka's insurance plan capitated (Policy 1 tab)?

_____

6. What is the entry in the Copayment Amount box for Hiro Tanaka (Policy 1 tab)?

_____

7. What code is entered in the Insurance 1 box for Hiro Tanaka (Policy 1 tab)?

_____

8. What is entered in the Description box for Lisa Wright (Personal tab)?

_____

9. What is the entry in the Price Code box for Lisa Wright (Account tab)?

_____

10. Has Lisa Wright met her deductible for the year (Policy 1 tab)?

_____

CHAPTER REVIEW

USING TERMINOLOGY

Match the terms on the left with the definitions on the right.

_____ **1.** capitated plan

_____ **2.** case

_____ **3.** chart

_____ **4.** primary insurance carrier

_____ **5.** record of treatment and progress

_____ **6.** referring provider

_____ **7.** sponsor

a. A folder that contains a patient's medical records.

b. Physician's notes about a patient's condition and diagnosis.

c. A physician who recommends that a patient make an appointment with a particular doctor.

d. An insurance plan in which payments are made to primary care providers whether patients visit the office or not.

e. The insurance company that receives claims before they are submitted to any other payer.

f. A grouping of transactions organized around a patient's condition.

g. The active-duty service member on the TRICARE government insurance program.

CHECKING YOUR UNDERSTANDING

Answer the questions below in the space provided.

8. Sarina Bell has no insurance of her own but is covered by her father's insurance policy. How would this be indicated in the Policy 1 tab for Sarina Bell?

_____

_____

9. Where in the Case dialog box can you find information about a patient's allergies?

_____

_____

10. Is it necessary to set up a new case when a patient changes insurance carriers? Why?

_____

_____

11. In the Case dialog box, where would you enter information about a work-related accident?

_____

_____

12. Where is information needed to complete the Diagnosis tab usually found?

_____

_____

13. A patient has been seeing the doctor regularly for treatment of diabetes. She was hospitalized yesterday, and the doctor saw her in the hospital for treatment. Do you need to set up a new case for the hospitalization?

_____

_____

APPLYING KNOWLEDGE

Answer the questions below in the space provided.

14. While you are entering case information for a new patient, you realize that the patient's referring provider is not one of the choices in the Referring Provider box in the Account tab. What should you do?

_____

_____

15. An established patient has changed insurance carriers from Blue Cross and Blue Shield to OhioCare HMO. What specific boxes need to be changed in the Case dialog box?

_____

_____

AT THE COMPUTER

Answer the following questions at the computer.

16. Using the information contained in the Case dialog box, list Randall Klein's primary and secondary insurance carriers.

_____

_____

17. Who is the guarantor for Janine Bell's account?

_____

_____

Entering Charge Transactions and Patient Payments

6

WHAT YOU NEED TO KNOW

To use this chapter, you need to know how to:

◆ Start Medisoft, use menus, and enter and edit text.

◆ Enter patient information in Medisoft.

◆ Work with chart and case numbers.

LEARNING OUTCOMES

In this chapter, you will learn how to:

◆ Enter charges for procedures.

◆ Edit and delete charge transactions.

◆ Use Medisoft's Search features to find specific transaction data.

◆ Record and apply payments received from patients.

◆ Process a refund for a patient who has overpaid.

◆ Print walkout receipts.

KEY TERMS

adjustments
charges
MultiLink codes
payments

TRANSACTION ENTRY OVERVIEW

Three types of transactions are recorded in Medisoft: charges, payments, and adjustments. **Charges** are the amounts a provider bills for the services performed. **Payments** are monies received from patients and insurance carriers. **Adjustments** are changes to patients' accounts. Examples of adjustments include returned check fees, insurance write-offs, Medicare adjustments, and changes in treatment. This chapter covers charge transactions and patient copayments. Chapter 8 covers insurance payment and adjustment transactions.

charges amounts a provider bills for the services performed

payments monies received from patients and insurance carriers

adjustments changes to patients' accounts that alter the amounts charged or paid

The primary document needed to enter charge transactions in Medisoft is a patient's encounter form. Typically, the physician circles or checks the appropriate procedure and diagnosis codes on the encounter form during or just after the patient visit. Charges and payments listed on an encounter form are later entered in the Transaction Entry dialog box in Medisoft by an insurance billing specialist. After the information is entered, it is checked for accuracy. If all the information is correct, the transaction data are saved, and a walkout receipt is printed for the patient. If it is incorrect, the data are edited and then saved.

Transactions are entered in the Transaction Entry dialog box, which is accessed by selecting Enter Transactions on the Activities menu. The Transaction Entry dialog box consists of three main sections (see Figure 6-1):

1. The top third contains information about the patient, the insurance coverage, and the patient's account.

2. The middle section lists charge transactions.

3. The bottom third lists payments and adjustments.

PATIENT/ACCOUNT INFORMATION

The Patient/Account Information section consists of the top third of the Transaction Entry dialog box (see Figure 6-2). It contains two critical pieces of information: chart number and case number. Boxes for entering these numbers are found at the top left of the dialog box.

CHART

The Chart drop-down list includes all patients in the practice. In large practices, the list of chart numbers could be very long, so it is important to know how to search for a chart number. One way to

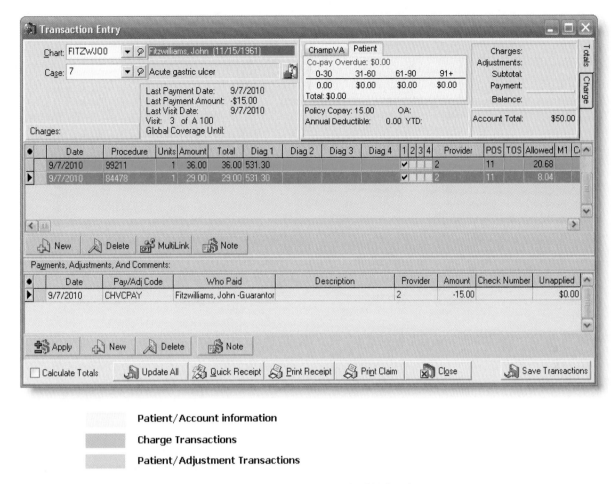

Figure 6-1   Transaction Entry dialog box with three sections highlighted

- Patient/Account information
- Charge Transactions
- Patient/Adjustment Transactions

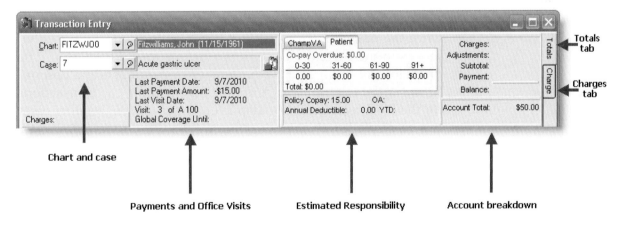

Figure 6-2   The Patient/Account Information section of the Transaction Entry dialog box

locate a chart number is to key the first several letters of a patient's last name. As the letters are keyed, the first chart number in the list that matches is highlighted. In the example in Figure 6-3, the letter *F* was keyed. The program highlights the first patient with a chart number beginning with *F*—in this case, John Fitzwilliams. If this is the correct patient, pressing Tab selects the patient and closes the

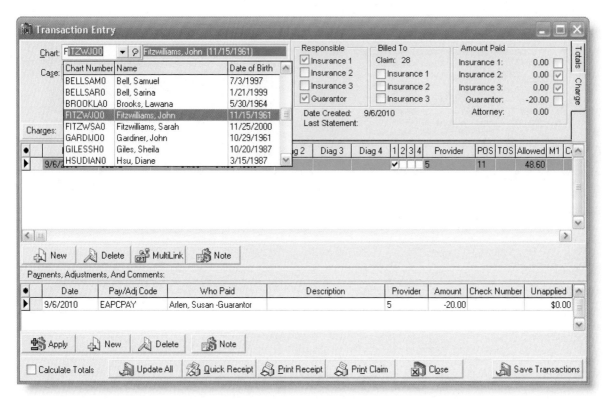

Figure 6-3   Chart drop-down list after *F* is keyed

drop-down list. If a different patient is desired, the up and down arrow keys are used to move up or down in the list.

CASE

Once the patient's chart number has been located, the Case that relates to the current charges or payments must be selected. The drop-down list in the Case box displays case numbers and descriptions for the patient (see Figure 6-4). By default, the transactions for the most recent case are displayed. Transactions for other cases can be displayed by changing the selection in the Case box. Only one case can be opened at a time.

TOTALS AND CHARGE TABS

The remaining areas in the Patient/Account Information section of the Transaction Entry dialog box include the Totals and Charge tabs. Information in these fields is entered automatically by the program, and no changes can be made. The figures are automatically updated after a new transaction is entered and saved.

Totals Tab

The Totals tab displays information for the insurance carrier and for the patient. In Figure 6-2 on page 137, the Totals tab is currently selected.

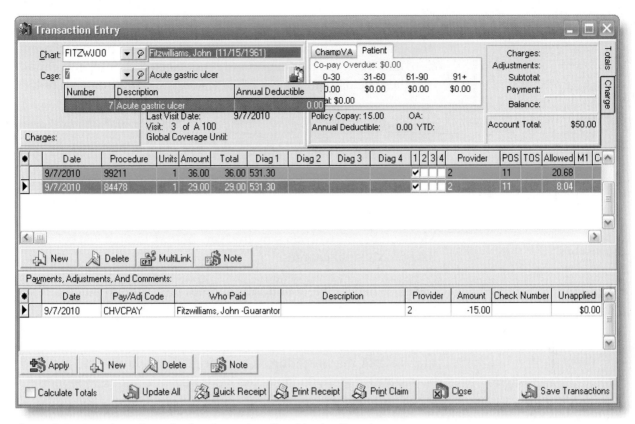

Figure 6-4 Case drop-down list for the patient listed in the Chart box

Account Aging This section displays the case's insurance carriers and the aging information for each. It also displays the patient aging information.

Total This field displays the total aging amount for the patient's account.

TNB This is the total not billed—the amount that has not been billed to the insurance carrier.

Policy Copay and OA The amount of the patient's copayment and any other arrangements (OA) for payment that may be in effect appear here.

Annual Deductible and YTD These fields list the patient's annual insurance deductible. The year-to-date (YTD) field calculates how much of the deductible has been met for the year.

Charges, Adjustments, Subtotal, Payment, Balance These fields display financial information for the case.

Account Total This field displays the patient's total account balance for all cases.

Charge Tab

The Charge tab shows responsibility information, billing information, and payment information for the selected charge. You cannot edit these fields. The Charge tab is visible in Figure 6-3 on page 138.

CHARGE TRANSACTIONS

Charges for procedures performed by a provider are entered in the Charges section in the middle of the Transaction Entry dialog box (see Figure 6-5). The process of entering a charge transaction in Medisoft begins with clicking the New button, located just below the list of individual charges.

Date When the New button is clicked, the program automatically enters the current date (the date that the Medisoft Program Date is set to) in the Date box (see Figure 6-6). If this is not the date on which the procedures were performed, it must be changed to reflect the actual date of the procedures. To change the default date for these boxes, any of these methods can be used:

◆ The Set Program Date command on the File menu can be clicked.

◆ The date button in the lower-right corner of the screen can be clicked. (This must be done before the New button is clicked in the Transaction Entry dialog box.)

◆ The information that is already in the Date box can be keyed over.

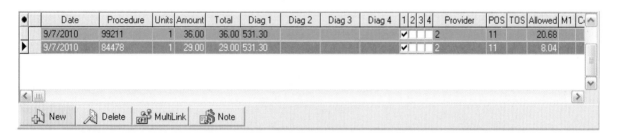

Figure 6-5 Charges area in the Transaction Entry dialog box, with the New button highlighted

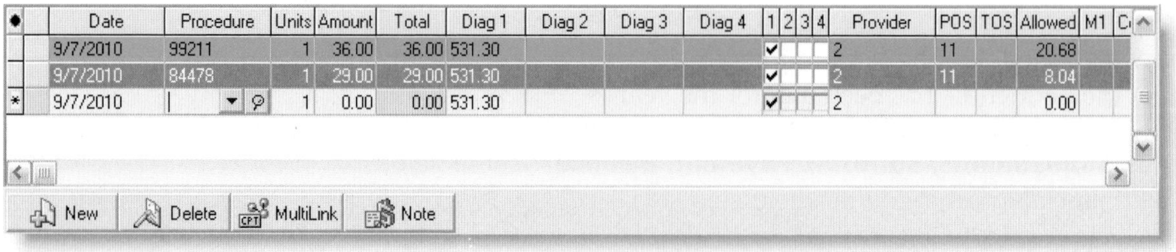

Figure 6-6 After the New button is clicked, the date is displayed in the Date column (new entry highlighted in yellow)

Procedure   After the date is entered, the next information required is the code for the procedure performed by the provider. The procedure code is selected from a drop-down list of CPT codes already in the database. Again, it is more efficient to locate a code by entering the full code number or the first several digits than to scroll through the entire list of codes. In the example in Figure 6-7, the numbers *800* were entered, and the first CPT code that matches is highlighted. To select the code, press Tab. If a different code is desired, use the up or down arrow keys on the keyboard to move up or down in the list.

Only one procedure code can be selected for each transaction. If multiple procedures were performed for a patient, each one must be entered as a separate transaction (unless a MultiLink code, which is discussed later in the chapter, is used).

If a CPT code for a procedure is not listed, it can be added to the database by pressing the F8 key or by clicking Procedure/Payment/Adjustment Codes on the Lists menu. This may be done without exiting the Transaction Entry dialog box.

After the code is selected and the Tab key is pressed, the program automatically enters data in the other columns (see Figure 6-8). These entries are described in the paragraphs that follow.

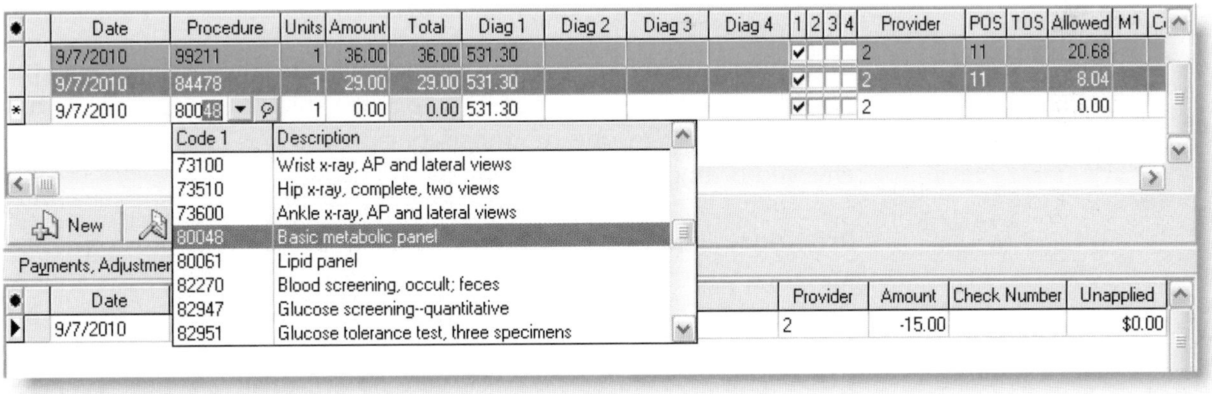

Figure 6-7   Procedure drop-down list after the numbers *800* are entered

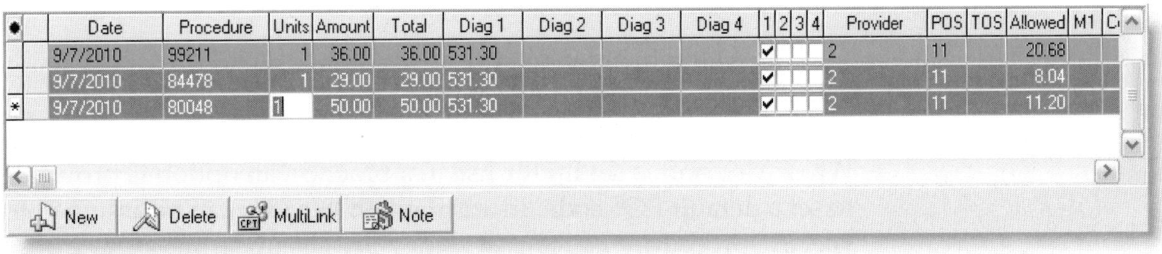

Figure 6-8   Charges section of the Transaction Entry dialog box after a procedure code is selected

Units   The Units box indicates the quantity of the procedure. Normally, the number of units is one. In some cases, however, it may be more than one. For example, if a patient had three skin tags removed, the CPT code is selected, and 3 is entered in the Units box.

Amount   The Amount box lists the charge amount for a procedure. The amount is entered automatically by the system based on the CPT code and insurance carrier. Each CPT code stored in the system has a charge amount associated with it. The charge amount can be edited if necessary.

Total   To the right of the Amount box is the Total box. This field displays the total charges for the procedure(s) performed. The amount is calculated by the system; the number in the Units box is multiplied by the number in the Amount box. For example, suppose a patient had three X-rays done at a charge of $45.00 per X-ray. The Units box would read "3," and the Amount box would read "$45.00." The Total box would read "$135.00," which is 3 × $45.00.

Diagnosis   The Diag 1, 2, 3, and 4 boxes correspond to the information in the Diagnosis tab of the Case folder. If a patient has several different diagnoses, the diagnosis that is most relevant to the procedure is used.

1, 2, 3, 4   The 1, 2, 3, and 4 boxes to the right of the Diag 1, 2, 3, and 4 boxes indicate which diagnoses should be used for this charge. A check mark appears in each Diagnosis box for which a diagnosis was entered in the Diag 1, 2, 3, 4 boxes. Some insurance carriers do not permit more than one diagnosis per procedure. Diagnoses can be checked or unchecked as needed.

Provider   The Provider box lists the code number of a patient's assigned provider. If a patient sees a different provider for a visit, the Provider box can be changed to list that provider instead.

POS   The POS, or place of service box, indicates where services were performed. The standard numerical codes used are:

11	Provider's office
21	Inpatient hospital
22	Outpatient hospital
23	Hospital emergency room

When Medisoft is set up for use in a practice, an option is provided to set a default POS code. In addition, POS codes can be assigned to specific procedure codes when they are set up in the Procedure/

Payment/Adjustment Codes List. For purposes of this book, the default code has been set to 11 for provider's office.

TOS   *TOS* stands for "type of service." Medical offices may set up a list of codes to indicate the type of service performed. For example, 1 may indicate an examination, 2 a lab test, and so on. The TOS code is specified in the Procedure/Payment/Adjustment entry for each CPT code.

Allowed   This is the amount allowed by the payer for this procedure. This value comes from the Allowed Amounts tab of the Procedure/Payment/Adjustment dialog box.

M1   The M1 box is for a CPT code modifier. The grid in the Transaction Entry dialog box can be changed to allow entry of up to four modifiers per line.

Co-Pay   A check mark in this box indicates that the code entered in the Procedure column requires a copayment.

BUTTONS IN THE CHARGES AREA OF THE TRANSACTION ENTRY DIALOG BOX

Four buttons are provided at the bottom of the Charges area: New, Delete, MultiLink, and Note. The New button, used to create a new charge entry, has already been discussed.

Delete Button   To delete a charge transaction, it is necessary to select the particular charge that is to be deleted. This is accomplished by clicking in any of the boxes associated with that transaction (Date, Procedure, Units, Amount, and so on). Clicking in a box selects the transaction, indicated by the black triangle pointer at the far left box on the line (see Figure 6-9).

Once the desired transaction is selected, it is ready for deletion. Clicking the Delete button causes a confirmation message to be

	Date	Procedure	Units	Amount	Total	Diag 1	Diag 2	Diag 3	Diag 4	1	2	3	4	Provider	POS	TOS	Allowed	M1	C
	9/7/2010	99211	1	36.00	36.00	531.30				✓				2	11		20.68		
▶	9/7/2010	84478	1	29.00	29.00	531.30				✓				2	11		8.04		
	9/7/2010	80048	1	50.00	50.00	531.30				✓				2	11		11.20		

New   Delete   MultiLink   Note

Figure 6-9   Transaction selected for deletion indicated by line pointer at left

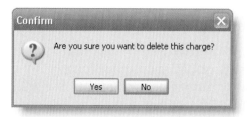

Figure 6-10 Confirm dialog box displayed after clicking the Delete button

displayed (see Figure 6-10). To continue with the deletion, click the Yes button. To cancel the deletion, click the No button.

> **WARNING!** All transactions can be deleted from within the Transaction Entry dialog box. Caution should be exercised when using the Delete feature. Deleted data cannot be recovered!

MultiLink Button Medisoft provides a feature that saves time when entering multiple CPT codes that are related to the same activity. **MultiLink codes** are groups of procedure code entries that relate to a single activity. For example, a MultiLink code could be created for the procedures related to diagnosing a strep throat: 99211 OF— Established patient, minimal; 87430 Strep test; and 85025 Complete CBC w/auto diff. WBC.

MultiLink codes groups of procedure code entries that relate to a single activity

When the MultiLink button is clicked, the code STREPM is selected from a drop-down list of MultiLink codes already in the database (see Figures 6-11 and 6-12). All three procedure codes associated with diagnosing a strep throat are entered automatically by the system, eliminating the need to enter each CPT code separately. The MultiLink feature saves time by reducing the number of procedure code entries, and it also reduces omission errors. When procedure codes are entered as a MultiLink, it is impossible to forget to enter a procedure, since all the codes that are in the MultiLink group are entered automatically.

Clicking the MultiLink button (see Figure 6-11) in the Transaction Entry dialog box displays the MultiLink dialog box (see Figure 6-12). After a MultiLink code is selected from the MultiLink drop-down list, the Create Transactions button is clicked.

Figure 6-11 MultiLink button

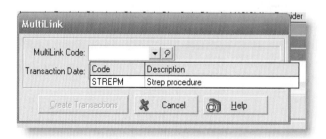

Figure 6-12 MultiLink code drop-down list

♦	Date	Procedure	Units	Amount	Total	Diag 1	Diag 2	Diag 3	Diag 4	1	2	3	4	Provider	POS	TOS	Allowed	M1	C
	9/7/2010	99211	1	36.00	36.00	531.30				✓				2	11		20.68		
	9/7/2010	84478	1	29.00	29.00	034.0				✓				2	11		8.04		
	9/21/2010	99211	1	36.00	36.00	034.0				✓				2	11		20.68		
	9/21/2010	87430	1	29.00	29.00	034.0				✓				2	11		16.01		
I	9/21/2010	85025	1	13.60	13.60	034.0				✓				2	11		10.79		

Figure 6-13 Charge transactions created with STREPM MultiLink code

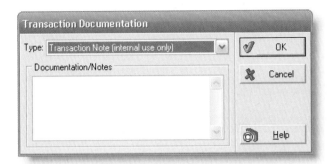

Figure 6-14 Transaction Documentation dialog box, where notes about a transaction are entered

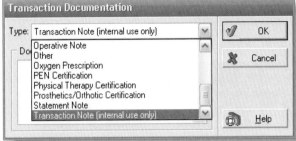

Figure 6-15 Some of the many types of transaction documentation available in Medisoft

The codes and charges for each procedure are automatically added to the list of transactions at the bottom of the Transaction Entry dialog box (see Figure 6-13).

Note Button The Note button is used to enter additional information about a particular procedure. To use this feature, click the Note button. The Transaction Documentation dialog box is displayed (see Figure 6-14).

In the Type field, Medisoft provides a list of types of documentation in the drop-down list (see Figure 6-15). Some of the information entered here is transmitted with an insurance claim when claims are transmitted electronically.

SAVING CHARGES

When all the charge information has been entered and checked for accuracy, the transaction must be saved. Transactions are saved by clicking the Save Transactions button, which is located at the bottom of the Transaction Entry dialog box (see Figure 6-16).

Transactions can also be saved by clicking the Update All button, located in the same row of buttons. When Update All is clicked, the transactions are saved, and the program checks all fields for missing or invalid information and displays various messages, such as a warning that the date entered is in the future.

The other buttons located in this row, Quick Receipt and Print Receipt, are used to print a walkout receipt for a patient (covered later in this

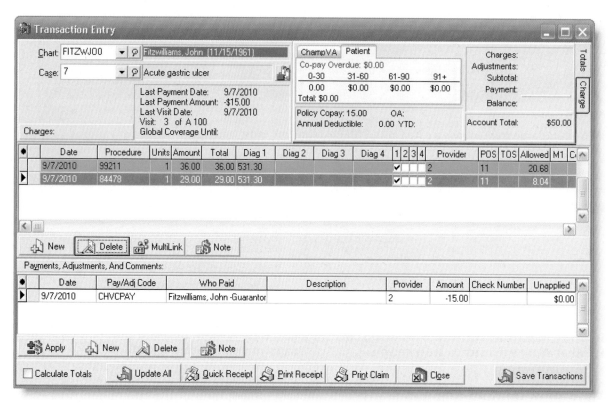

Figure 6-16   Transaction Entry window with Save Transactions button highlighted

chapter). The Print Claim button is discussed in Chapter 7. The Close button simply closes the Transaction Entry dialog box.

EDITING TRANSACTIONS

The most efficient way to edit a transaction is to click in the field that needs to be changed and enter the correct information. For example, to change the procedure code, click in the Procedure box, and either key a new code or select a new code from the drop-down list. After changes are made, the data must be saved. To view the updated amounts in the Patient/Account Information area, click the Update All button near the bottom of the Transaction Entry dialog box.

Depending on the type of edit, the program may display several message boxes. For example, if an attempt is made to change the Payment Type or Who Paid fields, a message is displayed to confirm the change. If someone tries to change a diagnosis code that is already included in a claim, the program asks whether to remove the transaction from the existing claim and create a new claim, or to replace the original diagnosis code in the transaction.

COLOR CODING IN TRANSACTION ENTRY

Transactions in Medisoft are color-coded, making it easy to determine the status of a charge or payment. No color can be assigned to

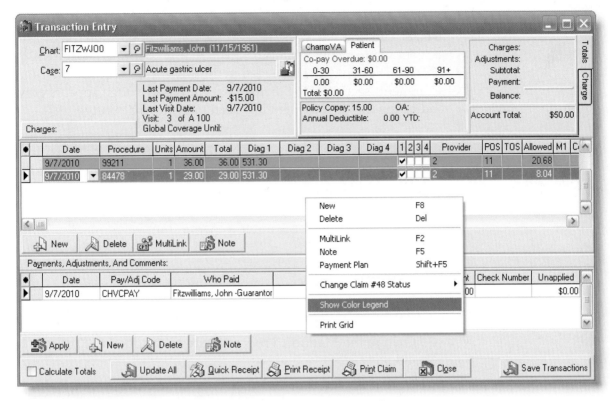

Figure 6-17 Submenu with Show Color Legend option highlighted

more than one transaction type at the same time. Color codes are set up using the Program Options selection on the File menu.

In the medical practice used in this textbook, the codes have already been determined. Three color codes are applied to the status of a charge:

1. No payment (gray)

2. Partially paid charge (aqua)

3. Overpaid charge (yellow)

Charges that have been paid in full are not colored and appear white.

To display a list of color codes used in Transaction Entry, click the right mouse button in the white area below the list of transactions, and a menu is displayed (see Figure 6-17).

When the Show Color Legend option is selected, the Color Coding Legend box appears on the screen (see Figure 6-18). The box lists the meaning of the color codes used in Transaction Entry—three for charges, and three for payments. The color codes used to indicate the status of a payment are discussed later in the chapter.

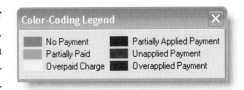

Figure 6-18 Color-Coding Legend box

In Figure 6-17, there are two charge entries on 9/7/2010: 99211 and 84478. The first entry, 99211, is color-coded as partially paid. The patient made a copayment of $15.00 that was applied to the 99211 charge. The copayment is listed in the Payments, Adjustments, and Comments section of the dialog box. The 84478 charge appears gray, indicating that no payment has been made on that charge.

EXERCISE 6-1

Using Source Document 3, enter a charge transaction for Hiro Tanaka's accident case.

Date: October 4, 2010

1. Start Medisoft and restore the data from your last work session.

2. Change the Medisoft Program Date to October 4, 2010, if it is not already set to that date.

3. On the Activities menu, click Enter Transactions. The Transaction Entry dialog box is displayed.

4. Key *T* in the Chart box, and then press Tab to select Hiro Tanaka. An Information dialog box is displayed with a message about Tanaka's allergies. Click the OK button to close the box.

5. Verify that the Accident—back pain case is the active case in the Case box.

6. In the Charges section of the dialog box, click the New button.

7. Verify that the entry in the Date box is 10/4/2010.

8. Click in the Procedure box, and enter *99202* to select the procedure code for the service checked off on the encounter form. Press Tab. Notice that the Diagnosis box and the Units box have been automatically completed. The Amount box is also automatically completed ($88.00). If necessary, these entries can be edited by clicking in the box and entering new data.

9. Review the entries in the Provider (1) and POS (11) boxes. Since there are no modifiers to the procedure code, the M1 box is left blank.

10. Check your entries for accuracy.

11. Click the Save Transactions button. A message appears that a $20.00 copayment is due. This will be entered in the section on payments in this chapter. Click the OK button.

12. Click the Save Transactions button again to save the transaction. When the Date of Service Validation message appears, click the Yes button, since you want to save the transaction. Notice that the Co-pay Overdue field in red now lists $20.00 and the Account Total field displays $88.00.

EXERCISE 6-2

Using Source Document 5, enter a charge transaction for Elizabeth Jones's diabetes case.

Date: October 4, 2010

1. If necessary, open the Transaction Entry dialog box.

2. Click in the Chart field; key *JO* in the Chart box; and press Tab to select Elizabeth Jones. Click the Case drop-down list, and select the Diabetes case.

3. Click the New button in the Charges section of the window.

4. Accept the default in the Date box (10/4/2010).

5. Key *99213* in the Procedure box to select the procedure code for the services checked off on the encounter form. Press Tab.

6. Keep "1" in the Units box.

7. Accept the charge for the procedure that is displayed in the Amount box ($72.00).

8. Review the entries in the other boxes, and check your entries for accuracy.

9. Click the Save Transactions button. When the Date of Service Validation box appears, click Yes.

PAYMENT/ADJUSTMENT TRANSACTIONS

Payments are entered in two different areas of the Medisoft program: the Transaction Entry dialog box, and the Deposit List dialog box, which will be discussed in Chapter 8. Practices may have different preferences for how payments are entered, depending on their billing procedures. In this book, you will be introduced to both methods of payment entry.

Patient payments made at the time of an office visit are entered in the Transaction Entry dialog box. Payments that are received electronically or by mail, such as insurance payments and mailed patient payments, are entered in the Deposit List dialog box. The Deposit List feature is very efficient for entering large insurance payments that must be split up and applied to a number of different patients.

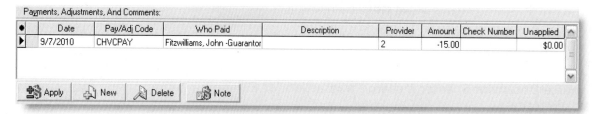

●	Date	Pay/Adj Code	Who Paid	Description	Provider	Amount	Check Number	Unapplied	
▶	9/7/2010	CHVCPAY	Fitzwilliams, John -Guarantor		2	-15.00		$0.00	

Apply | New | Delete | Note

Figure 6-19 Payments, Adjustments, and Comments area of the Transaction Entry dialog box

●	Date	Pay/Adj Code	Who Paid	Description	Provider	Amount	Check Number	Unapplied	
	9/7/2010	CHVCPAY	Fitzwilliams, John -Guarantor		2	-15.00		$0.00	
*	9/7/2010					0.00		$0.00	

Apply | New | Delete | Note

Figure 6-20 Payments, Adjustments, and Comments area after clicking the New button

ENTERING PAYMENTS MADE DURING OFFICE VISITS

The first step when entering a patient payment is to select a patient's chart number and case number in the Transaction Entry dialog box. After the chart and case numbers have been selected, a payment transaction can be entered. Payments are entered in the Payments, Adjustments, and Comments section of the Transaction Entry dialog box (see Figure 6-19).

The process of creating a payment transaction begins with clicking the New button. When the New button is clicked, the program automatically enters the current date (the date that the Medisoft program date is set to) in the Date box (see Figure 6-20).

If this is not the date on which the payment was received, the date must be changed to reflect this date. To change the default date for these boxes, any of these methods can be used:

◆ The Set Program Date command on the File menu can be clicked.

◆ The Date button in the lower-right corner of the screen can be clicked. (This must be done before the New button is clicked in the Transaction Entry dialog box.)

◆ The date that is already in the Date box can be keyed over.

Payment/Adjustment Code Once the correct date is entered, pressing the Tab key moves the cursor to the Payment/Adjustment Code box. The code for a payment is selected from the drop-down list of payment codes already entered in the system (see Figure 6-21).

If a payment code is not listed, it can be added to the database by pressing the F8 key or by clicking Procedure/Payment/Adjustment Codes on the Lists menu. This may be done without exiting the Transaction Entry dialog box.

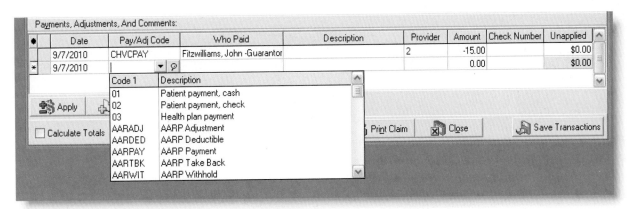

Figure 6-21 Payment/Adjustment Code drop-down list

Figure 6-22 Payments, Adjustments, and Comments area after Payment/Adjustment Code is entered

Who Paid   After the code is selected and the Tab key is pressed, the program automatically completes the Who Paid box based on information stored in the database (see Figure 6-22). The Who Paid field displays a drop-down list of guarantors and carriers that are assigned in the patient case folder.

Description   The Description field can be used to enter other information about the payment, if desired.

Provider   The Provider column lists the code number of the provider.

Amount   The Amount field contains the amount of payment received. If the payment is a copayment from a patient, this box is completed automatically when a Payment/Adjustment code is selected. Again, the program uses information stored in the database.

Check Number   The Check Number field is used to record the number of the check used for payment.

Unapplied   The dollar value in the Unapplied box is the amount that has not yet been applied to a charge transaction.

Applying Payments to Charges

Payments are color-coded to indicate payment status (see Figure 6-23). Three color codes are applied to the status of a payment:

1. Partially applied payment (blue)

2. Unapplied payment (red)

3. Overapplied payment (pink)

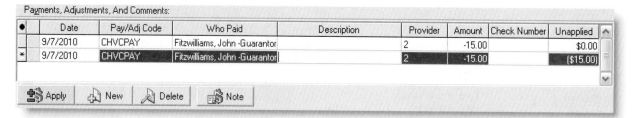

Payments, Adjustments, And Comments:

●	Date	Pay/Adj Code	Who Paid	Description	Provider	Amount	Check Number	Unapplied
	9/7/2010	CHVCPAY	Fitzwilliams, John -Guarantor		2	-15.00		$0.00
*	9/7/2010	CHVCPAY	Fitzwilliams, John -Guarantor		2	-15.00		($15.00)

Apply   New   Delete   Note

Figure 6-23   Payments, Adjustments, and Comments area with a color-coded unapplied payment

Payments that have been fully applied are not colored and appear white.

Once all the necessary information is entered, it is time to apply the payment to specific charges. This is accomplished by clicking the Apply button, which causes the Apply Payment to Charges dialog box to be displayed. The Apply Payment to Charges dialog box lists information about all unpaid charges for a patient, including the date of the procedure, the document number, the procedure code, the charge, the balance, and the total amount paid (see Figure 6-24).

In the upper-right corner of the dialog box, the amount of payment that has not yet been applied to charges is listed in the Unapplied box.

The first step in applying a payment is to determine the charge(s) to which the payment should be applied. Payments may be applied to charges that require a copayment, charges that are the oldest, or any other charges.

If the payment is a copayment, then the Apply to Co-pay button is clicked. When the Apply to Co-pay button is clicked, the program automatically applies the payment to the charge on that date that

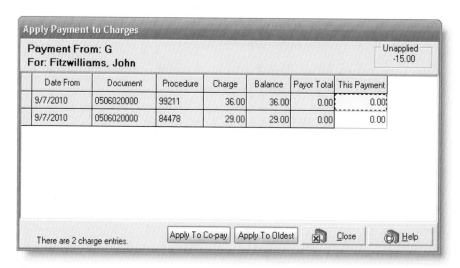

Figure 6-24   Apply Payment to Charges dialog box with This Payment box highlighted

requires a copayment. Information about whether a procedure code requires a copayment is located in the General tab of Procedure/Payment/Adjustment dialog box for that code.

If the payment should be applied to the oldest charge, then the Apply to Oldest button is clicked. When the Apply to Oldest button is used, the program automatically applies the payment to the oldest charge.

Payments may also be manually applied by clicking in the box in the This Payment column on the line that contains the charge. To select a box, click in it; a dotted rectangle appears around the outside of the box. Enter the amount of the payment (without a decimal point), and press the Enter key. The payment is applied, and the Unapplied Amount entry is lowered by the amount of the payment.

Notice in Figure 6-25 that the payment amount has been entered in the appropriate This Payment box.

Payments can be applied to more than one charge. For example, suppose that the payment is $200.00 and three charges have not been paid. The $200.00 payment can be applied to one, two, or all three of the charges.

Once the box is closed, the payment appears in the Payments, Adjustments, and Comments area of the Transaction Entry dialog box (see Figure 6-26).

SAVING PAYMENT INFORMATION

When all the information on a payment has been entered and checked for accuracy, it must be saved. Payment transactions are saved in the manner described earlier for charge transactions, by clicking the Save Transactions button.

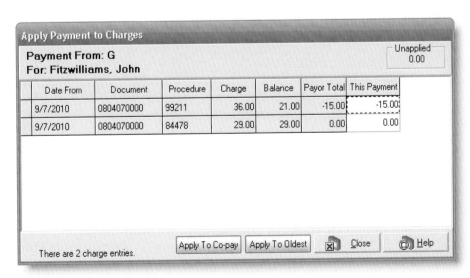

Figure 6-25 Apply Payment to Charges with payment entered

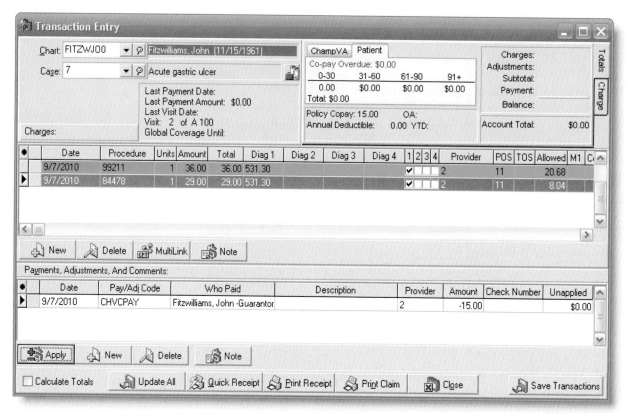

Figure 6-26   Payments, Adjustments, and Comments area with payment listed and charges color-coded as partially paid (aqua) and no payment (gray)

EXERCISE 6-3

Using Source Document 3, enter the copayment made by Hiro Tanaka for her October 4, 2010, office visit.

Date: October 4, 2010

1. Open the Transaction Entry dialog box if it is not already open.

2. In the Chart box, key *T,* and press Tab to select Hiro Tanaka. An Information box is displayed with information about Tanaka's allergies. Click the OK button.

3. Verify that Accident—back pain is the active case in the Case box.

4. Click the New button in the Payments, Adjustments, and Comments section of the dialog box.

5. Accept the default entry of 10/4/2010 in the Date box.

6. Click in the Pay/Adj Code box. From the drop-down list, select OHCCPAY (the code for OhioCare HMO copayment), and press Tab. Notice that some of the boxes have been completed by the program.

7. Verify that Tanaka, Hiro—Guarantor is listed in the Who Paid box.

8. Notice that –20.00 has already been entered in the Amount box. Confirm that this is the correct amount of the copay by looking at Source Document 1.

9. The Unapplied Amount box should read (20.00).

10. Click in the Check Number box; enter *123;* and press Tab.

11. Click the Apply button. The Apply Payment to Charges dialog box is displayed.

12. Notice that the amount of this payment (–20.00) is listed in the Unapplied box at the upper-right of the dialog box.

13. Click the Apply to Co-pay button. When the box appears that states "The payment has been fully applied," click OK. The program automatically enters –20.00 in the box in the This Payment column for the 99202 procedure charge. The Unapplied Amount column is now zero. (*Note:* If zero is not displayed yet, click once in the empty space below the This Payment box, and the program will update the unapplied column amount.)

14. Click the Close button. If an information box appears with the message "This case requires a $20.00 copay for each visit," click OK.

15. Click the Save Transactions button. When the date warning boxes appear, click Yes.

16. Notice that the line listing the procedure charge has changed from gray (not paid) to aqua (partially paid), indicating that a portion of the charge has been paid.

EXERCISE 6-4

Using Source Document 6, enter the procedure charges and copayment for John Fitzwilliams's acute gastric ulcer case.

Date: October 4, 2010

1. Click in the Chart box, and key *F.* Notice that the chart number for John Fitzwilliams is highlighted on the drop-down list. Press the Tab key. Verify that Acute gastric ulcer is the active case in the Case box.

2. Notice that there are already charges and payments listed for this case, since this is an existing medical condition for which the patient has been treated in the past.

3. Click the New button in the Charges section of the dialog box.

4. Accept the default in the Date box (10/4/2010).

5. Select the procedure code for the services checked off on the encounter form. There is more than one procedure. Enter the first procedure code (99212). Press Tab.

6. Accept the default entries in the other boxes.

7. Check your entries for accuracy.

Now enter the second procedure code marked on the encounter form by following these steps.

8. Click the New button. If an information box appears with a message about a $15.00 copay, click OK.

9. Accept the default in the Date box.

10. Select the procedure code for the second service checked off on the encounter form (82270). Press Tab.

11. Accept the default entries in the other boxes.

12. Check your entries for accuracy.

13. Click the Save Transactions button. Two Date of Service Validation boxes appear, one for each transaction. Click Yes each time a box is displayed.

Now enter the copayment listed on the encounter form by completing the remaining steps.

14. Click the New button in the Payments, Adjustments, and Comments section of the dialog box.

15. Accept the default entry of 10/4/2010 in the Date box.

16. On the Pay/Adj Code drop-down list, click CHVCPAY (ChampVA Copayment), and press Tab. Notice that all the remaining boxes except Check Number and Description are once again filled in. Verify that the entries are correct.

17. Enter *456* in the Check Number box, and press Tab.

18. Click the Apply button. The Apply Payment to Charges dialog box is displayed.

19. Notice that the amount of this payment (–15.00) is listed in the Unapplied box at the upper-right of the dialog box.

20. Click the Apply to Co-pay button. When the box appears that states "The payment has been fully applied," click OK.

21. Click the Close button.

22. Notice that the amount listed in the Unapplied Amount column is now zero. Also notice that the line listing the 99212 charge on 10/4/2010 is now aqua rather than gray, indicating that the charge has been partially paid.

23. Click the Save Transactions button. When the date warning boxes are displayed, click the Yes button.

PRINTING WALKOUT RECEIPTS

After a patient payment has been entered in the Transaction Entry dialog box, a walkout receipt is printed and given to the patient before he or she leaves the office. A walkout receipt, also known as a walkout statement, includes information on the procedures, diagnosis, charges, and payments for a visit. If there is a balance due, the receipt serves as a reminder to the patient of the amount owed.

In the Transaction Entry dialog box, walkout receipts are created via the Print Receipt or Quick Receipt button (see Figure 6-27). The Quick Receipt option remembers the user's preferred report format and eliminates several steps in the creation of a receipt. (*Note:* A Print Claim button also appears in the Transaction Entry dialog box; claim management is discussed in detail in Chapter 7.)

When the Print Receipt button is clicked, the Open Report window appears with the first report highlighted Walkout Receipt (All Transactions), as shown in Figure 6-28.

After clicking the OK button in the Open Report window, the Print Report Where? dialog box is displayed, and three options are provided (see Figure 6-29):

1. Previewing the report on the screen

2. Sending the report directly to the printer

3. Exporting the report to a file

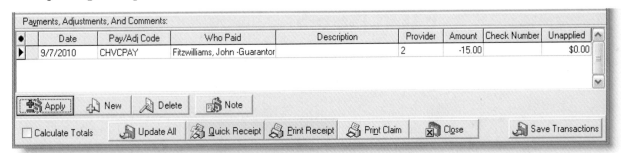

Figure 6-27   Print Receipt button highlighted in yellow

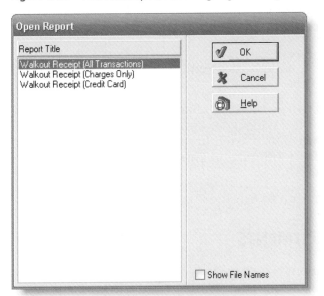

Figure 6-28   Open Report window with Walkout Receipt (All Transactions) selected

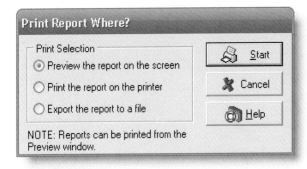

Figure 6-29   Print Report Where? dialog box

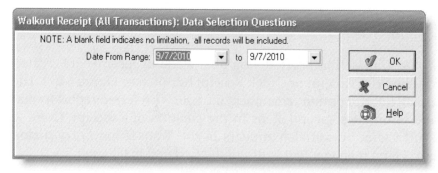

NOTE: A blank field indicates no limitation, all records will be included.

Date From Range: 9/7/2010 ▾ to 9/7/2010 ▾

OK

Cancel

Help

Walkout Receipt (All Transactions): Data Selection Questions

Figure 6-30   Data Selection Questions window

Once a printing choice is made, clicking the Start button causes the Data Selection Questions window to open (see Figure 6-30). This is where the date for the receipt is selected.

Finally, when the OK button is clicked, the report is sent to its destination (on screen, to the printer, to a file; see Figure 6-31).

EXERCISE 6-5

Create a walkout receipt for John Fitzwilliams.

Date: October 4, 2010

1. With the Transaction Entry dialog box open to John Fitzwilliams's acute gastric ulcer case, click the Quick Receipt button. The Print Report Where? dialog box is displayed.

2. In the Print Report Where? dialog box, accept the default selection to preview the report on the screen. Click the Start button. The Preview Report window opens, displaying the walkout receipt.

3. Review the charge and payment entries listed in the top half of the receipt.

4. Scroll down and review the total charges, payments, and adjustments listed at the lower-right area of the receipt. Compare the total account balance listed here with the amount listed in the Totals tab of the Transaction Entry dialog box. The numbers should be the same.

5. Click the Close button to exit the Preview Report window.

ENTERING ADJUSTMENTS

Adjustments to patient accounts are entered in the same manner as payments are recorded, in the lower third of the Transaction Entry dialog box. Clicking the New button begins the process of entering an adjustment. When the New button is clicked, the

Family Care Center

285 Stephenson Boulevard
Stephenson, OH 60089
(614)555-0000

Patient: John Fitzwilliams 1627 Forest Avenue Jefferson, OH 60093	**Instructions:** Complete the patient information portion of your insurance claim form. Attach this bill, signed and dated, and all other bills pertaining to the claim. If you have a deductible policy, hold your claim forms until you have met your deductible. Mail directly to your insurance carrier.
Chart #: FITZWJO0 **Case #:** 7	

Date	Description	Procedure	Modify	Dx 1	Dx 2	Dx 3	Dx 4	Units	Charge
9/7/2010	OF--established patient, minimal	99211		531.30				1	36.00
9/7/2010	Triglycerides test	84478		531.30				1	29.00
9/7/2010	ChampVA Copayment	CHVCPAY						1	-15.00

Provider Information		
Provider Name:	John Rudner MD	
License:	84701	
Champ VA PIN:		
SSN or EIN:	339-67-5000	

Total Charges:	$ 65.00
Total Payments:	-$ 15.00
Total Adjustments:	$ 0.00
Total Due This Visit:	**$ 50.00**
Total Account Balance:	$ 50.00

Assign and Release: I hereby authorize payment of medical benefits to this physician for the services described above. I also authorize the release of any information necessary to process this claim.

Patient Signature: _____   Date: _____

Figure 6-31 Sample walkout receipt

program automatically enters the current date (the date that the Medisoft program date is set to) in the Date box. The other fields include:

Payment/Adjustment Code   This code indicates the type of adjustment transaction, such as PTREFUND (patient refund).

Who Paid   In the case of a refund, the chart number of the patient who is receiving the refund is entered.

Description   The reason for the refund, such as "patient payment more than expected," is described.

Amount   The amount of the refund is shown.

Check Number   The number of the check used for the refund is entered.

Unapplied   The dollar value in the Unapplied box is the amount that has not yet been applied to a transaction.

If the patient's account has a positive balance because the patient overpaid, the patient's charge in the Transaction Entry box is color-coded yellow (see Figure 6-32). This indicates the patient is due a refund, and an adjustment needs to be made.

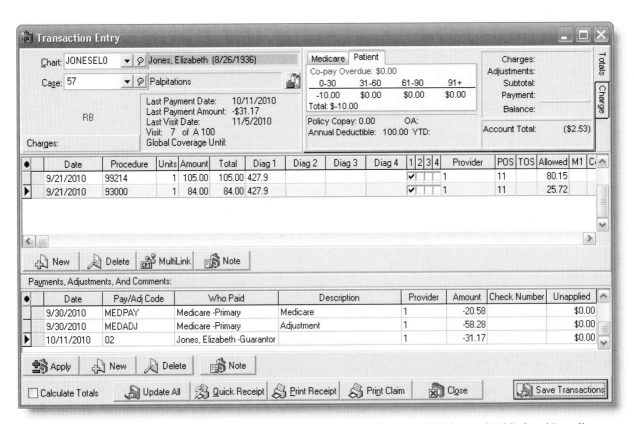

Figure 6-32   Payments, Adjustments, and Comments section with the overpaid charge highlighted in yellow

EXERCISE 6-6

Process a refund for a patient who has overpaid on his account.

Date: October 4, 2010

1. Open the Transaction Entry dialog box, if it is not already open.

2. In the Chart box, key **SM,** and press Tab to select James L. Smith.

3. Verify that Facial nerve paralysis is displayed in the Case box.

4. Notice that the entry in the Charges section of the window is highlighted in yellow, indicating that this is an overpaid charge. According to the patient's insurance plan, the plan pays 80 percent of charges and the patient pays 20 percent. In this case, 20 percent of the charges ($210.00) would be $42.00. However, the patient paid $52.00, and is therefore due a refund of $10.00.

5. Click the New button in the Payments, Adjustments, and Comments section of the dialog box.

6. Accept the default entry of 10/4/2010 in the Date box.

7. Click in the Pay/Adj Code box. Select PTREFUND (the code for a patient refund), and press Tab.

8. Select Smith, James—Guarantor in the Who Paid box.

9. Enter **Overpaid—refund** in the Description box, and press Tab twice to get to the Amount box.

10. Enter **10** in the Amount box, and press Tab. Notice that the amount is listed as a positive amount.

11. The Unapplied Amount box should read $10.00.

12. Click in the Check Number box; enter **456;** and press Tab.

13. Click the Apply button. The Apply Payment to Charges dialog box is displayed.

14. Notice that the amount of this refund ($10.00) is listed in the Unapplied box at the upper-right of the dialog box.

15. Click in the white box in the This Adjust. column. Enter **10,** and press Tab.

16. Click the Close button.

17. Click the Save Transactions button. When the date warning boxes appear, click Yes.

18. Notice that the line listing the procedure charge has changed from yellow (overpaid) to white (fully paid), indicating that the expected amount has been paid.

ON YOUR OWN EXERCISE 3 Enter Procedure Charges and a Patient Payment

October 4, 2010

Lisa Wright has just been seen by Dr. Jessica Rudner. Using Source Document 7, enter the diagnosis in the Case folder, and then enter the procedure charges in the Transaction Entry dialog box.

ON YOUR OWN EXERCISE 4 Print a Walkout Receipt

October 4, 2010

Print a walkout receipt to give to Hiro Tanaka before she leaves the office.

Remember to create a backup of your work before exiting Medisoft! To help you keep track of your work, name the backup file after the chapter you are working on, for example, StudentID-c6.mbk.

Electronic Medical Record Exchange

Importing Transactions

Transactions imported from an electronic medical record can be reviewed before they are posted in Medisoft. In the illustration below, the window at the top left lists the two charge transactions waiting to be posted. Once a billing specialist reviews the charges, they are imported and appear as posted charges in the Transaction Entry dialog box in Medisoft.

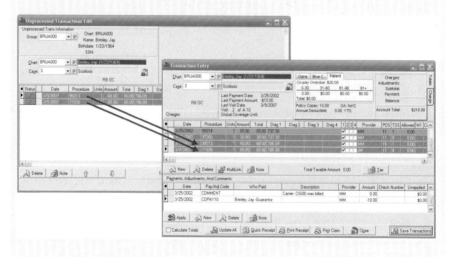

Name: _____   **Date:** _____

CHAPTER 6 WORKSHEET

After completing all the exercises in the chapter, answer the following questions in the spaces provided.

1. What are the total charges listed on John Fitzwilliams's walkout receipt?

   _____

2. What is entered in the Pay/Adj Code box for Hiro Tanaka's copayment on 10/4/2010 (Transaction Entry dialog box)?

   _____

3. What is listed as the annual deductible for John Fitzwilliams (Transaction Entry dialog box)?

   _____

4. What is listed in the Allowed Amount box for procedure 99212 on 10/4/2010 for John Fitzwilliams (Transaction Entry dialog box)?

   _____

5. What is entered in the Total box for procedure 99213 on 10/4/2010 for Elizabeth Jones (Transaction Entry dialog box)?

   _____

6. What is entered in the Diag 1 box for procedure 99202 on 10/4/2010 for Hiro Tanaka (Transaction Entry dialog box)?

   _____

7. What is entered in the Provider box for procedure 99202 on 10/4/2010 for Hiro Tanaka (Transaction Entry dialog box)?

   _____

8. What is entered in the Allowed box for procedure 99213 on 10/4/2010 for Elizabeth Jones (Transaction Entry dialog box)?

   _____

9. What is entered in the Amount box for procedure 99203 on 10/4/2010 for Lisa Wright (Transaction Entry dialog box)?

   _____

10. What two procedure codes are listed for Lisa Wright on 10/4/2010 (Transaction Entry dialog box)?

   _____

CHAPTER REVIEW

USING TERMINOLOGY

Match the terms on the left with the definitions on the right.

_____ **1.** adjustments

_____ **2.** charges

_____ **3.** MultiLink codes

_____ **4.** payments

a. Changes to patients' accounts.

b. The amounts billed by a provider for particular services.

c. Monies paid to a medical practice by patients and insurance carriers.

d. Groups of procedure code entries that are related to a single activity.

CHECKING YOUR UNDERSTANDING

Answer the questions below in the space provided.

5. What are the two key pieces of information you must have before entering a procedure charge?

_____

_____

6. List two advantages of using MultiLink codes.

_____

_____

7. When is it appropriate to print a walkout receipt?

_____

_____

8. What color code indicates that no payment has been made on a charge transaction?

_____

_____

9. What is the color code for an unapplied payment?

_____

_____

APPLYING KNOWLEDGE

Answer the questions below in the space provided.

10. After you have entered a charge for procedure code 99393, you realize it should have been 99394. What should you do?

_____

_____

11. The receptionist working at the front desk phones to tell you that Maritza Ramos has just seen the physician and would like to know—before she leaves the office—what the charges were for her September 8, 2010, office visit. You are in the middle of entering charges from an encounter form for another patient. What should you do first? What is your reasoning?

_____

_____

12. After you have entered a patient copayment for $20.00, you realize it should have been $30.00. What should you do?

_____

_____

AT THE COMPUTER

Answer the following questions at the computer.

13. What are the procedure codes and charges for Randall Klein for September 7, 2010?

_____

_____

14. What is the amount of the procedure charge entered on September 10, 2010, for patient Jo Wong?

_____

_____

15. What is the total amount that John Fitzwilliams paid in copayments in September 2010? (*Hint:* Include his daughter Sarah in the calculation.)

_____

_____

Creating Claims

7

WHAT YOU NEED TO KNOW

To use this chapter, you need to know how to:

◆ Start Medisoft, use menus, and enter and edit text.

◆ Work with chart numbers and codes.

LEARNING OUTCOMES

When you finish this chapter, you will be able to:

◆ Create claims.

◆ Review claims for errors and omissions.

◆ Edit claims.

◆ Add attachments to electronic claims.

KEY TERMS

filter
navigator buttons

INTRODUCTION TO HEALTH CARE CLAIMS

Once the services a patient has received from a provider have been entered into the practice management program, the next step is to create insurance claims. The insurance claim is the most important document for correct reimbursement. Claims communicate information about a patient's diagnosis and procedures and the charges to a payer.

A physician practice depends on the billing specialist to submit clean claims—claims with all the information necessary for payer processing. An error on a claim may cause the claim to be delayed or denied. Rejected claims can cost the practice twice as much as clean claims and can result in reduced cash flow. Claims that are not paid in full also have a negative effect on the practice's bottom line.

Today, almost all claims are sent electronically. The HIPAA standard transaction for electronic claims is the HIPAA X12 837 Health Care Claim or Equivalent Encounter Information (837P). The paper format is known as the CMS-1500 claim form. Both types of insurance claims are prepared in the practice management program.

The National Uniform Claim Committee (NUCC), led by the American Medical Association, determines the content of both the 837P and the CMS-1500. The CMS-1500 claim has 33 numbered boxes representing about 150 discrete data elements, while the 837P has a maximum of 244 segments representing about 1,054 elements. However, many of these data elements are conditional and apply to particular specialties only. The CMS-1500 is pictured in Figure 7-1.

A listing of the data elements on the CMS-1500 and the corresponding location of those data in Medisoft is provided in Table 7-1 (on pages 170–171).

CREATING CLAIMS

Within the Claim Management area of Medisoft, insurance claims are created, edited, and submitted for payment.

The Claim Management dialog box is displayed by clicking Claim Management on the Activities menu or by clicking the Claim Management shortcut button on the toolbar (see Figure 7-2 on page 172). The dialog box (see Figure 7-3 on page 172) lists all claims that have already been created. In this dialog box, several actions can be performed: existing claims can be reviewed and edited, new claims can be created, the status of existing claims can be changed, and claims can be printed or submitted electronically.

Figure 7-1   The CMS-1500 claim form

1500

HEALTH INSURANCE CLAIM FORM

APPROVED BY NATIONAL UNIFORM CLAIM COMMITTEE 08/05

PICA   PICA

1. MEDICARE (Medicare #)   MEDICAID (Medicaid #)   TRICARE CHAMPUS (Sponsor's SSN)   CHAMPVA (Member ID#)   GROUP HEALTH PLAN (SSN or ID)   FECA BLK LUNG (SSN)   OTHER (ID)   1a. INSURED'S I.D. NUMBER (For Program in Item 1)

2. PATIENT'S NAME (Last Name, First Name, Middle Initial)   3. PATIENT'S BIRTH DATE MM DD YY   SEX M F   4. INSURED'S NAME (Last Name, First Name, Middle Initial)

5. PATIENT'S ADDRESS (No., Street)   6. PATIENT RELATIONSHIP TO INSURED Self Spouse Child Other   7. INSURED'S ADDRESS (No., Street)

CITY   STATE   8. PATIENT STATUS Single Married Other   CITY   STATE

ZIP CODE   TELEPHONE (Include Area Code) (   )   Employed Full-Time Student Part-Time Student   ZIP CODE   TELEPHONE (Include Area Code) (   )

9. OTHER INSURED'S NAME (Last Name, First Name, Middle Initial)   10. IS PATIENT'S CONDITION RELATED TO: 11. INSURED'S POLICY GROUP OR FECA NUMBER

a. OTHER INSURED'S POLICY OR GROUP NUMBER   a. EMPLOYMENT? (Current or Previous) YES NO   a. INSURED'S DATE OF BIRTH MM DD YY   SEX M F

b. OTHER INSURED'S DATE OF BIRTH MM DD YY   SEX M F   b. AUTO ACCIDENT? YES NO   PLACE (State)   b. EMPLOYER'S NAME OR SCHOOL NAME

c. EMPLOYER'S NAME OR SCHOOL NAME   c. OTHER ACCIDENT? YES NO   c. INSURANCE PLAN NAME OR PROGRAM NAME

d. INSURANCE PLAN NAME OR PROGRAM NAME   10d. RESERVED FOR LOCAL USE   d. IS THERE ANOTHER HEALTH BENEFIT PLAN? YES NO If yes, return to and complete item 9 a-d.

READ BACK OF FORM BEFORE COMPLETING & SIGNING THIS FORM.
12. PATIENT'S OR AUTHORIZED PERSON'S SIGNATURE I authorize the release of any medical or other information necessary to process this claim. I also request payment of government benefits either to myself or to the party who accepts assignment below.

SIGNED _____   DATE _____

13. INSURED'S OR AUTHORIZED PERSON'S SIGNATURE I authorize payment of medical benefits to the undersigned physician or supplier for services described below.

SIGNED _____

14. DATE OF CURRENT: MM DD YY   ILLNESS (First symptom) OR INJURY (Accident) OR PREGNANCY(LMP)   15. IF PATIENT HAS HAD SAME OR SIMILAR ILLNESS. GIVE FIRST DATE MM DD YY   16. DATES PATIENT UNABLE TO WORK IN CURRENT OCCUPATION MM DD YY   FROM   TO MM DD YY

17. NAME OF REFERRING PROVIDER OR OTHER SOURCE   17a.   17b. NPI   18. HOSPITALIZATION DATES RELATED TO CURRENT SERVICES MM DD YY FROM   TO MM DD YY

19. RESERVED FOR LOCAL USE   20. OUTSIDE LAB? YES NO $ CHARGES

21. DIAGNOSIS OR NATURE OF ILLNESS OR INJURY (Relate Items 1, 2, 3 or 4 to Item 24E by Line)
1. ____ . ____   3. ____ . ____
2. ____ . ____   4. ____ . ____

22. MEDICAID RESUBMISSION CODE   ORIGINAL REF. NO.

23. PRIOR AUTHORIZATION NUMBER

24. A. DATE(S) OF SERVICE From MM DD YY To MM DD YY | B. PLACE OF SERVICE | C. EMG | D. PROCEDURES, SERVICES, OR SUPPLIES (Explain Unusual Circumstances) CPT/HCPCS   MODIFIER | E. DIAGNOSIS POINTER | F. $ CHARGES | G. DAYS OR UNITS | H. EPSDT Family Plan | I. ID. QUAL. | J. RENDERING PROVIDER ID. #

1   NPI
2   NPI
3   NPI
4   NPI
5   NPI
6   NPI

25. FEDERAL TAX I.D. NUMBER   SSN EIN   26. PATIENT'S ACCOUNT NO.   27. ACCEPT ASSIGNMENT? (For govt. claims, see back) YES NO   28. TOTAL CHARGE $ 29. AMOUNT PAID $ 30. BALANCE DUE $

31. SIGNATURE OF PHYSICIAN OR SUPPLIER INCLUDING DEGREES OR CREDENTIALS (I certify that the statements on the reverse apply to this bill and are made a part thereof.)   SIGNED   DATE   32. SERVICE FACILITY LOCATION INFORMATION   a. NPI   b.   33. BILLING PROVIDER INFO & PH # (   )   a. NPI   b.

NUCC Instruction Manual available at: www.nucc.org   APPROVED OMB-0938-0999 FORM CMS-1500 (08/05)

CARRIER

PATIENT AND INSURED INFORMATION

PHYSICIAN OR SUPPLIER INFORMATION

Box	CMS-1500 Field Name	Data Source in Medisoft	Dialog Box/Field Name in Medisoft
Top 1	Insurance Name/Address	Insurance	*Insurance Carrier,* Address, *Name, etc.*
Top 2	Primary, Secondary, Tertiary	Insurance	Determined by claim form selected
1	Insurance Type	Insurance	*Insurance Carrier,* Options, *Type*
1a	Insured's ID No.	Case	*Case,* Policy 1, 2, 3, *Policy No.*
2	Patient's Name	Patient	*Patient/Guarantor,* Name, Address, *Last Name, First Name, Middle Initial*
3	Patient Birth Date, Sex	Patient	*Patient/Guarantor,* Name Address, *Birth Date, Sex*
4	Insured's Name	Case	*Case,* Policy 1, 2, 3, *Policy Holder 1, 2, 3*
5	Patient's Address	Patient	*Patient/Guarantor,* Name, Address, *Street, City, State, Zip*
6	Patient Relation to Insured	Case	*Case,* Policy 1, 2, 3, *Relationship to Insured*
7	Insured's Address	Patient	*Patient/Guarantor,* Name, Address, *Street, City, State, Zip*
8	Patient Status	Case	*Case,* Personal, *Marital Status, Student Status, Employment Status*
9	Other Insured's Name	Case	*Case,* Policy, *Policy Holder 2, 3*
9a	Other Insured's Policy/Group No.	Case	*Case,* Policy 2, 3, *Policy Number, Group Number*
9b	Other Insured's Date of Birth, Sex	Patient	*Patient/Guarantor,* Name, Address, *Birth Date, Sex*
9c	Employer/School	Patient	*Patient/Guarantor,* Other Information, *Employer*
9d	Insurance Plan Name, Program	Insurance	*Insurance Carrier,* Options, *Plan Name;* if empty, prints carrier name
10a	Condition Related to Employment	Case	*Case,* Condition, *Employment Related* check box
10b	Condition Related to Auto Accident	Case	*Case,* Condition, *Accident, Related To*
10c	Condition Related to Other Accident	Case	*Case,* Condition, *Accident, Related To*
10d	Local Use	Case	*Case,* Miscellaneous, *Local Use A*
11	Insured's Policy Group/FECA#	Case	*Case,* Policy 1, *Policy Number, Group Number*
11a	Insured's Date of Birth, Sex	Patient	*Patient/Guarantor,* Name, Address, *Birth Date, Sex*
11b	Employer/School	Patient	*Patient/Guarantor,* Other Information, *Employer*
11c	Insurance Plan Name/Program	Insurance	*Insurance Carrier,* Options, *Plan Name;* if empty, prints carrier name
11d	Another Health Benefit Plan?	Case	*Case,* Policy 2, 3
12	Patient Signature or Authorized Signature	Patient	*Patient/Guarantor,* Other Information, *Signature on File; Insurance Carrier,* Options, *Patient Signature on File*
13	Insured's Signature or Authorized Signature	Patient	*Patient/Guarantor,* Other Information, *Signature on File; Insurance Carrier,* Options, *Insured Signature on File*

Box	CMS-1500 Field Name	Data Source in Medisoft	Dialog Box/Field Name in Medisoft
14	Date Current Ill/Inj/LMP	Case	*Case,* Condition, *Injury/Illness/LMP Date*
15	Same/Similar Date	Case	*Case,* Condition, *Date Similar Symptoms*
16	Dates Unable to Work	Case	*Case,* Condition, *Dates—Unable to Work*
17	Referring Provider	Case	*Case,* Account, *Referring Provider*
17a	Referring Provider, Other Identifier, Qualifier	Referring Provider	*Referring Provider,* Default Pins, *Extra 1* OR *Extra 2*
17b	Referring Provider NPI	Referring Provider	*Referring Provider,* Default PINs, *National Identifier*
18	Hospitalization Dates	Case	*Case,* Condition, *Dates—Hospitalization*
19	Local Use	Case	*Case,* Miscellaneous, *Local Use B*
20	Outside Lab? $ Charges	Case	*Case,* Miscellaneous, *Outside Lab Work*
21	Diagnosis	Case	*Case,* Diagnosis, *Default Diagnosis 1, 2, 3, 4*
22	Medicaid Resubmission	Case	*Case,* Medicaid and Tricare, *Resubmission No., Original Reference*
23	Prior Authorization #	Case	*Case,* Miscellaneous, *Prior Authorization Number*
24A	Dates of Service	Transaction	*Transaction Entry,* Date From, Date To
24B	Place of Service	Transaction	*Transaction Entry,* Place of Service
24C	EMG		*Payer Specific Code*
24D	Procedures, Services, or Supplies	Transaction	*Transaction Entry,* Procedure, M1, M2, M3, M4
24E	Diagnosis Pointer	Transaction	*Transaction Entry,* Diag 1, Diag 2, Diag 3, Diag 4
24F	$ Charges	Transaction	*Transaction Entry,* Amount
24G	Days or Units	Transaction	*Transaction Entry,* Units
24H	EPSDT	Case	*Case,* Medicaid and Tricare, *EPSDT*
24I	Rendering Provider, Other ID, Qualifier	Provider	*Provider,* Default Pins, *Extra 1 or Extra 2*
24J	Rendering Provider ID#	Provider	*Provider,* Default PINs, *National Identifier*
25	Federal Tax ID	Practice	*Provider,* Default Pins, *SSN/Federal Tax ID*
26	Patient's Account No.	Patient	*Patient/Guarantor,* Name, Address, *Chart No.*
27	Accept Assignment?	Case	*Case,* Policy 1, 2, 3, *Assignment of Benefits/Accept Assignment*
28	Total Charge	Transaction	Calculated field
29	Amount Paid	Transaction	*Transaction Entry,* Payment
30	Balance Due	Transaction	Calculated field
31	Physician's Signature	Provider	*Provider,* Address, *Signature on File; Insurance Carrier,* Options, *Physician Signature on File*
32	Facility Address	Practice	*Case,* Account, *Facility*
32A	Facility NPI	Address	*Address,* ID, *Identifier*
33	Billing Provider Information	Provider	*Provider,* Address, *First Name, Middle Initial, Last Name, Street, City, State, Zip*
33A	Billing Provider NPI	Provider	*Provider,* Default Pins, *National Identifier*

Figure 7-2
Claim Management
shortcut button

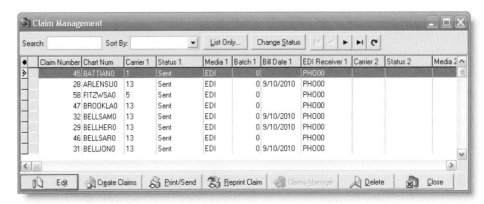

Figure 7-3   Claim Management dialog box

The upper-right corner of the Claim Management dialog box contains five **navigator buttons** that simplify the task of moving from one entry to another (see Figure 7-4). The First Claim button selects the first claim in the list and makes it active. The Previous Claim button reactivates the claim that was most recently active. The Next Claim button makes the next claim in the list active. The Last Claim button makes the last claim in the list active. The Refresh Data button is used to restore data when necessary.

navigator buttons   buttons that simplify the task of moving from one entry to another

Figure 7-4
Navigator buttons

The bottom of the Claim Management dialog box contains a number of buttons that are used for various functions (see Figure 7-3).

Edit   Opens a claim for editing.

Create Claims   Opens the Create Claims dialog box.

Print/Send   Begins the process of sending electronic claims or printing paper claims.

Reprint Claim   Reprints a claim that has already been printed.

Claims Manager (grayed out)   This button is available only to medical offices that have enrolled in Claims Manager, an online electronic claims service.

Delete   Deletes the selected claim and releases the transactions bound to the claim.

Close   Closes the Claim Management dialog box.

CREATE CLAIMS DIALOG BOX

Claims are created in the Create Claims dialog box. The Create Claims dialog box (see Figure 7-5) is accessed by clicking the Create Claims button in the Claim Management dialog box. This dialog box provides several filters to customize the creation of claims. A **filter** is a condition that data must meet to be selected. For example, claims can be created

filter   a condition that data must meet to be selected

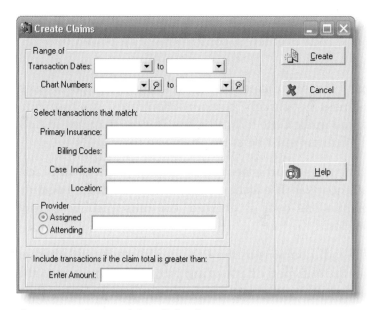

Figure 7-5   Create Claims dialog box

for services performed between the first and the fifteenth of the month. In this case, the filter is the condition that services must have been performed between the first and fifteenth of the month. Transactions that meet this criterion are included in the selection; transactions that do not fall within the date range are not be included. Filters can be used to create claims for a specific patient, for a specific insurance carrier, and for transactions that exceed a certain dollar amount, among others. The following filters can be applied within the Create Claims dialog box.

Range of   The options in this section of the dialog box provide filters for establishing the starting and ending dates as well as the starting and ending chart numbers for the claims that will be created.

Transaction Dates   The Transaction Dates boxes are used to specify the starting and ending dates for which claims will be created. If the boxes are left blank, transactions for all dates will be included.

Chart Numbers   In the Chart Numbers boxes, the starting and ending chart numbers for which claims will be created are entered. If the boxes are left blank, all chart numbers will be included.

Select Transactions That Match   The options in this section of the dialog box provide filters for matching the exact primary insurance carrier(s), billing code(s), case indicator(s), and location(s).

Primary Insurance   The carrier code for the insurance company is entered in the Primary Insurance box. If claims are being sent to a clearinghouse, more than one insurance carrier code can be entered. When more than one code is entered, commas must be placed between the codes. If claims are being sent directly to the carrier, only that carrier's code is entered.

Billing Codes   The billing code is entered in the Billing Codes box. If more than one code is entered, commas must be placed between the codes.

Case Indicator   If case indicators are used to classify patients (such as by type of illness for workers' compensation cases), the case indicator can be listed in the Case Indicator box. If more than one indicator is entered, commas must be placed between them.

Location   Sometimes a sort is needed by location, such as all procedures done at a hospital. The location code is entered in the Location box. If more than one code is entered, commas must be placed between the codes.

Provider   The radio buttons in the Provider box indicate whether the provider is the assigned or attending provider. In the box to the right of the radio buttons, the provider code is entered. If more than one code is entered, commas must be placed between the codes.

Include Transactions if the Claim Total is Greater Than   The dollar amount entered in this box is the minimum total amount required for a case before a claim can be created.

Any box that is not filled in will default to include all data, and claims with any entry in that box will be included. When all necessary information has been entered, clicking the Create button creates the claims. Medisoft will create a file of matching claims but will include only those that have not yet been billed.

EXERCISE 7-1

Create insurance claims for all patients with last names beginning with the letters *A* through *L*.

Date: November 5, 2010

1. Start Medisoft and restore the data from your last work session.

2. Set the Medisoft Program Date to November 5, 2010. On the Activities menu, click Claim Management. The Claim Management dialog box is displayed.

3. Click the Create Claims button.

4. In the first Chart Numbers box, enter *A,* and press Tab. In the second box, enter *L,* and press Tab. Leave the remaining boxes in the Create Claims dialog box blank.

5. Click the Create button.

6. Use the scroll bars to view the claims just created. New claims will have the status of Ready to Send in the Status 1 column.

7. Click the Close button.

CLAIM SELECTION

At times it is necessary to select and view specific claims that have already been created. For example, any claims prepared for submission to an insurance carrier must be selected and then reviewed for completeness and accuracy. In addition, all claims that have been rejected by insurance carriers are selected and reviewed before resubmission.

Medisoft's List Only feature is used when it is necessary to list claims that match certain criteria. Filters are applied in the List Only Claims That Match dialog box. They can be used to view claims selectively, such as claims for a specific insurance carrier and claims created on a certain date. Unlike the filters in the Create Claims dialog box, those in the List Only Claims That Match dialog box do not create claims; they simply list existing claims that meet the specified criteria.

Once the filters have been applied, only those claims that match the criteria are listed at the bottom of the main Claim Management dialog box. Claims can be sorted by chart number, date the claim was created, insurance carrier, electronic claim (EDI) receiver, billing method, billing date, batch number, and claim status. Not all the boxes need to be filled in, only the ones that will be used to select the desired claims.

The List Only feature is activated by clicking the List Only . . . button in the Claim Management dialog box. This causes the List Only Claims That Match dialog box to be displayed (see Figure 7-6).

The following filters are available in the List Only Claims That Match dialog box.

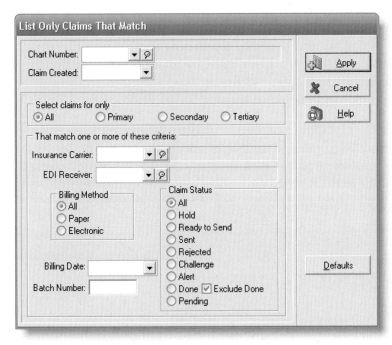

Figure 7-6   List Only Claims That Match dialog box

Chart Number A patient's chart number is selected from the drop-down list of patients' chart numbers.

Claim Created The date that a claim was created is entered in MMDDCCYY format.

Select Claims for Only A radio button is clicked for either all insurance carriers, primary insurance carrier only, secondary insurance carrier only, or tertiary insurance carrier only. When a patient has insurance coverage with more than one carrier, the primary carrier is billed first, and then, if appropriate, the second and third (tertiary) carriers are billed.

Insurance Carrier An insurance carrier is selected from the drop-down list of choices.

EDI Receiver An EDI receiver is selected from the choices on the drop-down list.

Billing Method In the Billing Method box, the radio button for All, Paper, or Electronic is clicked.

Billing Date The date of billing is entered in the Billing Date box.

Batch Number A batch number is entered in the Batch Number box.

Claim Status A claim status is selected from the list of radio buttons provided. If claims that have been billed and accepted (not rejected) are to be excluded from the search, the Exclude Done box is clicked. This causes a check mark to be displayed beside the option.

When the desired boxes have been filled in, clicking the Apply button applies the selected filters to the claims data. The Claim Management dialog box is displayed, listing only those claims that match the criteria selected in the List Only Claims That Match dialog box. From the Claim Management dialog box, the claims can now be edited, printed, and mailed or transmitted electronically.

To restore the List Only Claims That Match dialog box to its original settings (that is, to remove the filters selected), this dialog box is reopened; the Defaults button is clicked; and the Apply button is clicked. All the boxes in the dialog box will become blank, and the full list of claims is again displayed in the Claim Management dialog box.

EDITING CLAIMS

Medisoft's Claim Edit feature allows claims to be reviewed and verified on screen before they are submitted to insurance carriers for payment. With careful checking, problems can be solved before

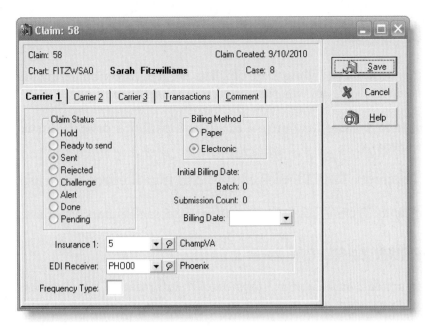

Figure 7-7 Claim dialog box

claims are sent to insurance carriers. When a claim is active in the Claim Management dialog box, it can be edited by clicking the Edit button or by double-clicking the claim itself. The Claim dialog box is displayed (see Figure 7-7). The top section of the Claim dialog box lists the claim number, the date the claim was created, the chart number, the patient's name, and the case number. This information cannot be edited, although the information in the five tabs can be edited.

CARRIER 1 TAB

The Carrier 1 tab displays information about claims being submitted to a patient's primary insurance carrier. The following boxes are listed in the Carrier 1 tab:

Claim Status   The Claim Status box indicates the status of a particular claim: Hold, Ready to send, Sent, Rejected, Challenge, Alert, Done, and Pending. The radio button that reflects a claim's status should be clicked.

Billing Method   The Billing Method box displays two choices: Paper or Electronic. The radio button that describes the billing method should be clicked.

Initial Billing Date   If the claim was sent more than once, this box automatically displays the initial billing date.

Batch   If the claim has been assigned to a batch, the batch number is displayed.

Submission Count The Submission Count area lists the number of claims submitted.

Billing Date The Billing Date box lists the most recent date the bill was sent (if the claim was submitted more than once).

Insurance 1 The Insurance 1 box lists a patient's primary insurance carrier.

EDI Receiver The EDI receiver is selected from the drop-down list.

Frequency Type This field is required by some insurance carriers.

CARRIER 2 AND CARRIER 3 TABS

The Carrier 2 and Carrier 3 tabs display information about claims being submitted to a patient's secondary (Carrier 2) and tertiary (Carrier 3) insurance carriers. The boxes in these tabs are the same as the boxes in the Carrier 1 tab, with the exception of the Claim Status box and the Frequency Type box. In the Carrier 2 and Carrier 3 tabs, there is no Pending radio button in the Claim Status box, and there is no Frequency Type box. Otherwise the three tabs are the same.

TRANSACTIONS TAB

The Transactions tab lists information about the transactions included in a claim. The scroll bars can be used to view all the information in the Transactions tab (see Figure 7-8).

Diagnosis The diagnosis for the listed transactions is displayed.

Date From The Date From box lists the date on which service was provided.

Document The Document box lists the document number of a transaction.

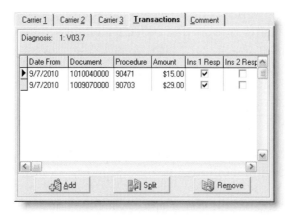

Figure 7-8 Transactions tab

Procedure   The Procedure box displays the procedure code for a performed procedure.

Amount   In the Amount box, the dollar cost of a service is displayed.

Ins 1 Resp   If this box is checked, the primary insurance carrier is responsible for the claim.

Ins 2 Resp   If this box is checked, the secondary insurance carrier is responsible for the claim.

Ins 3 Resp   If this box is checked, the tertiary insurance carrier is responsible for the claim.

The Transactions tab also contains three buttons at the bottom of the dialog box:

Add   The Add button is used to add a transaction to an existing claim.

Split   The Split button removes a single transaction from an existing claim and places it on a new claim.

Remove   The Remove button deletes a transaction from the claim database.

COMMENT TAB

The Comment tab provides a place to include any specific notes or comments about the claim (see Figure 7-9).

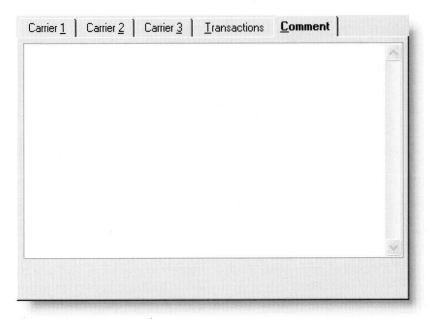

Figure 7-9   Comment tab

EXERCISE 7-2

Review insurance claims for patients with East Ohio PPO as their insurance carrier.

Date: November 5, 2010

1. Open the Claim Management dialog box.

2. Click the List Only . . . button.

3. Click 13 East Ohio PPO on the drop-down list in the Insurance Carrier box.

4. Click the Apply button. You are returned to the Claim Management dialog box. Notice that only claims for patients who have East Ohio PPO as their insurance carrier are listed.

5. Click on the claim for Lawana Brooks (chart number BROOKLAØ).

6. Click the Edit button to review the claim. The Claim dialog box is displayed.

7. Review the information in the Carrier 1 tab.

8. Review the information in the Transactions tab.

9. Click the Cancel button to exit the Claim dialog box without saving any changes. (The Cancel button does not cancel the claim; it just cancels any changes that may have been made.)

10. To restore the full list of claims in the Claim Management box, click the List Only . . . button, and then click the Defaults button.

11. Click the Apply button.

12. Close the Claim Management dialog box.

ELECTRONIC CLAIMS

Before the implementation of the HIPAA Electronic Health Care Transactions and Code Sets standards in 2003, physician practices used many different electronic data interchange (EDI) systems to submit electronic claims. The HIPAA standards describe a particular electronic format that providers and payers must use to send and receive health care transactions. They also establish standard medical code sets, such as ICD-9 and CPT-4, for use in health care transactions. Most of the setup and data entry requirements for electronic claims are handled by the medical office's systems manager.

STEPS IN SUBMITTING ELECTRONIC CLAIMS

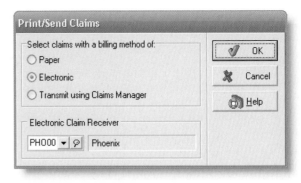

1. Click Claim Management on the Activities menu. The Claim Management dialog box is displayed.

2. Click the Print/Send button.

3. The Print/Send Claims dialog box appears (see Figure 7-10). Click the Electronic button to change the billing method to electronic, if it is not already selected. Leave the Electronic Claim Receiver box set to select Phoenix on the Electric Claim Receiver drop-down list. Click the OK button.

Figure 7-10   Print/Send Claims dialog box set up for electronic claims

4. The ANSI X12 dialog box is displayed, with PHX (Phoenix) displayed as the receiver (see Figure 7-11). Click the Send Claims Primary Now button.

5. The Data Selection Questions dialog box appears. The various range boxes provide options for filtering the claims (see Figure 7-12). Once these selections are made, click the OK button.

6. An Information dialog box appears, asking whether to display a Verification report (see Figure 7-13). After clicking Yes, the Preview Report window appears with a copy of a batch verification report displayed. The report displays the details of each claim in the batch (see Figures 7-14a and 7-14b). Click the Close button when finished viewing the report.

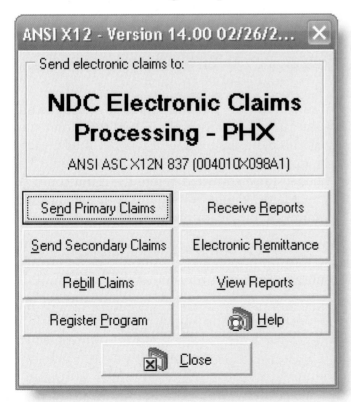

Figure 7-11   ANSI X12 dialog box for sending electronic claims

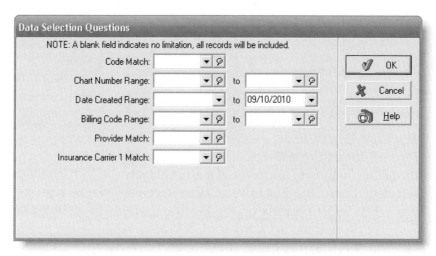

Figure 7-12 Data Selection Questions dialog box

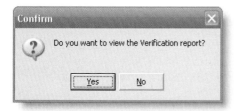

Figure 7-13 Information dialog box

7. The Preview Report window closes, and an Information box appears, asking if you want to continue with the transmission. If you were in a medical office, you would click the Yes button, and the claim would be sent from your computer to a computer at the clearinghouse. Because you are in a school setting and are not set up to submit electronic claims at this time, you will not be able to transmit electronic claims. Click the No button, and then click the Close button on the ANSI X12 dialog box to end the electronic claims processing procedure.

8. If you had been able to transmit claims, the clearinghouse would send back a claim submission report, indicating that the claim file had been received. Figure 7-15 (on page 184) displays a sample report.

The clearinghouse would then perform an edit—a check to see that all necessary information is included in the claim file. After the edit was complete, an audit/edit report would be sent from the clearinghouse to the practice. This report would list problems that needed to be corrected before the claim could be sent to the health plan. Any claims that required correction would have to be resubmitted to the clearinghouse.

Once this step was complete, the clearinghouse would transmit the claim files to the appropriate payers, and the payers would send back transmission reports. A transmission report communicates what happened to a claim once it left the clearinghouse. The appearance of this report varies from payer to payer, but the report usually includes the following information:

- Date the report was run
- Payer name
- Provider ID number

EDI Primary Insurance Verification

EDI Batch Verification Report

Claim #	Chart#	Patient Name		Policy#	Group#	Referring Provider	Facility	
	Date From	Proc. Code	Modifiers	Pos Tos	Units	Diagnoses		Amount

---

EDI Receiver: Phoenix (PHO00)
File name: C:\MediData\FCC14\EMC\16.TCH

Provider: Katherine Yan (1)   Group Control Number Suffix: 1

58	FITZWSA0	Sarah Fitzwilliams		457091	3265	Wood Janet	Not Found	

Insurance Carrier: ChampVA (5)

Diagnoses: 1: V03.7   Immunization against tetanus

| | 09/07/2010 | 90471 | | 11 | 1 | Diagnosis: 1 | | $15.00 |
| | 09/07/2010 | 90703 | | 11 | 1 | Diagnosis: 1 | | $29.00 |

Claim 58 Total: $44.00

Provider Katherine Yan (1) Total: $44.00

Provider: John Rudner (2)   Group Control Number Suffix: 1

| 32 | BELLSAM0 | Samuel Bell | | 50632 | 6209 | Not Found | Not Found | |

Insurance Carrier: East Ohio PPO (13)

Diagnoses: 1: 072.9   Epidemic parotitis

| | 09/06/2010 | 99212 | | 11 | 1 | Diagnosis: 1 | | $54.00 |

Claim 32 Total: $54.00

| 29 | BELLHER0 | Herbert Bell | | 50632 | 6209 | Brown Bertram | Not Found | |

Insurance Carrier: East Ohio PPO (13)

Diagnoses: 1: 072.9   Epidemic parotitis

| | 09/06/2010 | 99211 | | 11 | 1 | Diagnosis: 1 | | $36.00 |

Claim 29 Total: $36.00

Provider John Rudner (2) Total: $90.00

Provider: Jessica Rudner (3)   Group Control Number Suffix: 1

| 46 | BELLSAR0 | Sarina Bell | | 50632 | 6209 | Brown Bertram | Not Found | |

Insurance Carrier: East Ohio PPO (13)

Diagnoses: 1: 382.9   Unspecified otitis media

| | 09/06/2010 | 99213 | | 11 | 1 | Diagnosis: 1 | | $72.00 |

3:
4:
5:

Figure 7-14a   Sample first page of an electronic claims verification report

- Claim acceptance/rejection status

- Location in the claim that is causing the rejection

An example of this report appears in Figure 7-16 (on page 185).

9. Click the Close button to close the Claim Management dialog box and return to the main Medisoft window.

Family Care Center

EDI Primary Insurance Verification

EDI Batch Verification Report

Claim #	Chart#	Patient Name		Policy#	Group#	Referring Provider	Facility	
	Date From	Proc. Code	Modifiers	Pos Tos	Units	Diagnoses		Amount

Provider: Dana Banu (6)　　　　　　　　　　　　　　　　　　Group Control Number Suffix: 1

53	PATELRA0	Raji Patel		5789	334U	Wood Janet	Not Found	
	Insurance Carrier: East Ohio PPO (13)							
	Diagnoses: 1: 724.2	Low back pain						
	10/29/2010	99212		11	1	Diagnosis: 1		$54.00

　　　　　　　　　　　　　　　　　　　　　　　　　　　　　　Claim 53 Total:　　$54.00

56	SYZMAMI0	Michael Syzmanski		996782	8463	Wood Janet	Not Found	
	Insurance Carrier: East Ohio PPO (13)							
	Diagnoses: 1: 706.1	Acne						
	10/29/2010	99212		11	1	Diagnosis: 1		$54.00

　　　　　　　　　　　　　　　　　　　　　　　　　　　　　　Claim 56 Total:　　$54.00

　　　　　　　　　　　　　　　　　　　　　　Provider Dana Banu (6) Total:　　$108.00

　　　　　　　　　　　　　　　EDI Receiver: Phoenix (PHO00) Total:　　**$1,434.00**

Total Transaction(s):	22		
Total Claim(s):	14	Batch Total:	$1,434.00

Figure 7-14b　Sample last page of an electronic claims verification report

---

Fri Jan 16 (Date Downloaded) 10:07:00 2010

6401C0040312081199702553NDC CLAIMS SUBMISSION REPORT MAIL-CLAIMS-SUMMARY NDC CARRIER CLAIMS SUBMISSION REPORT DEC 08, 2009 (Inbound Date)

38377 PRACTICE NAME

RECEIVED | RECEIVED AMT | REJECT | REJECT AMT | FORWARDED | FORWARD AMT

------- -------- ------------ ------ ---------- --------- -----------

MEDICARE OH 11 2,574.00 0 0.00 11 2,574.00

BCBS OH 2 340.00 0 0.00 2 340.00

------ ------------ ------ ------------ ----- ------------

TOTAL 13 2,914.00 0 0.00 13 2,914.00

Figure 7-15　Example of a claim submission report

```
6401C0040403091978006957D E L A Y E D R E S P O N S E ---


PROXYMED MU020 Accepted Claims: 03/08/10 Page: 3
62308 PROVIDER CODE - #########


Patient Name Account No Insured ID Dates of Service Proc Total Chg Transaction Cntl #
------------------------ ---------------- --------------- ----------------- -------- -------- --------------------
*******,****** ********* 20100227 20100227 98.00 0*************5
A21 Claim/encounter has been accepted for processing by the payer


PROXYMED MU030 Rejected Claims: 03/08/10 Page: 4
BS028 PROVIDER CODE - #########


Patient Name Account No Insured ID Dates of Service Proc Total Chg Transaction Cntl #
------------------------ ---------------- --------------- ----------------- -------- -------- --------------------
*********,**** ********* 20100223 20100223 98.00 0*************5
LOOP: 2420E SEG ID: REF MSG: ORD PVDR SCNDRY ID MUST=1B,1G,EI,SY,0B
```

Figure 7-16   Example of a transmission report from a payer

SENDING ELECTRONIC CLAIM ATTACHMENTS

When sending a claim electronically, an attachment that needs to accompany the claim, such as radiology films, must be referred to in the claim. In Medisoft, the EDI Report area within the Diagnosis tab of the Case dialog box is used to indicate to the payer when an attachment will accompany the claim and how the attachment will be transmitted (see Figure 7-17).

The EDI Report section contains three boxes:

1. **Report Type Code box** This entry indicates the type of report that is to be attached (for example, a diagnostic report).

2. **Report Transmission Code** This indicates the means by which the report will be transmitted to the payer (for example, via mail, e-mail, or fax).

3. **Attachment Control Number** This box contains the attachment's reference number (up to seven digits, assigned by the practice).

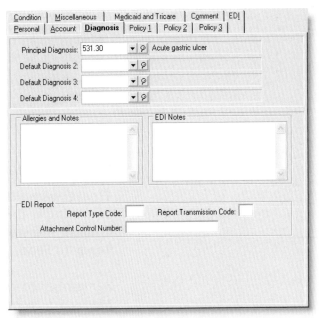

Figure 7-17   Diagnosis tab with EDI Report fields

Refer to the Medisoft Help feature for a list of possible codes for the Report Type and Report Transmission boxes.

CHANGING THE STATUS OF CLAIMS

If claims were transmitted electronically, the Claim Status for each claim would automatically change from Ready to Send to Sent once the claims were sent. Since it is not possible to actually send electronic claims during these exercises, for the purposes of this text/workbook, you will be asked to change the claim status manually from Ready to Send to Sent for claims you create. In the next exercise, you change the claim status for the claims created earlier in the chapter.

EXERCISE 7-3

Change the Claim Status for the claims created on November 5, 2010, from Ready to Send to Sent.

Date: November 5, 2010

1. In the Claim Management dialog box, click the Change Status button. The Change Claim Status/Billing Method dialog box appears.

2. Click Batch, and accept the default entry of "0."

3. Select Ready to Send in the Status From column.

4. Select Sent in the Status To column.

5. Click the OK button. The dialog box closes, and the Claim Management dialog box reappears with the Claim Status column displaying Sent for the two new claims at the bottom of the list.

ON YOUR OWN EXERCISE 5 Create Insurance Claims

November 5, 2010

Create insurance claims for all patients with last names beginning with the letter *P* through the end of the alphabet. Change the status of the claims just created to Sent from Ready to Send.

Remember to create a backup of your work before exiting Medisoft! To help you keep track of your work, name the backup file after the chapter you are working on, for example, StudentID-c7.mbk.

Name: _____ **Date:** _____

CHAPTER 7 WORKSHEET

After completing all the exercises in the chapter, answer the following questions in the spaces provided.

1. Claims were created for which patients in Exercise 7-1?

_____

_____

2. After completing Exercise 7-1, what was listed in the Status 1 column for the claims created?

_____

_____

3. What transactions are listed on Lawana Brooks's insurance claim?

_____

_____

4. After completing Exercise 7-3, what is listed in the Status 1 column for the claims for John Fitzwilliams and Elizabeth Jones?

_____

_____

5. Claims were created for which patients in On Your Own Exercise 5?

_____

_____

CHAPTER REVIEW

USING TERMINOLOGY

Define the terms below.

1. filter

_____

_____

2. navigator buttons

_____

_____

CHECKING YOUR UNDERSTANDING

Answer the questions below in the space provided.

3. A claim needs to be submitted for John Fitzwilliams. How would you select only those claims pertaining to John Fitzwilliams?

_____

_____

4. If an error is found on a claim, how is it corrected?

_____

_____

5. What is meant by a "clean" claim?

_____

_____

6. What is HIPAA X12 837?

_____

_____

7. What is the List Only feature in the Claim Management dialog box used for?

_____

_____

8. In Medisoft, where is information about electronic claim attachments entered?

_____

_____

APPLYING KNOWLEDGE

Answer the questions below in the space provided.

9. Suppose you were asked to create claims for Samuel Bell. After entering his chart number in the Create Claims dialog box, you receive the message "No new claims were created." Why were no claims created for Samuel Bell?

_____

_____

10. How would you create claims for one specific insurance carrier?

_____

_____

11. You are not sure whether an electronic claim for a particular patient was transmitted. How would you find out?

_____

_____

12. A new billing specialist in the office tells you it is less costly to submit electronic claims directly to insurance carriers without using a clearinghouse. Why do you think offices use clearinghouses? What are the benefits?

_____

_____

AT THE COMPUTER

Answer the following questions at the computer.

13. How many claims were created on November 5, 2010?

_____

_____

14. What transactions were included on the September 10, 2010, claim for Sheila Giles?

_____

_____

Posting Insurance Payments and Creating Patient Statements

8

WHAT YOU NEED TO KNOW

To use this chapter, you need to know how to:

◆ Start Medisoft, use menus, and enter and edit text.

◆ Edit information in an existing case.

◆ Work with chart and case numbers.

◆ Select patients and cases for transaction entry.

LEARNING OUTCOMES

When you finish this chapter, you will be able to:

◆ Record and apply payments received from insurance carriers.

◆ Record insurance adjustments.

◆ Enter capitation payments.

◆ Create statements.

◆ Edit statements.

◆ Print statements.

KEY TERMS

capitation payments
cycle billing
electronic remittance
    advice (ERA)
fee schedule

once-a-month billing
patient statement
payment schedule
remainder statements
standard statements

THIRD-PARTY REIMBURSEMENT OVERVIEW

fee schedule a document that specifies the amount the provider bills for provided services

payment schedule a document that specifies the amount the payer agrees to pay the provider for a service, based on a contracted rate of reimbursement

The amount a physician is reimbursed for a service depends on the patient's insurance benefits and the provider's agreement with the third-party payer. Providers establish a list of standard fees, known as a **fee schedule,** for procedures and services—this is the amount the provider bills the payer. Payers also develop a list of standard fees, but this **payment schedule** is based on a rate established in a contract with the provider. Most of the time, the amount the provider bills and the rate specified in the contract with the payer differ. The difference between the amount billed (the fee schedule) and the amount paid per contract (the payment schedule) is an adjustment that is entered in the billing area of the practice management program.

The following examples illustrate how reimbursement is calculated for an indemnity plan, a managed care plan, and a Medicare plan.

INDEMNITY PLAN EXAMPLE

In an indemnity plan, insurers often reimburse 80 percent of "reasonable charges," and the patient pays the remaining 20 percent.

Provider's usual fee	$100.00
Allowed charge	$100.00
Insurance payment	$80.00
Patient coinsurance	$20.00

In this example, the amount allowed by the payer is the same as the provider's charge. The payer reimburses at 80 percent, and the patient is responsible for the remaining 20 percent. The provider is paid for the entire billed amount; no adjustment is necessary.

MANAGED CARE PLAN EXAMPLE

Providers enter into contracts with managed care companies in which they agree to accept reduced fees for services. A managed care plan may require the patient to pay a fixed copayment, usually between $10.00 and $30.00.

Provider's usual fee	$100.00
Allowed charge	$90.00
Patient copayment	$20.00
Insurance payment	$70.00
Adjustment	$10.00

In this example, the provider charges $100.00. However, the provider has a contract with the payer requiring that 90 percent of the usual and customary charge be accepted as payment. This amount is known as the approved amount. The provider must enter an adjustment to write off the $10.00 difference between the amount charged and the amount approved per the contract. The patient pays a fixed copayment of $20.00, which is subtracted from the approved charge.

MEDICARE PARTICIPATING EXAMPLE

Medicare uses its own payment schedule, known as the Medicare Fee Schedule (MFS), which is updated annually. Providers who agree to participate in Medicare must accept the fee listed in the MFS as payment in full. Medicare is responsible for paying 80 percent of this amount, and the patient is responsible for the other 20 percent (after a deductible has been met).

Provider's usual fee	$100.00
Medicare allowed charge	$64.00
Medicare pays 80 percent	$51.20
Patient pays 20 percent	$12.80
Adjustment	$36.00

In this example, the provider charges $100.00. The maximum allowed amount in the Medicare Fee Schedule is $64.00. The difference between $100.00 and $64.00 must be written off by the provider. Medicare pays 80 percent of the allowed amount, and the patient is billed for the remaining 20 percent, or $12.80.

Note: Providers who do not participate in the Medicare program may accept assignment on a claim-by-claim basis, but they are paid 5 percent less than providers who participate. Providers who do not participate and who do not accept assignment of a claim are subject to Medicare's limiting charge. This rule limits the amount a provider can charge to 115 percent of the fee listed in the Medicare nonparticipating fee schedule.

The chart displayed in Figure 8-1 contains the fee schedules for the providers and payers used in the exercises in this book. The information on the chart includes:

◆ **CPT code** The procedure code for the service provided

◆ **Provider's usual fee** The usual amount the provider bills for the service

◆ **Managed care allowed charge** The discounted fee specified by contract

◆ **Medicare allowed charge** The maximum fee a participating provider can collect for the service

CPT Code	Provider's Usual Fee	Managed Care Allowed	Medicare Allowed
12011	$202.00	$181.80	$148.70
29125	$99.00	$89.10	$61.21
29425	$229.00	$206.10	$87.55
50390	$551.00	$495.90	$101.47
71010	$91.00	$81.90	$26.77
71020	$112.00	$100.80	$34.71
71030	$153.00	$137.70	$45.25
73070	$102.00	$91.80	$27.06
73090	$99.00	$89.10	$27.44
73100	$93.00	$83.70	$26.37
73510	$124.00	$111.60	$32.56
73600	$96.00	$86.40	$26.37
80048	$50.00	$45.00	$11.20
80061	$90.00	$81.00	$18.72
82270	$19.00	$17.10	$4.54
82947	$25.00	$22.50	$5.48
82951	$63.00	$56.70	$16.12
83718	$43.00	$38.70	$11.44
84478	$29.00	$26.10	$8.04
85007	$21.00	$18.90	$4.81
85018	$13.00	$11.70	$3.31
85025	$13.60	$12.24	$10.79
85651	$24.00	$21.60	$4.96
86580	$25.00	$22.50	$6.86
87076	$75.00	$67.50	$11.29
87077	$60.00	$54.00	$11.29
87086	$51.00	$45.90	$11.28
87430	$29.00	$26.10	$16.01
87880	$24.00	$21.60	$16.01
90471	$15.00	$13.50	$17.82
90703	$29.00	$26.10	$14.30

CPT Code	Provider's Usual Fee	Managed Care Allowed	Medicare Allowed
90772	$40.00	$36.00	$18.74
92516	$210.00	$189.00	$59.32
93000	$84.00	$75.60	$25.72
93015	$401.00	$360.90	$103.31
96900	$39.00	$35.10	$16.42
99070	$0.00	$0.00	$0.00
99201	$66.00	$59.40	$35.58
99202	$88.00	$79.20	$63.28
99203	$120.00	$108.00	$94.28
99204	$178.00	$160.20	$133.56
99205	$229.00	$206.10	$169.28
99211	$36.00	$32.40	$20.68
99212	$54.00	$48.60	$37.36
99213	$72.00	$64.80	$51.03
99214	$105.00	$94.50	$80.15
99215	$163.00	$146.70	$116.96
99381	$210.00	$189.00	$100.27
99382	$218.00	$196.20	$108.13
99383	$224.00	$201.60	$106.00
99384	$262.50	$236.25	$115.30
99385	$247.50	$222.75	$115.30
99386	$267.00	$240.30	$135.69
99387	$298.50	$268.65	$147.13
99391	$165.00	$148.50	$76.39
99392	$184.50	$166.05	$85.69
99393	$192.00	$172.80	$84.63
99394	$222.00	$199.80	$93.56
99395	$204.00	$183.60	$94.63
99396	$222.00	$199.80	$104.64
99397	$236.00	$212.40	$115.37

Figure 8-1   Fee schedule/payment schedule for payers in contract with the Family Care Center

REMITTANCE ADVICE PROCESSING

Once a claim has been received and accepted, it is processed, and the appropriate payment is determined. The payer then generates a remittance advice (RA) and sends it to the provider. A remittance advice lists patients, dates of service, charges, and the amount paid or denied by the insurance carrier. A sample RA is illustrated in Figure 8-2.

electronic remittance advice (ERA) an electronic document that lists patients, dates of service, charges, and the amount paid or denied by the insurance carrier

The RA may be sent in electronic format, called an **electronic remittance advice (ERA),** or in paper format. Although similar information is featured on the ERA and the paper RA, the ERA offers additional data not available on a paper RA. The ERA that is mandated for use by HIPAA is called the ASC X12 835 Remittance Advice Transaction, or simply the 835. In addition to physicians, other health care providers receiving the 835 include hospitals, nursing homes, laboratories, and dentists.

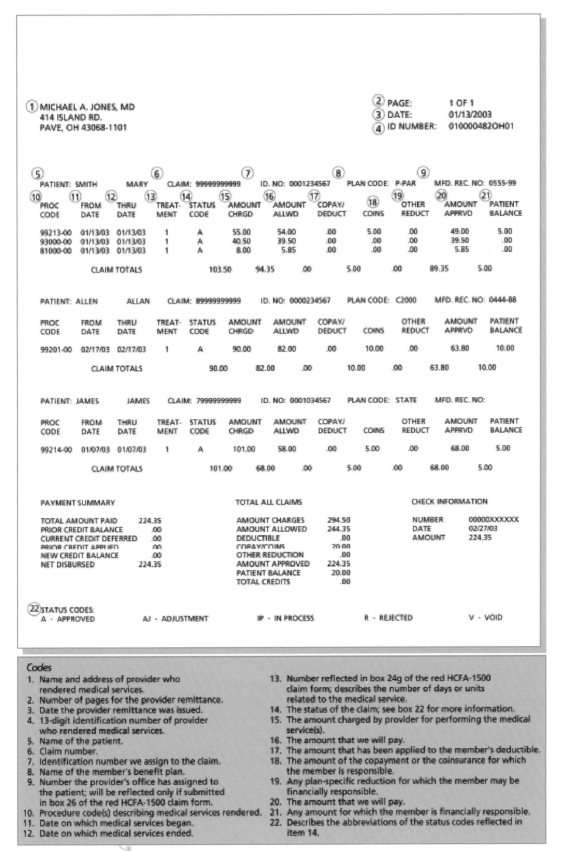

① MICHAEL A. JONES, MD
414 ISLAND RD.
PAVE, OH 43068-1101

② PAGE: 1 OF 1
③ DATE: 01/13/2003
④ ID NUMBER: 010000482OH01

⑤ PATIENT: SMITH MARY ⑥ CLAIM: 99999999999 ⑦ ID. NO: 0001234567 ⑧ PLAN CODE: P-PAR ⑨ MFD. REC. NO: 0555-99

⑩ PROC CODE	⑪ FROM DATE	⑫ THRU DATE	⑬ TREAT-MENT	⑭ STATUS CODE	⑮ AMOUNT CHRGD	⑯ AMOUNT ALLWD	⑰ COPAY/ DEDUCT	⑱ COINS	⑲ OTHER REDUCT	⑳ AMOUNT APPRVD	㉑ PATIENT BALANCE
99213-00	01/13/03	01/13/03	1	A	55.00	54.00	.00	5.00	.00	49.00	5.00
93000-00	01/13/03	01/13/03	1	A	40.50	39.50	.00	.00	.00	39.50	.00
81000-00	01/13/03	01/13/03	1	A	8.00	5.85	.00	.00	.00	5.85	.00
	CLAIM TOTALS				103.50	94.35	.00	5.00	.00	89.35	5.00

PATIENT: ALLEN ALLAN CLAIM: 89999999999 ID. NO: 0000234567 PLAN CODE: C2000 MFD. REC. NO: 0444-88

PROC CODE	FROM DATE	THRU DATE	TREAT-MENT	STATUS CODE	AMOUNT CHRGD	AMOUNT ALLWD	COPAY/ DEDUCT	COINS	OTHER REDUCT	AMOUNT APPRVD	PATIENT BALANCE
99201-00	02/17/03	02/17/03	1	A	90.00	82.00	.00	10.00	.00	63.80	10.00
	CLAIM TOTALS				90.00	82.00	.00	10.00	.00	63.80	10.00

PATIENT: JAMES JAMES CLAIM: 79999999999 ID. NO: 0001034567 PLAN CODE: STATE MFD. REC. NO:

PROC CODE	FROM DATE	THRU DATE	TREAT-MENT	STATUS CODE	AMOUNT CHRGD	AMOUNT ALLWD	COPAY/ DEDUCT	COINS	OTHER REDUCT	AMOUNT APPRVD	PATIENT BALANCE
99214-00	01/07/03	01/07/03	1	A	101.00	58.00	.00	5.00	.00	68.00	5.00
	CLAIM TOTALS				101.00	68.00	.00	5.00	.00	68.00	5.00

PAYMENT SUMMARY

TOTAL AMOUNT PAID	224.35
PRIOR CREDIT BALANCE	.00
CURRENT CREDIT DEFERRED	.00
PRIOR CREDIT APPLIED	.00
NEW CREDIT BALANCE	.00
NET DISBURSED	224.35

TOTAL ALL CLAIMS

AMOUNT CHARGES	294.50
AMOUNT ALLOWED	244.35
DEDUCTIBLE	.00
COPAY/COINS	20.00
OTHER REDUCTION	.00
AMOUNT APPROVED	224.35
PATIENT BALANCE	20.00
TOTAL CREDITS	.00

CHECK INFORMATION

NUMBER	00000XXXXXX
DATE	02/27/03
AMOUNT	224.35

㉒ STATUS CODES:
A - APPROVED   AJ - ADJUSTMENT   IP - IN PROCESS   R - REJECTED   V - VOID

Codes

1. Name and address of provider who rendered medical services.
2. Number of pages for the provider remittance.
3. Date the provider remittance was issued.
4. 13-digit identification number of provider who rendered medical services.
5. Name of the patient.
6. Claim number.
7. Identification number we assign to the claim.
8. Name of the member's benefit plan.
9. Number the provider's office has assigned to the patient; will be reflected only if submitted in box 26 of the red HCFA-1500 claim form.
10. Procedure code(s) describing medical services rendered.
11. Date on which medical services began.
12. Date on which medical services ended.
13. Number reflected in box 24g of the red HCFA-1500 claim form; describes the number of days or units related to the medical service.
14. The status of the claim; see box 22 for more information.
15. The amount charged by provider for performing the medical service(s).
16. The amount that we will pay.
17. The amount that has been applied to the member's deductible.
18. The amount of the copayment or the coinsurance for which the member is responsible.
19. Any plan-specific reduction for which the member may be financially responsible.
20. The amount that we will pay.
21. Any amount for which the member is financially responsible.
22. Describes the abbreviations of the status codes reflected in item 14.

Figure 8-2   Example of a payer's remittance advice

STEPS FOR PROCESSING A REMITTANCE ADVICE

1. Compare the RA to the original insurance claim. Make sure that all procedures listed on the claim are represented on the RA and that the CPT codes have not changed.

2. Review the payment amount against the expected amount.

3. Identify the reasons for denials or payment reductions; resubmit claim or appeal if necessary.

4. Post payment information for individual claims to the appropriate patient accounts.

5. Bill the patient's secondary health care plan (if appropriate).

In most cases, insurance carriers do not fully pay the amount billed by the provider. The provider bills according to the provider's fee schedule, while the payer's rate is determined by a contract with the provider. When the RA is reviewed, the billing specialist checks to see that the amount paid is the expected amount, per the provider's contract with the payer. If a payment is not as expected, the specialist must determine the reason for the discrepancy.

Charges may be denied by insurance carriers for a number of reasons. For example, a procedure may not be covered by the patient's plan, or a procedure or diagnosis may be coded incorrectly. If the reimbursement on an RA is lower than the amount expected, it is important to determine the reason and to take action to collect the correct amount. The problem could have originated in the provider's office, or it could have occurred during processing by the payer. When an error has been made in the provider's office, the billing staff member must correct the error in the billing software and resubmit the claim to the payer. If the error occurs during processing by the third-party payer, an appeal process may be started. Table 8-1 lists common errors that result in reduced or denied payments.

Table 8-1	Common Claim Errors
Remittance Advice Result	**Possible Reasons**
Reimbursement is made at a reduced rate.	• Clerical error was made. • Precertification or preapproval guidelines were not followed.
Reimbursement is denied.	• Clerical error was possibly made. • Precertification or preapproval guidelines were not followed. • Insufficient documentation was provided to establish medical necessity. • All information required by payer was not included. • The wrong payer was billed.
Payment is not received.	• Claim is missing or lost in the system.
Multiple procedures were not paid.	• Payer either missed the additional procedures or grouped them with the primary procedure.

ENTERING INSURANCE CARRIER PAYMENTS IN MEDISOFT

Payment information located on the remittance advice is entered in Medisoft through the Enter Deposits/Payments option on the Activities menu. The Deposit/Payments area of the program is very efficient for entering large insurance payments that must be split up and applied to a number of different patients.

Deposits are created within the Deposit List dialog box (see Figure 8-3). The Deposit List dialog box is opened by clicking Enter Deposits/Payments on the Activities menu or by clicking the Enter Deposits and Apply Payments shortcut button.

The Deposit List dialog box contains the following information:

Deposit Date   The program displays the current date (the Medisoft Program Date). The date can be changed by keying over the default date.

Show All Deposits   If this box is checked, all payments are displayed, regardless of the date entered.

Show Unapplied Only   If the Show Unapplied Only box is checked, only payments that have not been fully applied to charge transactions are displayed. If the box is not checked, all payments—both applied and unapplied—are listed.

Sort By   The Sort By drop-down list offers several choices for how payment information is listed. The default is sorting payments by

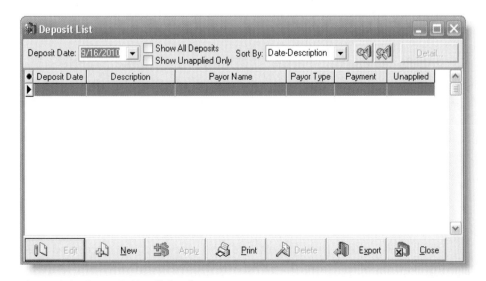

Figure 8-3   Deposit List dialog box

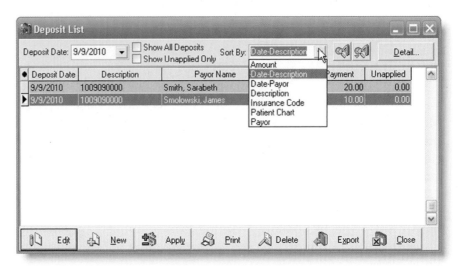

Figure 8-4   Deposit List dialog box with Sort By drop-down list displayed

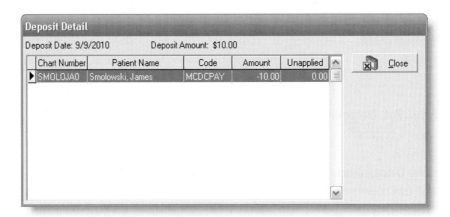

Figure 8-5   Deposit Detail dialog box

amount, from lowest to highest. Payments can also be sorted by other data fields (see Figure 8-4).

Locate Buttons   The Locate and Locate Next buttons, indicated by the two magnifying glass icons, are used to search for a deposit.

Detail   To view a specific deposit in more detail, highlight the deposit, and click the Detail button. A dialog box opens with more information about the selected deposit (see Figure 8-5).

In the middle section of the Deposit List window, information is listed for each deposit and payment, including:

Deposit Date   Lists the date of the deposit or payment.

Description   Displays whatever was entered in the Description or Check Number box in the Deposit dialog box. The Deposit dialog box is where new payments and deposits are recorded (see Figure 8-6). It is accessed by clicking the New button in the Deposit List dialog box.

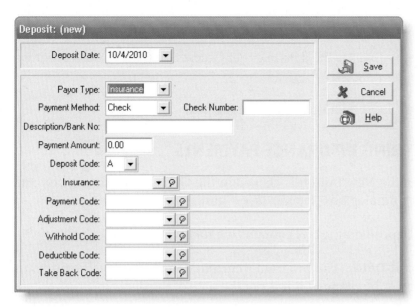

Figure 8-6 Deposit dialog box

Payor Name Lists the name of the insurance carrier or individual who made the payment.

Payor Type A classification column that lists whether the payment is an insurance payment, a patient payment, or a capitation payment. **Capitation payments** are made to physicians on a regular basis (such as monthly) for providing services to patients in a managed care insurance plan. In traditional insurance plans, physicians are paid based on the specific procedures they perform and the number of times the procedures are performed. Under a capitated plan, a flat fee is paid to the physician no matter how many times a patient receives treatment, up to the maximum number of treatments allowed per year. For example, a primary care physician with fifty patients may receive a payment of $2,500 per month for those patients, regardless of whether the physician has seen them during that month.

capitation payments payments made to physicians on a regular basis (such as monthly) for providing services to patients in a managed care insurance plan

Payment Lists the amount of the payment.

Unapplied The amount of the deposit that has not been applied to a charge.

At the bottom of the Deposit List dialog box are buttons that perform the following actions:

Edit Opens the highlighted payment or deposit for editing.

New Opens the Deposit dialog box, where new payments and deposits are recorded.

Apply Applies payments to specific charge transactions.

Print Sends a command to print the deposit list.

Delete   Deletes the highlighted transaction.

Export   Exports the data in either Quicken or Quick Books program formats.

Close   Exits the Deposit List dialog box.

ENTERING INSURANCE PAYMENTS

When the New button is clicked in the Deposit List dialog box, the Deposit dialog box appears (see Figure 8-6).

The Deposit dialog box contains the following fields:

Deposit Date   The program's current date is displayed by default and must be changed if it is not the date of the deposit.

Payor Type   This selection in this box indicates whether the payer is an insurance carrier, a capitation plan, or a patient (see Figure 8-7). Some of the boxes at the bottom of the Deposit dialog box change based on the selection in this box. If Insurance is selected, the dialog box is as illustrated in Figure 8-6. If capitation is selected, all the boxes below Insurance disappear. If Patient is chosen, the boxes listed below Deposit Code become Chart Number, Payment Code, and Adjustment Code.

Payment Method   This box lists whether the payment is check, cash, credit card, or electronic.

Check Number   The number of the check (if a check payment) is selected in this box.

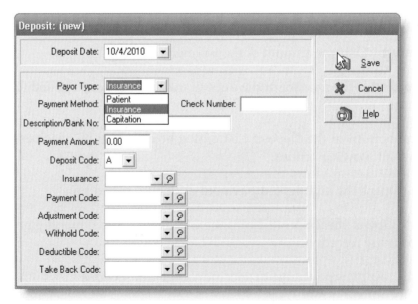

Figure 8-7   Payor Type options in the Deposit dialog box

Description/Bank No. This box can be used to enter a description of the payment, if desired.

Payment Amount The total amount of the payment is entered in this box.

Deposit Code This field can be used by practices to sort deposits according to user-defined categories.

Insurance The insurance carrier that is making the payment is selected.

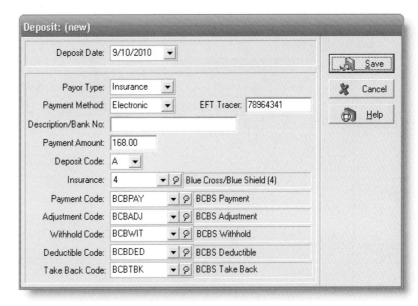

Figure 8-8 Deposit dialog box with information entered

Payment Code, Adjustment Code, Withhold Code, Deductible Code, and Take Back Code The appropriate codes for the insurance carrier are selected.

Once all the information has been entered and checked for accuracy, the deposit is saved by clicking the Save button (see Figure 8-8). When the deposit entry is saved, the Deposit dialog box closes, and the Deposit List dialog box reappears, with the new deposit listed (see Figure 8-9).

APPLYING INSURANCE PAYMENTS TO CHARGES

After a deposit has been entered, the next step is to apply the payment to the applicable transactions for each patient. To apply a

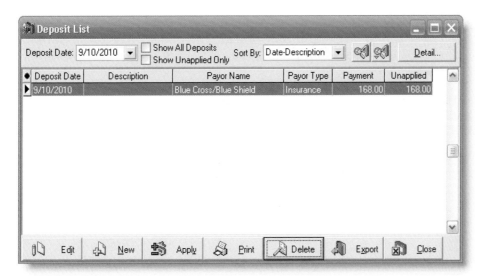

Figure 8-9 Deposit List dialog box with deposit entered

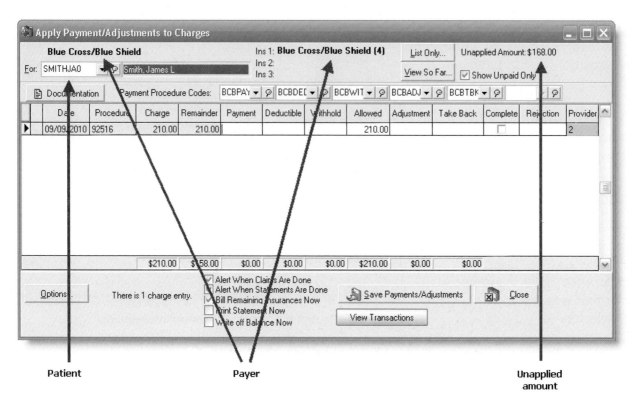

Patient
Payer
Unapplied amount

Figure 8-10   Apply Payment/Adjustments to Charges dialog box

deposit, highlight the payment in the Deposit List, and click the Apply button. The Apply Payment/Adjustments to Charges window opens (see Figure 8-10).

The top section of the dialog box contains information about the payer, the patient, and the amount of the payment that is unapplied.

The upper-left corner of the dialog box displays the payer's name in bold type, and it is also listed in the Ins 1 field. In Figure 8-10, the payer is Blue Cross and Blue Shield. The patient who has a transaction listed on the remittance advice is selected from the drop-down list in the For box.

The upper-right area of the dialog box lists the amount of the deposit that has not yet been applied.

Note: If a patient is selected who does not have coverage with the insurance carrier that is making the deposit, a Select Payor window opens (see Figure 8-11) with the message that the payer does not match any case for the patient. Clicking the Cancel button closes the dialog box.

The middle section of the Apply Payments to Charges window is where payments are entered and applied (see Figure 8-12).

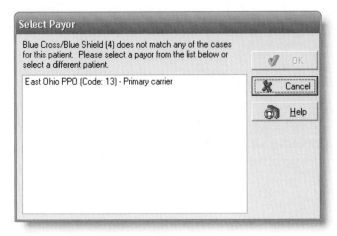

Figure 8-11 Select Payor dialog box

	Date	Procedure	Charge	Remainder	Payment	Deductible	Withhold	Allowed	Adjustment	Take Back	Complete	Rejection	Provider
▶	09/09/2010	92516	210.00	210.00				210.00			☐		2
			$0.00	$210.00	$0.00	$0.00	$0.00	$210.00	$0.00	$0.00			

Figure 8-12 Payment entry area of the Apply Payments to Charges window

Date, Procedure, Charge, Remainder   These fields show the date of service, procedure code, charge amount, and amount remaining for each transaction, as already entered in the database. This information cannot be edited in this dialog box.

Payment   The amount of the payment for this procedure is entered. The program automatically makes this a negative sum, so it is not necessary to enter a minus sign.

Deductible   If applicable, enter the amount of the deductible listed on the RA.

Withhold   Some insurance companies may withhold money for multiple charges and then pay out all at once. If applicable, enter the withholding amount in this field.

Allowed   This is the amount allowed by the payer for this procedure. These values are located in the Allowed Amounts tab of the Procedure/Payment/Adjustment dialog box (see Figure 8-13).

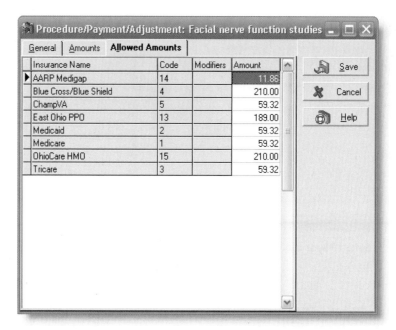

Figure 8-13 Allowed Amounts tab in the Procedure/Payment/Adjustment dialog box

Adjustment   The amount entered here is the charge amount minus whatever is entered in the Allowed field. This amount is calculated by the program.

Take Back   This field contains only positive adjustment amounts. It is provided for situations in which the insurance company over-pays on one charge and then indicates that the overpayment should be applied as a payment. Most times, the take back should be applied to the same charge that had the overpayment.

Complete   The program places a check in this box to indicate that the payer's responsibility is complete for this transaction.

Rejection   If desired, a rejection message from the RA can be entered.

Provider   This field lists the provider assigned to the transaction.

Figure 8-14 shows an Apply Payment/Adjustments to Charges dialog box with a payment entered.

The lower third of the Apply Payment/Adjustments to Charges window contains several options that affect claims and statements (see Figure 8-15).

Options   The Options button is used to change the default settings for patient payment application codes.

Alert When Claims are Done   This field determines whether a message appears as notification that a claim is done for a payer.

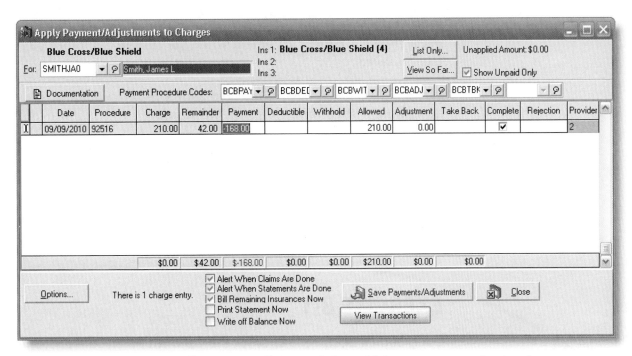

Figure 8-14   Apply Payment/Adjustments to Charges window with insurance payment entered

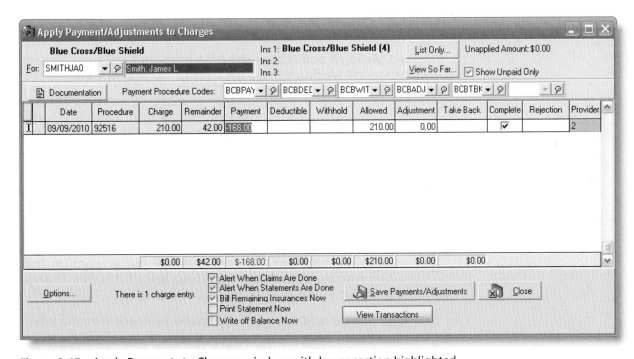

Figure 8-15   Apply Payments to Charges window with lower section highlighted

Alert When Statements are Done   This field determines whether a message appears as notification that a statement is done for a patient.

Bill Remaining Insurances Now   If this box is checked, claims for any secondary or tertiary payer associated with the claim are created when the current insurance payment is saved.

Print Statement Now   If a check mark appears in this box, the program creates a patient statement when the current insurance payment is saved.

Write Off Balance Now   This field allows patient remainder balances to be written off from within this window.

Save Payments/Adjustments   Clicking this button saves the payment currently being applied. Once the payment is saved, another patient can be selected in the For field, or the dialog box can be closed.

View Transactions   Clicking this button displays the transactions for the selected patient.

EXERCISE 8-1

Using Source Document 8, enter the payment received from John Fitzwilliams's insurance carrier for services provided on September 7, 2010. Note that John is guarantor for his daughter Sarah, so her charges and payments are included on the remittance advice.

Date: October 4, 2010

1. Start Medisoft and restore the data from your last work session. Change the Medisoft Program Date to October 4, 2010.

2. Click Enter Deposits/Payments on the Activities menu. The Deposit List dialog box is displayed. Verify that 10/4/2010 is displayed in the Deposit Date box, that the two check boxes—Show All Deposits and Show Unapplied Only—are not checked, and that Date-Payor is displayed in the Sort By box.

3. Click the New button. Click No in response to the message that is displayed about changing the date because it is in the future. Click the New button again. The Deposit dialog box is displayed. Verify that the Deposit Date is 10/4/2010.

4. Since this is a payment from an insurance carrier, confirm that Insurance is selected in the Payor Type box. If it is not, change the selection in the Payor Type box to Insurance.

5. Accept the default entry (Check) in the Payment Method box.

6. Enter *214778924* in the Check Number box, and press Tab twice. (The Description/Bank No. field can be left blank.)

7. Enter the amount of the payment (*28.02*) in the Payment Amount box. Press Tab.

8. Accept the default entry (A) in the Deposit Code box. Press Tab.

9. Select the insurance carrier that is making the payment (5—ChampVA) from the Insurance drop-down list. Medisoft automatically enters the defaults for ChampVA in the Payment, Adjustment, Withhold, Deductible, and Take Back Code boxes.

10. Click the Save button to save the entry, and close the Deposit dialog box.

11. The Deposit List box reappears. The insurance payment appears in the list of deposits.

12. Now the payment must be applied to the specific procedure charges to which it corresponds. With the ChampVA payment entry highlighted, click the Apply button. The Apply Payment/ Adjustments to Charges dialog box appears.

13. Key *F* in the For box, and press Tab to select John Fitzwilliams, since a portion of this payment is for his account. All the charge entries for John Fitzwilliams that have not been paid in full are listed. Notice that the amount listed in the Unapplied box in the upper-right corner shows the full deposit amount, since nothing has been applied yet.

14. Enter the first payment, which is for the 99211 procedure completed on 09/07/2010. Notice that the cursor is blinking in Payment box for this charge.

15. Enter *5.68* in the Payment box, and press Tab. Medisoft automatically places a minus sign before the amount. Notice that once the payment is applied, the Complete box to the right of the dialog box is checked. This indicates that the transaction is complete for this payer. Also notice that the Unapplied amount has been reduced by $5.68. Press Tab to move through each column until you reach the end of the first row so that the program can update the amounts. When you tab past the end of row 1, notice the remainder amount (in column 4) changes to 0.00 and the adjustment amount (in column 9) now displays −15.32.

16. Now enter the payment for the 84478 charge. Enter *8.04* in the Payment box. Press Tab to move through each column until you reach the end of the first row so that the program can update the amounts. When you tab past the end of the row, the remainder amount (in column 4) changes to 0.00 and the adjustment amount (in column 9) now displays −20.96.

17. Click the Save Payments/Adjustments button to save your entry. When you click this button, an Information dialog box displays the message that the claim has been marked "done" for the primary insurance. Click OK. The dialog box is cleared of the current transaction and is ready for a new transaction.

18. Now enter a payment for Sarah Fitzwilliams. Key F in the For box, and then locate her name in the drop-down list. Click on her chart number to display her data. Notice on Source Document 8 and in the Apply Payment/Adjustment to Charges dialog box that her $15.00 co-payment was applied to the charge for procedure code 90471, which now has a 0.00 remainder balance. As a result, the payment from CHAMPVA must be applied to the second charge, which is for procedure code 90703. When you are finished, click the Save Payments/Adjustments button.

19. Click the Close button to exit the Apply Payment/Adjustments to Charges dialog box.

20. Without closing the Deposit List dialog box, open the Transaction Entry dialog box, select John Fitzwilliams, and verify that the insurance carrier payments appear in the list of transactions. Payments entered in the Deposit List dialog box also appear in the Transaction Entry dialog box. In the Totals tab area of the dialog box, notice that there is still a balance due on Fitzwilliams's account, for his office visit on 10/4/2010.

21. Now select Sarah Fitzwilliams. The payment from ChampVA appears in the Payments, Adjustments, And Comments section, and the Account Total balance in the Total tab area is now 0.00.

22. Close the Transaction Entry dialog box.

EXERCISE 8-2

The medical office has just received an ERA from East Ohio PPO (see Source Document 9). The total amount of the electronic funds transfer (EFT) is $450.60. This amount includes payments for a number of patients. Enter the insurance carrier payment, and apply it to the appropriate patients.

Date: October 4, 2010

1. Verify that the entry in the Deposit Date box in the Deposit List dialog box is 10/4/2010.

2. Click the New button. Click No in response to the message that is displayed about changing the date because it is in the future. Click the New button again. The Deposit dialog box is displayed. Verify that the Deposit Date is 10/4/2010.

3. Select Insurance in the Payor Type box.

4. Select Electronic in the Payment Method box. Press Tab twice.

5. Enter the ERA ID number, *00146972,* in the Description/Bank No. box.

6. Enter *450.60* in the Payment Amount box, and press Tab.

7. Accept the default entry in the Deposit Code box.

8. Select 13—East Ohio PPO in the Insurance box. Medisoft automatically completes the Payment, Adjustment, Withhold, Deductible, and Take Back Code boxes.

9. Click the Save button.

10. The payment entry appears in the Deposit List dialog box.

11. Now apply the payment to the specific transaction charges.

12. With the East Ohio PPO line highlighted, click the Apply button. The Apply Payment/Adjustments to Charges dialog box is displayed.

13. Key *A* in the For box, and press Tab to select Susan Arlen.

14. Locate the charge for procedure code 99212 on 09/6/2010. Key the amount of the payment, *28.60,* in the Payment box, and

press Tab. Notice that Medisoft automatically checks the Complete box, since Susan Arlen has only one insurance carrier (there is no payment forthcoming from any other carrier, so the charge is complete). Tab through to the end of the line to view the adjustment amount and the new remainder amount.

15. Click the Save Payments/Adjustments button, and then click the OK button when the Information box appears, reporting that the claim has been marked "done." The data for Susan Arlen that were visible in the Apply Payment/Adjustments to Charges dialog box are cleared, and the dialog box is ready for the next payment or adjustment. Notice also that the amount listed in the Unapplied column for East Ohio PPO has been reduced by the amount of the Arlen payment.

16. Now enter the payment for the next patient listed on the ERA, Herbert Bell.

17. Key *BE* in the For box, and press Tab to select Herbert Bell.

18. Enter the payment of *12.40* in the Payment box for the 99211 charge on 09/6/2010. Tab to the end of the line.

19. Click the Save Payments/Adjustments button, and then click the OK button.

20. Key *BELLSAM* in the For box, and press Tab to select Samuel Bell.

21. Enter the payment of *28.60* in the Payment box for the 99212 charge on 09/6/2010. Tab to the end of the line.

22. Click the Save Payments/Adjustments button, and then click the OK button.

23. Continue to apply the insurance payments for Janine Bell, Jonathan Bell, and Sarina Bell using the information on Source Document 9. Click the Save Payments/Adjustments button after you complete the payment entries for each patient. When you have applied all the payments, the amount in the Unapplied box for the East Ohio PPO payment should be 0.00.

24. Close the Apply Payment/Adjustments to Charges dialog box.

EXERCISE 8-3

The medical office has just received an ERA from Blue Cross and Blue Shield (see Source Document 10). The total amount of the remittance is $214.40. This amount includes payments for a number of patients. Enter the insurance carrier payment for each patient. You will need to enter a zero payment on a charge for Sheila Giles, as one of her procedures was denied.

Date: November 4, 2010

1. In the Deposit List dialog box, change the date in the Deposit Date box to 11/4/2010, and press the Tab key. A Confirm box is displayed, stating that the date entered is in the future, and asking if you want to change it. Click the No button to keep the new date.

2. Click the New button in the Deposit List dialog box.

3. Select Insurance in the Payor Type box. Press Tab.

4. Change the entry in the Payment Method box to Electronic, since this payment was sent electronically to the practice's bank account.

5. Enter the ERA number, *001234,* in the Description/Bank No. box.

6. Enter *214.40* in the Payment Amount box. Press Tab.

7. Accept the default entry in the Deposit Code box. Press Tab.

8. Select 4—Blue Cross/Blue Shield in the Insurance box. Medisoft automatically completes the Payment, Adjustment, Withhold, Deductible, and Take Back Code boxes.

9. Click the Save button.

10. The payment entry appears in the Deposit List dialog box.

11. Now apply the payment to the specific transaction charges.

12. With the Blue Cross/Blue Shield line highlighted, click the Apply button. The Apply Payment/Adjustments to Charges dialog box is displayed.

13. Key *GI* in the For box to select Sheila Giles, and then press Tab.

14. Three charges are listed. Locate the charge for procedure code 99213 on 10/29/2010. Key the amount of the payment, *57.60,* in the Payment box, and press Tab. Medisoft automatically checks the Complete box, since Giles has only one insurance carrier (no payment is forthcoming from any other carrier, so the charge is complete). Continue pressing the Tab key until the amount listed in the Remainder column changes to $14.40.

15. Now enter the payment for the next procedure listed on the ERA—71010. (*Note:* The order of procedures is different on the ERA than it is in the Apply Payment/Adjustment to Charges window. Be sure to apply the payment to the correct procedure.) Remember to click the Tab key until the amount in the Remainder column changes.

16. Look again at Source Document 10. Notice that the amount paid for the final procedure, 87430, is $0.00. Read the note listed to determine why the charge was not paid. This denial of payment must be entered in Medisoft so practice billing staff members will be aware that Giles is responsible for the entire amount of that charge, $29.00.

17. Click in the Payment box for the charge for procedure 87430. Enter *0,* and press Tab. Notice that the amount listed in the Remainder column is the full amount of the charge, $29.00. The charge has also been marked as complete, since the insurance carrier is not responsible for the remainder amount.

18. Click the Save Payments/Adjustments button. An Information box is displayed, indicating that the claim has been marked done for the primary insurance. Click the OK button.

19. This time, to verify the payment in the Transaction Entry dialog box without exiting the Apply Payment/Adjustment to Charges dialog box, click the View Transactions button.

20. The Transaction Entry dialog box appears. Locate Sheila Giles's upper respiratory infection case. In the Charges area, notice that two of the charges appear in an aqua color, which indicates that they have been partially paid. The charge that was denied by the insurance carrier—87430—is still in gray, indicating that no payment has been made.

21. Now look at the Account Total in the Totals tab area in the Transaction Entry dialog box. Sheila Giles is listed as being responsible for paying $61.60, which breaks down as follows:

Code	Charge Amount	Patient Responsible for
99213	$72.00	$14.40 (20% of charge)
71010	$91.00	$18.20 (20% of charge)
87430	$29.00	$29.00 (100% of charge)
Totals	**$192.00**	**$61.60**

22. Close the Transaction Entry dialog box.

23. You are returned directly to the Apply Payments/Adjustments to Charges dialog box with the rest of the Blue Cross/Blue Shield payment still displayed. Enter the payments for the next patient listed on Source Document 10, Jill Simmons.

24. Key **S** in the For box, and press Tab to select Jill Simmons.

25. Enter the payment of **43.20** in the Payment box for the 99212 charge on 10/29/2010. Tab to the end of the row.

26. Enter the other payment for Jill Simmons. Notice that the amount listed in the Unapplied area is now 0.00, indicating that the entire payment has been entered.

27. Click the Save Payments/Adjustments button.

28. Close the Apply Payment/Adjustments to Charges dialog box.

29. The Deposit List dialog box reappears, with the Blue Cross/Blue Shield deposit listed.

30. Close the Deposit List dialog box.

ENTERING CAPITATION PAYMENTS AND ADJUSTMENTS

Capitation payments are entered in the Deposit List dialog box. To indicate a capitation payment, Capitation is selected from the Payor Type drop-down list in the Deposit window (see Figure 8-16).

When a capitation payment is entered in Medisoft, the payment is not applied to the charges of individual patients. However, the charges in each patient's account must be adjusted to a zero balance

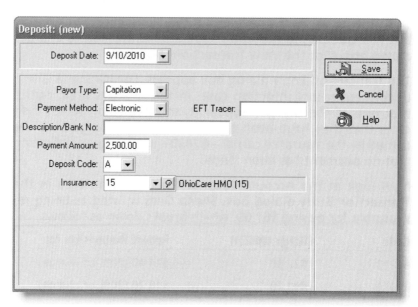

Figure 8-16   Deposit dialog box for a capitation payment

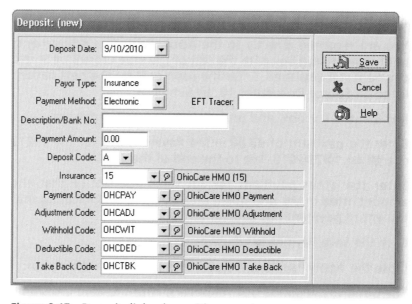

Figure 8-17   Deposit dialog box with a zero insurance payment amount

to indicate that the insurance company has met its obligation (through the capitation payment) and that the patient has also done so (by paying a copayment at the time of the office visit).

In order to adjust the patient accounts of those covered by the capitated plan, a second deposit is entered as an insurance payment with a zero amount (see Figure 8-17).

Once the zero amount deposit is saved, the deposit appears in the Deposit List window (see Figure 8-18). The Payment column lists "EOB Only," since there is no payment associated with the zero amount deposit.

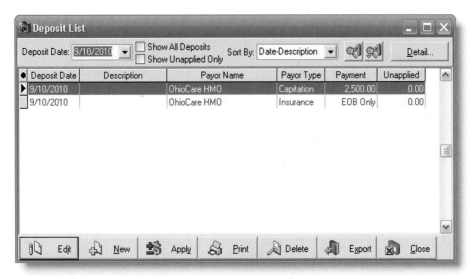

Figure 8-18 Deposit List dialog box with a capitation payment and a zero insurance payment entered

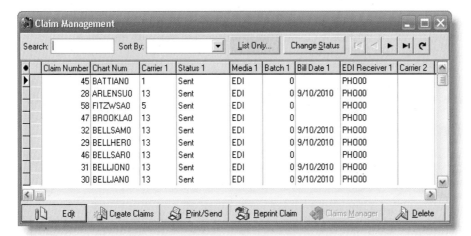

Figure 8-19 Claim Management dialog box with List Only button highlighted

The next step is to locate patients who have claims covered by the capitation payment. This is accomplished using the List Only button in the Claim Management dialog box (see Figure 8-19).

When the List Only button is clicked, the List Only Claims That Match dialog box appears. The List Only Claims That Match dialog box (see Figure 8-20) provides an option for searching for claims by insurance carrier. Using this option, patients with active capitated claims from a given carrier can be identified.

Once patients have been identified, the Claim Management dialog box is closed, and the Deposit List window is opened. To apply the zero amount payment to these patient accounts, select the line for the deposit and click the Apply button. In the Apply Payment/ Adjustments to Charges dialog box, select each patient chart number covered by the zero payment, and enter an adjustment equal to the outstanding balance (see Figure 8-21). In the example in

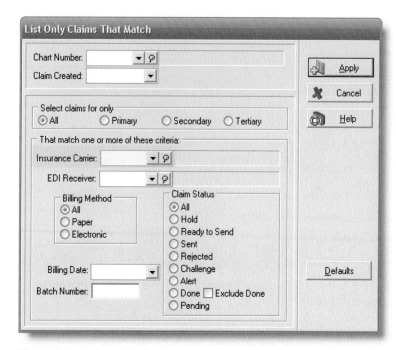

Figure 8-20 List Only Claims That Match dialog box with Insurance Carrier field highlighted

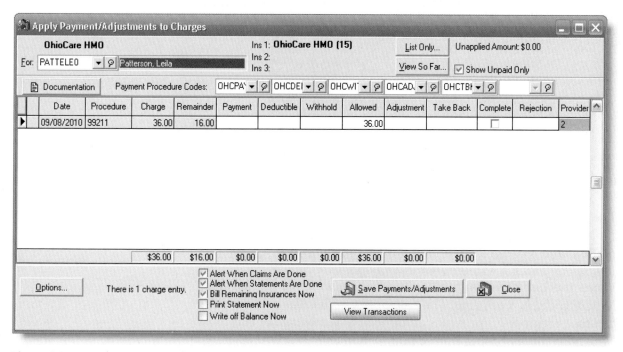

Figure 8-21 Apply Payment/Adjustments to Charges window with capitated patient account displayed

Figure 8-21, the amount in the Remainder column is $16.00. This is the amount that must be entered in the Adjustment column to adjust the account to a zero balance. Figure 8-22 shows the dialog box after the $16.00 adjustment has been applied. Notice that the amount in the Remainder column is now zero. This procedure must be followed for each patient covered by the capitation payment who has an outstanding balance.

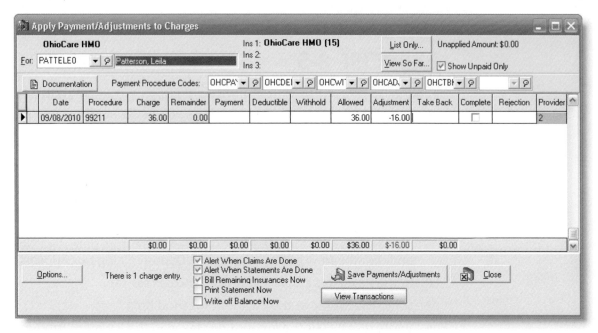

Figure 8-22 Apply Payment/Adjustments to Charges window after patient account is adjusted to a zero balance

EXERCISE 8-4

Using Source Document 11, enter a capitation payment from OhioCare HMO for the month of October 2010. The total amount of the electronic funds transfer is $2,500.00.

Date: November 4, 2010

1. In the Deposit List dialog box, verify that the date in the Deposit Date box is 11/4/2010. Click the New button. A Confirm box appears with a message about entering a future date. Click No. Click the New button again. The Deposit dialog box appears.

2. In the Payor Type box, select Capitation. Press Tab.

3. Select Electronic in the Payment Method box. Notice that the Check Number box becomes an EFT Tracer box. Press Tab twice.

4. Key *001006003* in the Description/Bank No. box. This is the ID number that is listed on the ERA. Press Tab.

5. Key *2500* in the Payment Amount box, and press Tab.

6. Accept the default entry of "A" in the Deposit Code box. Press Tab.

7. Click 15—OhioCare HMO in the Insurance drop-down list.

8. Click the Save button.

9. The Deposit List window reappears, displaying the payment just entered. Unlike other insurance payments, capitation payments are not applied to individual charges in the Deposit List dialog box. However, amounts do need to be adjusted in the patient accounts in the Transaction Entry dialog box.

EXERCISE 8-5

Enter a zero insurance payment amount deposit for OhioCare HMO. Using the List Only Claims That Match option in Claim Management, locate the patients with capitated plans who visited the practice in October 2010. Using the Apply Payment/Adjustments to Charges window, apply the zero amount deposit to adjust the patient accounts to a zero balance.

Date: November 4, 2010

1. In the Deposit List dialog box, click the New button. (If a Confirm box appears with a message about entering a future date, click No, and click the New button again.) The Deposit dialog box appears.

2. In the Payor Type box, select Insurance. Press Tab.

3. Select Electronic in the Payment Method box.

4. Verify that 0.00 is the amount displayed in the Payment Amount box, and press Tab.

5. Accept the default entry of "A" in the Deposit Code box. Press Tab.

6. Click 15—OhioCare HMO in the Insurance drop-down list.

7. Click the Save button. The Deposit List window reappears.

8. Open the Claim Management dialog box.

9. Click the List Only button.

10. In the List Only Claims That Match dialog box, select 15—OhioCare HMO in the Insurance Carrier drop-down list.

11. Click the Apply button. The Claim Management window appears with the capitated claims listed. In this case, there is only one capitated claim. (*Note:* Use the Edit button to view details of the claim, verifying that the transactions took place in October 2010.) Note the patient chart number for the claim, and close the Claim Management window.

12. You are returned to the Deposit List dialog box. With the zero insurance payment amount deposit selected, click the Apply button.

13. Select the capitated patient in the For field.

14. Identify the amount in the Remainder column, and enter an equal amount in the Adjustment column. Press tab to the end of the row, until the remainder amount changes to zero.

15. Click the Save Payments/Adjustments button. Then, to verify that the account has been adjusted to a zero balance, use the View Transactions button to open the Transaction Entry dialog box and display the capitated patient's transaction information. When finished viewing the data, close the Transaction Entry dialog box.

16. If there were other patients with capitated claims in October, you would repeat the process for each patient's account.

17. Close the Apply Payment/Adjustments to Charges dialog box.

18. Close the Deposit List dialog box.

CREATING STATEMENTS

A **patient statement** lists the amount of money a patient owes, organized by the amount of time the money has been owed, the procedures performed, and the dates the procedures were performed. Patient statements are created after an insurance claim has been filed and a remittance advice has been received. A patient statement is sent to collect the balance on an account that is the patient's responsibility. This may include coinsurance charges and charges for procedures that were not covered by the insurance company.

Statements are created using the Statement Management feature, which is listed on the Activities menu. Just as Claim Management provides a range of options for billing insurance carriers, Statement Management offers multiple choices for billing patients. Within the Statement Management area of Medisoft, statements are created and printed.

STATEMENT MANAGEMENT DIALOG BOX

The Statement Management dialog box is displayed by clicking Statement Management on the Activities menu or by clicking the Statement Management shortcut button on the toolbar (see Figure 8-23). The dialog box lists all statements that have already been created (see Figure 8-24). In this dialog box, several actions can be performed: existing statements can be reviewed and edited, new statements can be created, the status of existing statements can be changed, and statements can be printed.

Figure 8-23
Statement Management shortcut button

Stmt # The Stmt # column lists the statement number, which is generated by the program in sequential order.

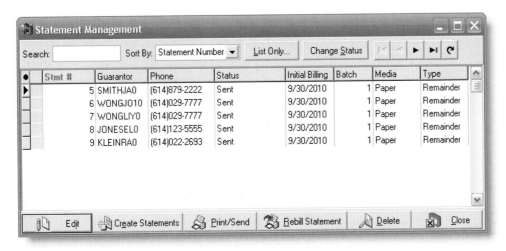

Figure 8-24   Statement Management dialog box

Guarantor In the Statement Management dialog box, guarantors rather than patients are listed because statements are created only for those financially responsible for accounts. For example, if a patient's father is the guarantor, a statement is created for the patient's father, not for the patient. In the Statement Management dialog box, the statement is listed under the father's chart number. If the father is also guarantor on his wife's account, his chart number will appear twice in the Statement Management window. When statements are printed, however, all transactions for the guarantor's child and wife are billed on one statement.

Phone The Phone column lists the guarantors' phone numbers.

Status The status assigned to each statement depends on whether the statement has been billed and whether the account has a zero balance:

♦ **Ready to Send** Transactions that have not been billed

♦ **Sent** Transactions that have been billed but not fully paid

♦ **Done** Transactions that have been billed and fully paid

Medisoft assigns status based on:

Initial Billing The date the statement was initially sent appears in the Initial Billing column. If a statement has been sent more than once, the most recent date is shown in the Billing Date field located in the General Tab of the Edit Statement dialog box.

Batch The batch number assigned by Medisoft is displayed.

Media The media format for the statement, either paper or electronic, is designated.

Type The type of statement, either Standard or Remainder, is listed.

CREATE STATEMENTS DIALOG BOX

The Create Statements dialog box is where information is entered that determines which statements are generated (see Figure 8-25).

The following filters can be applied in the Create Statements dialog box:

Transaction Dates A range of dates is entered to select transactions that occur within those dates. The dates can be entered directly by keying in the boxes, or they can be selected from the calendar that is displayed when clicking the drop-down arrow. To create statements for all available transactions, leave these two date boxes blank.

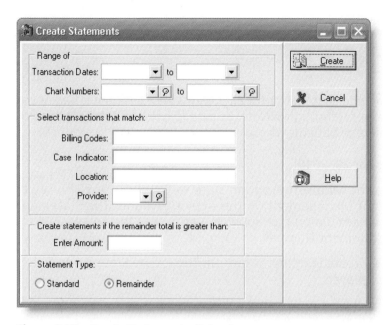

Figure 8-25   Create Statements dialog box

Chart Numbers   In the Chart Numbers boxes, the starting and ending chart numbers for which statements will be created are entered. If the boxes are left blank, all chart numbers will be included.

Select Transactions That Match   The options in this portion of the dialog box provide filters for creating statements for billing code(s), case indicator(s), location(s), and provider. In all instances except provider, commas must be placed between entries if more than one code is entered.

Create statements if the remainder total is greater than . . . Enter Amount   The dollar amount entered in this box is the minimum outstanding balance required for a statement to be created. For example, if 5.00 is entered in this box, the program will not create statements for accounts with a balance below $5.00. If this field is left blank, statements will be created for all accounts, regardless of the balance.

Statement Type   **Standard statements** show all available charges regardless of whether the insurance has paid on the transactions. **Remainder statements** list only those charges that are not paid in full after all insurance carrier payments have been received. Once a statement type is selected, the setting remains in effect until the other type of statement is selected.

After all selections are complete in the Create Statements dialog box, clicking the Create button instructs the program to generate statements. (*Note:* If you click the Create button and no statements can be created, the following message appears: "No new statements were created." Click OK to close the dialog box that contains the message.)

standard statements
statements that show all charges regardless of whether the insurance has paid on the transactions

remainder statements
statements that list only those charges that are not paid in full after all insurance carrier payments have been received

EXERCISE 8-6

Create remainder statements for all patients with last names beginning with the letters *H* through *S*. *Note:* Be sure to enter *SYZMAM* instead of just *S* to select all patients whose last names begin with the letter *S*.

Date: October 29, 2010

1. Change the Medisoft Program Date to October 29, 2010. Select Statement Management on the Activities menu. The Statement Management dialog box appears. Verify that the Sort By Field is set to Statement Number.

2. Click the Create Statements button. The Create Statements dialog box is displayed.

3. Enter the chart numbers that will select all patients with last names beginning with *H* through *S*. Note that you will need to select Michael Syzmanski in the second Chart Numbers field to include all patients with last names beginning with the letter "S."

4. Be sure the Statement Type field is set to Remainder. If it is not, click the Remainder button. Click the Create button to generate statements.

5. A message appears stating the number of statements that have been created. Click the OK button. Any new statements that were created are added to the list of statements in the Statement Management dialog box, with a Ready to Send status.

EDITING STATEMENTS

The Edit button in the Statement Management dialog box is used to perform edits on account statements (see Figure 8-26). The three tabs in the Statement dialog box contain important information about the statement.

GENERAL TAB

The following information is located in the General tab:

Status These buttons indicate the current status of the statement.

Billing Method The statement can be either paper or electronic.

Type The Type field indicates whether the statement is standard or remainder.

Initial Billing Date The Initial Billing Date is the date the statement was first created.

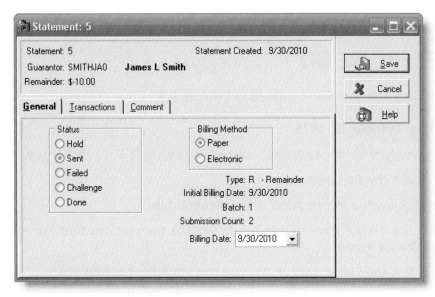

Figure 8-26   The Statement dialog box

Batch   The Batch number assigned to the statement appears.

Submission Count   This entry shows how many times a statement has been sent or printed.

Billing Date   The most current billing date is displayed.

TRANSACTIONS TAB

The Transactions tab lists the transactions placed on the statement (see Figure 8-27). The buttons at the bottom of the tab are used to add transactions to the statement, split transactions, or remove transactions from the statement.

COMMENT TAB

The Comment tab provides a place to include notes about the statement (see Figure 8-28).

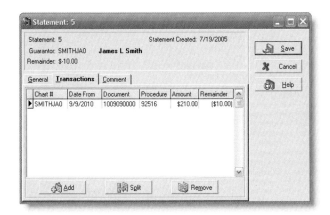

Figure 8-27   Transactions tab

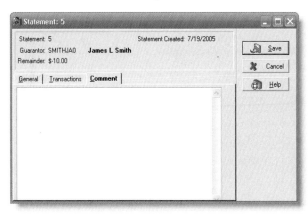

Figure 8-28   Comment tab

EXERCISE 8-7

Review the statement created in Exercise 8-6.

Date: October 29, 2010

1. Verify that the statement created in Exercise 8-6 is highlighted.

2. Click the Edit button.

3. Review the information in the General tab.

4. Click on the Transactions tab to see the transactions that are on the statement.

5. Click the Cancel button to close the Statement dialog box.

PRINTING STATEMENTS

Once statements have been created, the next step is to send them to a printer or to transmit them electronically. When the Print/Send button is clicked, the Print/Send Statements dialog box is displayed (see Figure 8-29). This box lists options for choosing the type of statement that will be created—Paper or Electronic. Paper statements are printed and mailed by the practice. Electronic statements are sent electronically to a processing center, which prints and mails them.

The Exclude Billed Paid Entries box designates whether transactions that have been billed and paid are left out of the statement processing.

When the Paper button is selected and the OK button is clicked, the Open Report dialog box appears (see Figure 8-30).

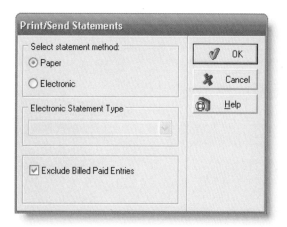

Figure 8-29   Print/Send Statements dialog box

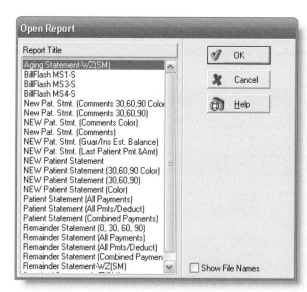

Figure 8-30   Open Report dialog box

SELECTING A FORMAT

The report selected in this dialog box must match the type of statement selected in the Statement Type field of the Create Statements dialog box—either Standard or Remainder. If Remainder was checked, statements will print only if one of the five Remainder Statement report formats is selected in the Open Report window:

1. Remainder Statement (0, 30, 60, 90)

2. Remainder Statement (All Payments)

3. Remainder Statement (All Pmts/Deduct)

4. Remainder Statement (Combined Payments)

5. Remainder Statement-WZ(SM)

Likewise, for Standard statements to print, one of the other patient statement report formats on the list must be chosen, such as Patient Statement [All Payments].

After the report format is selected, click the OK button to display the Print Report Where? dialog box, which asks whether to preview the report on screen, send the report directly to the printer, or export the report to a file format (see Figure 8-31).

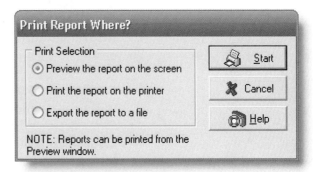

Figure 8-31   Print Report Where? dialog box

Once the Start button is clicked, the Remainder Statement (All Payments), Data Selection Questions dialog box appears (see Figure 8-32).

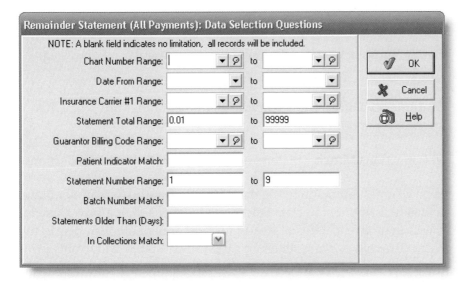

Figure 8-32   Remainder Statement (All Payments), Data Selection Questions dialog box

SELECTING THE FILTERS AND PRINTING STATEMENTS

The fields in the (Remainder Statements (All Payments), Data Selection Questions dialog box are used to filter statement selections. For example, to print statements for a certain group of patients, entries are made in the Chart Number Range field. In **once-a-month billing**, all statements are printed and mailed at once. Many practices use cycle billing instead. In a **cycle billing** system, patients are divided into groups, and statement printing and mailing is staggered throughout the month. For example, statements for guarantors whose last names begin with the letters *A* to *G* are mailed on the first of the month, those with last names that begin with *H* to *S* are mailed on the eighth of the month, and so on.

In addition to the Chart Number Range filter, other available filters include:

Date From Range   Statements within a range of dates.

Insurance Carrier #1 Range   Statements for a range of insurance carriers.

Statement Total Range   Statements for guarantors with a balance within a specified range.

Guarantor Billing Code Range   Statements for a range of guarantors assigned billing codes (from the Other Information tab in the Patient/Guarantor dialog box).

Patient Indicator Match   Statements for patients assigned a particular patient indicator (from the Other Information tab in the Patient/Guarantor dialog box).

Statement Number Range   Statements for a range of statement numbers (assigned by Medisoft).

Batch Number Match   Statements in a particular batch (assigned by Medisoft).

Statements Older Than (Days)   Statements that are older than a specified number of days.

In Collections Match   Statements for accounts that are in collections.

If no changes are made to the default entries in the Remainder Statements (All Payments), Data Selection Questions dialog box, all statements that have a status of Ready to Send or Sent are included in the batch. To avoid printing statements with a Sent status, and to only print those with a Ready to Send status, a zero is entered in the Batch Number Match field. All statements that are Ready to Send have a batch number of zero. Figure 8-33 displays a sample remainder statement.

once-a-month billing   a type of billing in which statements are mailed to all patients at the same time each month

cycle billing   a type of billing in which patients are divided into groups and statement printing and mailing is staggered throughout the month

Family Care Center
285 Stephenson Boulevard
Stephenson, OH 60089
(614)555-0000

Statement Date	Chart Number	Page
04/02/2008	SIMMOJI0	1

Make Checks Payable To:
Family Care Center
285 Stephenson Boulevard
Stephenson, OH 60089
(614)555-0000

Jill Simmons
30 Arbor Way
Stephenson, OH 60089

Date of Last Payment: 11/4/2010   Amount: -84.00   Previous Balance: 0.00

Patient: Jill Simmons   Chart Number: SIMMOJI0   Case: Urinary tract infection

Dates	Procedure	Charge	Paid by Primary		Paid By Guarantor	Adjustments	Remainder
10/29/10	99212	54.00	-43.20			0.00	10.80
10/29/10	87086	51.00	-40.80			0.00	10.20

Figure 8-33   Sample remainder statement

EXERCISE 8-8

Print remainder statements for all patients with last names beginning with the letter *H* and ending with the letter *S*. *Note:* Be sure to enter *SYZMAM* instead of just *S* to select all patients whose last names begin with the letter *S*.

Date: October 29, 2010

1. Click the Print/Send button in the Statement Management dialog box. The Print/Send Statements dialog box is displayed.

2. Select Paper as the statement method. Verify that the Exclude Billed Paid Entries box is checked. Click the OK button.

3. In the Open Report dialog box that appears, select Remainder Statement (All Payments). Click the OK button.

4. In the Print Report Where? dialog box, choose the option to preview the report on screen. Click the Start button. The Data Selection Questions dialog box is displayed.

5. In the Chart Number Range boxes, enter the chart numbers that will select all patients with last names beginning with *H* through *S*. Click the OK button.

6. Browse the statements in the Preview Report window. Notice that statements with a Sent status do not show any transactions, whereas newly created statements, with a Ready to Send status, list the transactions. Click the Print button. After printing, close the Preview window.

7. Notice that Jill Simmons's statement now has a status of Sent. Once a statement is printed, its status changes from Ready to Send to Sent. Close the Statement Management dialog box.

ON YOUR OWN EXERCISE 6 Enter Insurance Payments

October 29, 2010

Using Source Document 12, enter the payment information from the remittance advice, and apply payments to patient accounts.

ON YOUR OWN EXERCISE 7 Create Statements

October 29, 2010

Create remainder statements for all patients with last names beginning with *T* through the end of the alphabet. Print the statement(s) just created.

Remember to create a backup of your work before exiting Medisoft! To help you keep track of your work, name the backup file after the chapter you are working on, for example, StudentID-c8.mbk.

CHAPTER 8 WORKSHEET

After completing all the exercises in the chapter, answer the following questions in the spaces provided.

1. What is the amount the insurance carrier paid for procedure 99211 for John Fitzwilliams on 9/6/2010?

   _____

2. What is the amount the insurance carrier paid for procedure 99211 for Herbert Bell on 9/6/2010?

   _____

3. What is the amount the insurance carrier paid for procedure 90471 for Sarah Fitzwilliams on 9/7/2010?

   _____

4. What is listed as the Last Payment Amount on Herbert Bell's account after the East Ohio PPO payments were entered on 10/4/2010 (Transaction Entry dialog box)?

   _____

5. What is the remaining balance on Sheila Giles' account after the Blue Cross and Blue Shield payments were entered on 11/4/2010?

   _____

6. What is listed as the Last Payment Amount on John Fitzwilliams's account after the ChampVA payments were entered on 10/4/2010 (Transaction Entry dialog box)?

   _____

7. What is listed as the Last Payment Amount on Sheila Giles's account after the Blue Cross and Blue Shield payments were entered on 11/4/2010 (Transaction Entry dialog box)?

   _____

8. A statement was created for which patient(s) in Exercise 8-6?

   _____

9. What is the amount of the Blue Cross and Blue Shield payment for procedure 71020 for Lisa Wright on 10/4/2010 (Transaction Entry dialog box)?

   _____

10. What is listed as the amount due on Lisa Wright's statement created in On Your Own Exercise 7?

   _____

CHAPTER REVIEW

USING TERMINOLOGY

Match the terms on the left with the definitions on the right.

_____ 1. capitation payments

_____ 2. cycle billing

_____ 3. electronic remittance advice (ERA)

_____ 4. fee schedule

_____ 5. once-a-month billing

_____ 6. patient statement

_____ 7. payment schedule

_____ 8. remainder statements

_____ 9. standard statements

a. A list of the amount of money a patient owes, organized by the amount of time the money has been owed, the procedures performed, and the dates the procedures were performed.

b. A type of billing in which patients are divided into groups and statement printing and mailing is staggered throughout the month.

c. A document that specifies the amount the provider will be paid for each procedure.

d. Statement that shows all charges regardless of whether the insurance has paid on the transactions.

e. Payments made to physicians on a regular basis (such as monthly) for providing services to patients in a managed care insurance plan.

f. An electronic document that lists patients, dates of service, charges, and the amount paid or denied by the insurance carrier.

g. A document that specifies the amount the payer agrees to pay the provider for a service, based on a contracted rate of reimbursement.

h. A type of billing in which statements are mailed to all patients at the same time each month.

i. Statements that list only those charges that are not paid in full after all insurance carrier payments have been received.

CHECKING YOUR UNDERSTANDING

Answer the questions below in the space provided.

10. Why is it easier to enter large insurance payments in the Deposit List dialog box than in the Transaction Entry dialog box?

_____

_____

11. When all payments on a remittance advice have been successfully entered and applied to charges, what should appear in the Unapplied box in the upper-right corner of the Deposit List dialog box?

_____

_____

12. Why do charges need to be adjusted for patients who are covered under a capitated insurance plan?

_____

_____

13. If a practice did not want to create statements for patients with an account balance of less than $5.00, how would this be done?

_____

_____

APPLYING KNOWLEDGE

Answer the questions below in the space provided.

14. Randall Klein calls. He would like to know whether Medicare has paid any of the charges for his September office visit. How would you look up this information in Medisoft?

_____

_____

15. Why do many practices send out remainder statements rather than standard statements?

_____

_____

AT THE COMPUTER

Answer the following questions at the computer.

16. What is the total amount that John Fitzwilliams paid in copayments in September 2010? (*Hint:* Include his daughter Sarah in the calculation.)

_____

_____

17. On September 10, 2010, $168.00 was received from Blue Cross and Blue Shield as payment for James Smith's facial nerve function studies performed on September 9, 2010. How much should James Smith have paid, assuming he has met his annual deductible?

_____

_____

Printing Reports

9

WHAT YOU NEED TO KNOW

To use this chapter, you need to know how to:

◆ Start Medisoft, use menus, and enter and edit text.

◆ Work with chart numbers and codes.

LEARNING OUTCOMES

When you finish this chapter, you will be able to:

◆ Select the options available for different reports.

◆ Preview and print a variety of Medisoft reports.

◆ Access Medisoft's Report Designer.

KEY TERMS

aging report
day sheet
insurance aging report
patient aging report
patient day sheet
patient ledger
payment day sheet
practice analysis report
procedure day sheet

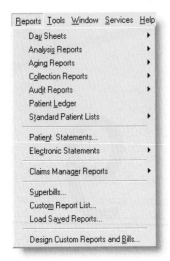

Figure 9-1   Reports menu

REPORTS IN THE MEDICAL OFFICE

Reports are an important tool in managing a medical office. They provide useful information about a practice and its patients. Providers and office managers ask for different reports at different times. Some providers want to see daily reports of each day's transactions. Others want to see reports on particular patients' accounts on a weekly or bimonthly basis.

Medisoft provides a variety of standard reports and also has the ability to create custom reports using the Report Designer. The Reports menu lists standard reports and also provides choices for designing custom reports using the Report Designer (see Figure 9-1).

DAY SHEETS

day sheet a report that provides information on practice activities for a twenty-four-hour period

A **day sheet** is a report that provides information on practice activities for a twenty-four-hour period. In Medisoft, there are three types of day sheet reports: patient day sheets, provider day sheets, and payment day sheets. Day sheets can be created for a single day or for a range of dates.

Patient Day Sheet

patient day sheet a summary of patient activity on a given day

At the end of the day, a medical practice often prints a **patient day sheet,** which is a summary of the patient activity on that day (see Figures 9-2a and 9-2b). Medisoft's version of this report lists the

---

Family Care Center
Patient Day Sheet

September 07, 2010
9/7/2010

Entry	Date	Document	POS	Description	Provider	Code	Modifiers	Amount
FITZWJO0 Fitzwilliams, John								
380	9/7/2010	1009070000	11	ChampVA Copayment	2	CHVCPAY		-15.00

Patient's Charges	Patient's Receipts	Insurance Receipts	Adjustments	Patient Balance
$0.00	-$15.00	$0.00	$0.00	$58.00

Entry	Date	Document	POS	Description	Provider	Code	Modifiers	Amount
GARDIJO0 Gardiner, John								
385	9/7/2010	1009070000	11	OF--established patient, minimal	1	99211		36.00
387	9/7/2010	1009070000	11	OhioCare HMO Copayment	1	OHCCPAY		-20.00

Patient's Charges	Patient's Receipts	Insurance Receipts	Adjustments	Patient Balance
$36.00	-$20.00	$0.00	$0.00	$0.00

Entry	Date	Document	POS	Description	Provider	Code	Modifiers	Amount
KLEINRA0 Klein, Randall								
388	9/7/2010	1009070000	11	OF--established patient, low	2	99212		54.00
389	9/7/2010	1009070000	11	Application of short leg cast, walking	2	29425		229.00
390	9/7/2010	1009070000	11	Supplies and materials provided	2	99070		20.00

Patient's Charges	Patient's Receipts	Insurance Receipts	Adjustments	Patient Balance
$303.00	$0.00	$0.00	$0.00	$5.80

Figure 9-2a   Page 1 of a Patient Day Sheet report

```
                        Family Care Center
                      Patient Day Sheet
                      September 07, 2010
                           9/7/2010

                   Total # Patients                      3
                   Total # Procedures                    4
                   Total Procedure Charges         $339.00
                   Total Global Surgical Procedures   $0.00
                   Total Product Charges              $0.00
                   Total Inside Lab Charges           $0.00
                   Total Outside Lab Charges          $0.00
                   Total Billing Charges              $0.00
                   Total Tax Charges                  $0.00
                                                 _____
                   Total Charges                   $339.00

                   Total Insurance Payments           $0.00
                   Total Cash Copayments              $0.00
                   Total Check Copayments           -$35.00
                   Total Credit Card Copayments       $0.00
                   Total Patient Cash Payments        $0.00
                   Total Patient Check Payments       $0.00
                   Total Credit Card Payments         $0.00
                                                 _____
                   Total Receipts                   -$35.00

                   Total Credit Adjustments           $0.00
                   Total Debit Adjustments            $0.00
                   Total Insurance Credit Adjustments $0.00
                   Total Insurance Debit Adjustments  $0.00
                   Total Insurance Withholds          $0.00
                   Total Adjustments                  $0.00
                                                 _____
                   Net Effect on Accounts Receivable $304.00

              Practice Totals:
                      Total # of Procedures          50
                      Total Charges            $4,085.50
                      Total Payments          -$2,127.19
                      Total Adjustments       -$1,019.29

                      Accounts Receivable        $939.02
```

Figure 9-2b   Page 2 of a Patient Day Sheet report

procedures for a particular day, grouped by patient, in alphabetical order by chart number. It includes:

- ◆ Procedures performed for a particular patient or group of patients

- ◆ Charges, receipts, adjustments, and balances for a particular patient or group of patients

- ◆ A summary of a practice's charges, payments, and adjustments

The option to view or print a patient day sheet is located on the Reports menu, within the Day Sheets submenu (see Figure 9-3). The first step in creating a day sheet after the option is selected on the Reports menu is to complete the Data Selection Questions dialog box. This dialog box is used to select the range of data that will be included in the report (see Figure 9-4). If any box is left blank, all

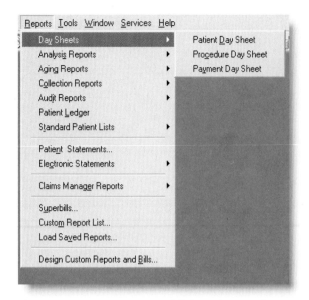

Figure 9-3 Reports menu with Day Sheets submenu displayed

values are included in the report. For example, if no chart numbers are entered, all patients will be included in the report. The selection options in the dialog box are as follows:

Chart Number Range In the Chart Number Range boxes, a range of chart numbers for patients is entered. If a report is needed for just one patient, that patient's chart number is entered in both boxes.

Date Created Range The Date Created Range refers to the actual date the information was entered in the computer. The date created may or may not be the same as the date a transaction took place. For example, suppose transactions from Friday, October 1, are entered in Medisoft on Monday morning, October 4. In this example, the Date Created is the date the transaction was entered—October 4. The transaction date is the date on which the patient was in the office—October 1.

By default, Medisoft enters the Windows System Date in both Date Created Range boxes. In the exercises in this chapter, the date displayed in both Date Created Range boxes must be changed in each exercise. You will always enter 01/01/2008 in the first box and 01/01/2018 in the second box. This broad range of dates was selected to make certain that all data entered by students was included in the report.

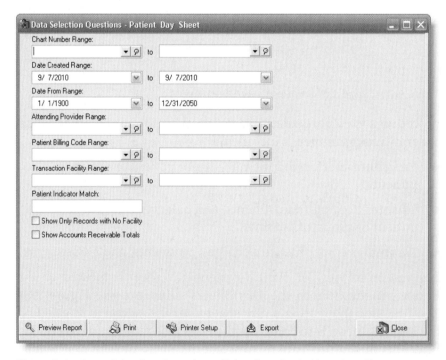

Figure 9-4 Data Selection Questions dialog box for Patient Day Sheet report

Date From Range   The Date From Range refers to the actual date of the transaction. In the example just described, the entry in both Date From Range boxes would be 10/1/2010. The default entries in the Date From Range boxes are 1/1/1900 and 12/31/2050. At the beginning of each exercise, these dates must also be changed to the date listed before Step 1 of the exercise.

Note: There are two ways of changing dates in the Data Selection Questions dialog box. You can enter the date using the keyboard, entering the numbers and slashes. For example, January 1, 2010 would be keyed as 01/01/2010. The slashes must be entered as well as the numbers. The other way of entering dates is to use the pop-up calendar. The pop-up calendar is displayed when you click on the down arrow at the right side of the box that contains the date (see Figure 9-5). Once this calendar is visible, clicking on the month in the blue banner at the top of the calendar displays a list of the months (see Figure 9-6). Clicking any month in the list changes the calendar to that month. Clicking on the year in the blue banner displays up and down arrows that can be clicked to advance the year forward or

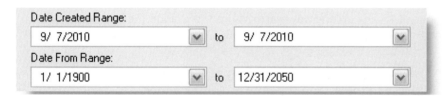

Figure 9-5   Down arrows (highlighted in yellow) used to display pop-up calendar

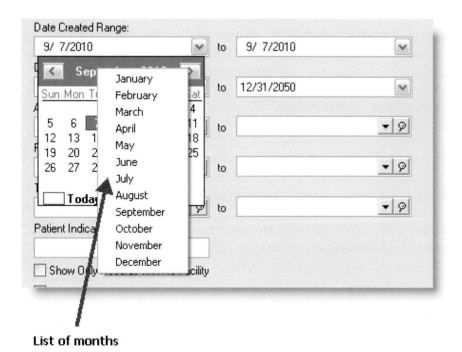

List of months

Figure 9-6   List of months in the pop-up calendar

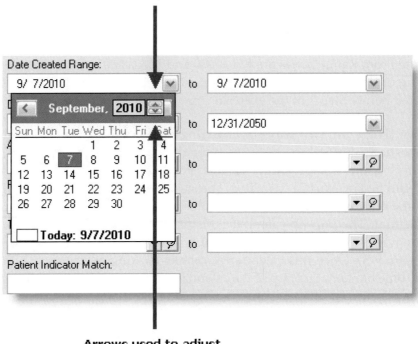

**Arrows used to adjust
year up or down**

Figure 9-7   The up and down arrows used to change the year in the pop-up calendar

backward (see Figure 9-7). The day is changed by clicking on the desired day in the calendar below the blue banner.

Attending Provider Range   A range of codes for the attending providers is entered in the Attending Provider Range boxes.

Patient Billing Code Range   If the practice uses Medisoft's Patient Billing Code feature, codes can be entered in this box to select only those patients with the designated billing code(s).

Transaction Facility Range   This field is used to select transactions that occurred at specific facilities.

Patient Indicator Match   If the practice has assigned a Patient Indicator code to each patient, an entry can be made to select only those patients who match a specific code.

Show Only Records with No Facility   If this box is checked, the report will limit the report to transactions with no facility selected in the Accounts tab of the Case folder.

Show Accounts Receivable Totals   If this box is checked, accounts receivable totals will appear at the end of the Patient Day Sheet report.

When these selection boxes have been completed, the next step in creating a report is to click one of the buttons in the lower section of the dialog box: Preview Report, Print, Printer Setup, Export, and Close.

Preview Report Creates the report and displays it in the Report Preview window.

Print Creates the report and displays the Print dialog box, which is used to send the report to the printer.

Printer Setup Specifies settings for the printer that is used for printing the reports.

Export Creates the report and provides options for selecting the format and destination of the saved file.

Close Closes the Data Selection Questions dialog box.

The Report Preview window, common to all reports, provides options for viewing or printing a report (see Figure 9-8). The buttons on the Report Preview toolbar control how a report is displayed on the screen and how to move from page to page within a report (see Figure 9-9). The buttons on the toolbar, from left to right, are as follows:

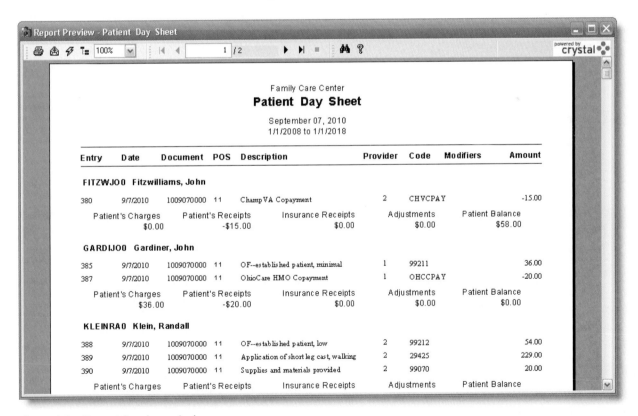

Figure 9-8 Report Preview window

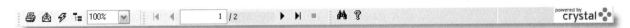

Figure 9-9 Buttons on Report Preview toolbar

Print   This button is used to print the report.

Export   The Export button exports the data in the report to a file format such as Microsoft Word, Microsoft Excel, Adobe PDF, HTML, or text.

Refresh   This button refreshes the page in order to show the most recent data.

Toggle Group Tree   This choice changes the display of the report, which makes it easier to locate specific information in a report.

Zoom   The Zoom button changes the size of the image in the preview window to any of several sizes, both larger and smaller.

Navigate   Four triangle buttons, two on the left and two on the right, are used to move through pages of a multipage report. The First Page button, farthest on the left, moves to the beginning of a report. The Previous Page button moves to the page that precedes the one currently displayed. The bar between the two sets of triangle buttons indicates how many pages are in a report and the number of the current page. To the right of the bar are the other two triangle buttons. The Next Page button moves to the page following the current one. The Last Page button moves to the end of a report.

Stop Loading   This stops a report from loading.

Search Text   The Search Text button performs a case-sensitive text search in the report displayed in the preview window.

Help   This button opens the Medisoft built-in Help feature.

EXERCISE 9-1

Print a patient day sheet report for October 4, 2010.

Date: October 4, 2010

1. Start Medisoft and restore the data from your last work session.

2. On the Reports menu, click Day Sheets and then Patient Day Sheet. The Data Selection Questions dialog box is displayed.

3. Leave the Chart Number Range boxes blank.

4. Today's date—that is, the date on which you are working on this exercise—will likely appear in both Date Created Range boxes. Enter *01/01/2008* in the first Date Created Range box, and enter *01/01/2018* in the second box. You may also use

the pop-up calendar to change the dates. If you type in the numbers rather than use the pop-up calendar, be sure to enter the slashes (/) between the day, month, and year.

5. Enter *10/04/2010* in both Date From Range boxes, or use the pop-up calendar to change the date to October 4, 2010. Leave all other boxes blank. This will select data for all patients and attending providers for October 4, 2010.

6. Check the Show Accounts Receivable Totals box.

7. Click the Preview Report button. The patient day sheet report is displayed.

8. If necessary, use the scroll bar to view additional entries on the first page of the report.

9. Click the Go to Next Page triangle button to advance to the second page of the report.

10. Click the Print button, and then click the OK button to print the report.

11. Click the red Close box at the top right of the window to exit the Report Preview window.

Procedure Day Sheet

A **procedure day sheet** lists all procedures performed on a particular day and gives the dates, patients, document numbers, places of service, debits, and credits relating to them (see Figure 9-10). Procedures are listed in numerical order. Procedure day sheets are printed by clicking Procedure Day Sheet on the Reports menu. The same Data Selection Questions dialog box used for a patient day sheet is displayed, except that a range of procedure codes rather than patients can be selected. A procedure day sheet will be generated only for data that meet the selection criteria. If any box is left blank, all values are included in the report. The report can be previewed on the screen, printed directly, or exported to a file.

procedure day sheet a report that lists all the procedures performed on a particular day, in numerical order

EXERCISE 9-2

Print a procedure day sheet report for October 4, 2010, with the entire range of procedure codes, dates from, and attending providers.

Date: October 4, 2010

1. On the Reports menu, click Day Sheets and then Procedure Day Sheet. The Data Selection Questions dialog box is displayed.

2. Leave the Procedure Code Range boxes blank.

3. Change the entry in the first Date Created Range box to 01/01/2008 and the entry in the second box to 01/01/2018.

Reminder: the dates can be entered using the keyboard to enter numbers and slashes, or by using the pop-up calendar.

4. Change the entries in both Date From Range boxes to 10/04/2010.

5. Check the Show Accounts Receivable Totals box.

6. Click the Report Preview button. The procedure day sheet report is displayed.

7. Send the report to the printer.

8. Exit the Report Preview window.

Family Care Center
Procedure Day Sheet
9/7/2010

Entry	Date	Chart	Name	Document	POS	Debits	Credits
29425		**Application of short leg cast, walking**					
389	9/7/2010	KLEINRA0	Klein, Randall	1009070000	11	$229.00	
		Total of 29425		Quantity: 1		$229.00	$0.00
99070		**Supplies and materials provided**					
390	9/7/2010	KLEINRA0	Klein, Randall	1009070000	11	$20.00	
		Total of 99070		Quantity: 1		$20.00	$0.00
99211		**OF --established patient, minimal**					
385	9/7/2010	GARDIJO0	Gardiner, John	1009070000	11	$36.00	
		Total of 99211		Quantity: 1		$36.00	$0.00
99212		**OF --established patient, low**					
388	9/7/2010	KLEINRA0	Klein, Randall	1009070000	11	$54.00	
		Total of 99212		Quantity: 1		$54.00	$0.00
CHVCPAY		**ChampVA Copayment**					
380	9/7/2010	FITZWJO0	Fitzwilliams, John	1009070000	11		-$15.00
		Total of CHVCPAY		Quantity: 1		$0.00	-$15.00
OHCCPAY		**OhioCare HMO Copayment**					
387	9/7/2010	GARDIJO0	Gardiner, John	1009070000	11		-$20.00
		Total of OHCCPAY		Quantity: 1		$0.00	-$20.00
				Total of Codes:		$339.00	-$35.00
				Balance:		$304.00	

Practice Totals:

Total # of Procedures	**50**
Total Charges	**$4,085.50**
Total Payments	**-$2,127.19**
Total Adjustments	**-$1,019.29**
Accounts Receivable	**$939.02**

Figure 9-10   Page 1 of Procedure Day Sheet

Payment Day Sheet

A **payment day sheet** lists all payments received on a particular day, organized by provider (see Figures 9-11a and 9-11b). It is printed by clicking Payment Day Sheet on the Reports menu. The same Data Selection Questions dialog box is displayed, but with fewer data fields. A payment day sheet will be generated only for data that meet the selection criteria. If any box is left blank, all values for that box are included in the report. Again, the report can be previewed on the screen, printed directly, or exported to a file.

payment day sheet a report that lists all payments received on a particular day, organized by provider

Family Care Center
Payment Day Sheet
9/7/2010

Entry	Date	Document	Description	Chart	Code	Amount
1	**Yan, Katherine**					
387	9/7/2010	1009070000		GARDIJO0	OHCCPAY	-20.00
			Count: 1		**Provider Total:**	-20.00
2	**Rudner, John**					
380	9/7/2010	1009070000		FITZWJO0	CHVCPAY	-15.00
			Count: 1		**Provider Total:**	-15.00

Figure 9-11a   Page 1 of Payment Day Sheet

Family Care Center
Payment Day Sheet
9/7/2010

Report Totals

Total # Payments	2
Total Payments	-$35.00

Practice Totals:

Total # of Payments	59
Total Payments	-$2,127.19
Total Applied Payments	-$2,127.19
Total Unapplied Payments	$0.00
Accounts Receivable	$939.02

Figure 9-11b   Page 2 of Payment Day Sheet

EXERCISE 9-3

Print a payment day sheet report for October 4, 2010, with the entire range of attending providers.

Date: October 4, 2010

1. On the Reports menu, click Day Sheets and then Payment Day Sheet. The Data Selection Questions dialog box is displayed.

2. Leave the Attending Provider Range boxes blank to include all providers on the report.

3. Change the entry in the first Date Created Range box to 01/01/2008 and the entry in the second box to 01/01/2018.

4. Change the entries in both Date From Range boxes to 10/04/2010.

5. If it is not already checked, be sure to check the Show Accounts Receivable Totals box.

6. Click the Preview Report button. The payment day sheet report is displayed.

7. Send the report to the printer.

8. Exit the Report Preview window.

ANALYSIS REPORTS

Medisoft includes a number of reports that provide detailed information about practice finances. These reports are known as analysis reports. The analysis reports submenu is shown in Figure 9-12. The following paragraphs provide a description of each report. Not all reports can be created in a student exercise, since data have not actually been sent to insurance carriers and patients.

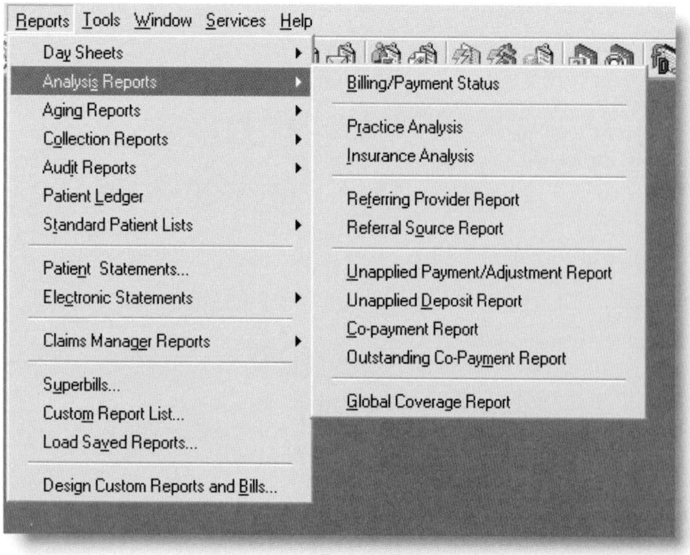

Billing/Payment Status Report

The Billing/Payment Status report lists the status of all transactions that have responsible insurance carriers, showing who has paid and who has not been billed (see Figures 9-13a and 9-13b). The report is in a column format sorted

Figure 9-12 The analysis reports submenu

Family Care Center

Family Care Center
Billing Payment Status
Ending 9/7/2010

Date	Document	Procedure	Amount	Policy 1	Policy 2	Policy 3	Guarantor	Adjustments	Balance

ARLENSU0   Susan Arlen   (614)315-2233

Case 24   1: East Ohio PP O (419)444-1505

Subtotal:	0.00
Unapplied Payments and Adjustments:	34.00
Case Balance:	34.00
Patient Balance:	34.00

BELLHER0   Herbert Bell   (614)030-1111

Case 21   1: East Ohio PP O (419)444-1505

Subtotal:	0.00
Unapplied Payments and Adjustments:	16.00
Case Balance:	16.00
Patient Balance:	16.00

BELLJAN0   Janine Bell   (614)030-1111

Case 22   1: East Ohio PP O (419)444-1505

Subtotal:	0.00
Unapplied Payments and Adjustments:	176.00
Case Balance:	176.00
Patient Balance:	176.00

BELLJON0   Jonathan Bell   (614)030-1111

Case 4   1: East Ohio PP O (419)444-1505

Subtotal:	0.00
Unapplied Payments and Adjustments:	202.00
Case Balance:	202.00
Patient Balance:	202.00

BELLSAM0   Samuel Bell   (614)030-1111

* indicates that this payment is complete
A date in the payment columns indicates the billing date

Figure 9-13a   Sample first page of a Billing/Payment Status report

Date	Document	Procedure	Amount	Policy 1	Policy 2	Policy 3	Guarantor	Adjustments	Balance
Case 40		1: Medicare (215)599-0000							
7/12/2010	1007120000	99212	54.00	-29.89*	0.00*	0.00*	5/4/2006	-16.64*	7.47
								Subtotal:	7.47
						Unapplied Payments and Adjustments:			46.53
								Case Balance:	54.00
								Patient Balance:	54.00
ZAPATKRO	Kristin Zapata (614)033-0044								
Case 60		1: Blue Cross/Blue Shield (614)024-9000							
8/28/2009	0803270000	99385	247.50	8/30/2010	0.00*	0.00*	Not Billed	0.00*	247.50
								Subtotal:	247.50
						Unapplied Payments and Adjustments:			0.00
								Case Balance:	247.50
								Patient Balance:	247.50
								Report Balance:	$1,310.50

Figure 9-13b   Sample last page of a Billing/Payment Status report

first by Chart Number and then by Case. Every chart number listed shows a patient balance and any unapplied payments or unapplied adjustments. An asterisk (*) next to a number indicates that the payer has made complete payment for that transaction. Information in this report can be used by practices to determine whether billing charges can be applied to a patient account.

Practice Analysis Report

practice analysis report a report that analyzes the revenue of a practice for a specified period of time, usually a month or a year

Medisoft's **practice analysis report** analyzes the revenue of a practice for a specified period of time, usually a month or a year (see Figures 9-14a and 9-14b). The report can be used to generate medical practice financial statements. It can also be used for profit analysis. The summary at the end of the report breaks down the information into total charges, total payments and copayments, and total adjustments.

Practice Analysis

From 9/1/2010 to 9/30/2010

Code	Modifiers	Description	Amount	Units	Average	Costs	Net
02		Patient payment, check	-52.00	1	-52.00	0.00	-52.00
29425		Application of short leg cast, walking	229.00	1	229.00	0.00	229.00
50390		Aspiration of renal cyst by needle	551.00	1	551.00	0.00	551.00
73510		Hip x-ray, complete, two views	124.00	1	124.00	0.00	124.00
92516		Facial nerve function studies	210.00	1	210.00	0.00	210.00
93000		Electrocardiogram--ECG with interp	84.00	1	84.00	0.00	84.00
99070		Supplies and materials provided	20.00	1	20.00	0.00	20.00
99201		OF--new patient, minimal	66.00	1	66.00	0.00	66.00
99211		OF--established patient, minimal	144.00	4	36.00	0.00	144.00
99212		OF--established patient, low	324.00	6	54.00	0.00	324.00
99213		OF--established patient, detailed	144.00	2	72.00	0.00	144.00
99214		OF--established patient, moderate	105.00	1	105.00	0.00	105.00
99394		Preventive est., 12-17 years	222.00	1	222.00	0.00	222.00
AARPAY		AARP Payment	-23.18	3	-7.73	0.00	-23.18
CHVCPAY		ChampVA Copayment	-15.00	1	-15.00	0.00	-15.00
EAPCPAY		East Ohio PPO Copayment	-160.00	8	-20.00	0.00	-160.00
OHCCPAY		OhioCare HMO Copayment	-40.00	2	-20.00	0.00	-40.00

Figure 9-14a   Page 1 of Practice Analysis report (page 2 is on page 246)

EXERCISE 9-4

Print a practice analysis report for October 2010.

Date: October 31, 2010

1. On the Reports menu, click Analysis Reports and then Practice Analysis. The Data Selection Questions dialog box appears.

2. Leave the Procedure Code Range boxes blank to include all procedure codes in the report.

3. Change the entry in the first Date Created Range box to 01/01/2008 and the entry in the second box to 01/01/2018.

4. Change the entry in the first Date From Range box to 10/01/2010, and the entry in the second box to 10/31/2010.

5. If it is not already checked, be sure to check the Show Accounts Receivable Totals box.

6. Leave the rest of the boxes blank. Click the Preview Report button.

7. View the report on the screen.

8. Go to the second page of the report.

9. Send the report to the printer.

10. Exit the Report Preview window.

Family Care Center

Practice Analysis

From 9/1/2010 to 9/30/2010

Code	Modifiers	Description	Amount	Units	Average	Costs	Net
		Total Procedure Charges					$2,223.00
		Total Global Surgical Procedures					$0.00
		Total Product Charges					$0.00
		Total Inside Lab Charges					$0.00
		Total Outside Lab Charges					$0.00
		Total Billing Charges					$0.00
		Total Tax Charges					$0.00
		Total Charges					$2,223.00
		Total Insurance Payments					-$23.18
		Total Cash Copayments					$0.00
		Total Check Copayments					-$215.00
		Total Credit Card Copayments					$0.00
		Total Patient Cash Payments					$0.00
		Total Patient Check Payments					-$52.00
		Total Credit Card Payments					$0.00
		Total Payments					-$290.18
		Total Deductibles					$0.00
		Total Debit Adjustments					$0.00
		Total Credit Adjustments					$0.00
		Total Insurance Debit Adjustments					$0.00
		Total Insurance Credit Adjustments					$0.00
		Total Insurance Withholds					$0.00
		Total Adjustments					0.00
		Net Effect on Accounts Receivable					$1,932.82

Practice Totals:

	Net
Total # of Procedures	50
Total Charges	$4,085.50
Total Payments	-$2,127.19
Total Adjustments	-$1,019.29
Accounts Receivable	$939.02

Figure 9-14b   Page 2 of Practice Analysis report

Insurance Analysis

The Insurance Analysis report tracks charges, insurance payments received during a specified period, and copayments applied to accounts that include those procedures. It is usually printed at the end of the month. The amount listed as the Outstanding Balance displays the total charges, subtracting the full amount of the charge if the insurance payment was made.

Referring Provider Report

This Referring Provider report enables a practice to determine the origins of revenue derived from providers who have referred patients to the practice. The report lists the percentage of total income that was generated by referring providers.

Referral Source Report

This report tracks the source of referrals that are not from other medical offices or providers, such as referrals from established patients.

Unapplied Payment/Adjustment Report

This report lists payments or adjustments that have not been fully applied. Information about the payment or adjustment includes the case, document number, posting date, code, code description, transaction amount, and unapplied amount.

Unapplied Deposit Report

The Unapplied Deposit Report lists deposits that have an unapplied amount. The report includes the date, code, payer name, payer type, amount of the deposit, and unapplied amount.

Co-Payment Report

This report lists patients who have copayment transactions. It shows the amount paid, how much was applied, and how much, if any, was left unapplied.

Outstanding Co-Payment Report

This report shows patients who have outstanding copayment transactions. The report shows the copayment amount expected, the actual amount paid, and the amount due.

Global Coverage Report

The Global Coverage Report displays the patients who fall under global coverage during a specific time frame. The report detail includes information on the patients, the date the coverage expires, and the total that would have been billed if global coverage did not apply.

AGING REPORTS

aging report a report that lists the amount of money owed to the practice, organized by the amount of time the money has been owed

Aging reports are of particular importance to medical billing specialists. An **aging report** lists the amount of money owed to the practice, organized by the amount of time the money has been owed. Medical practices use aging reports to determine which accounts require follow-up to collect past due balances. A **patient aging report** lists a patient's balance by age, date and amount of the last payment, and telephone number.

patient aging report a report that lists a patient's balance by age, date and amount of the last payment, and telephone number

insurance aging report a report that lists how long a payer has taken to respond to insurance claims

An **insurance aging report** shows how long a payer has taken to respond to each claim. This information is used to compare the response time with the terms of the contract the practice has with the payer. For example, a practice may discover that a payer is routinely responding to claims ten days later than the claim turnaround time specified in the contract. In that case, the practice manager might review the situation with the payer's customer service manager and ask the payer to adhere to its guidelines. The aging reports submenu is illustrated in Figure 9-15.

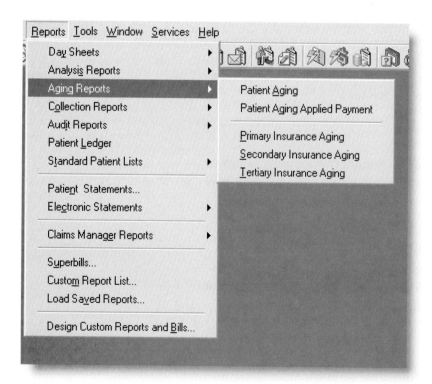

Figure 9-15   The aging reports submenu

Patient Aging Reports

Medisoft includes two different patient aging reports. The Patient Aging report includes payments that have not been applied to charges; the Patient Aging Applied Payments report excludes unapplied payments (see Figure 9-16). Both reports are listed on the Aging Reports submenu.

Patient aging reports are printed by clicking Aging Reports and then Patient Aging or Patient Aging Applied Payment on the Reports menu.

Insurance Aging Report

An insurance aging report permits tracking of claims

```
                          Family Care Center
              Patient Aging Applied Payment
                            by Date From
              From January 01, 2010 to September 30, 2010
```

Chart # Name	Birthdate	Current 0 - 30	Past 31 - 60	Past 61 - 90	Past 91 +	Total Balance
JONESEL0 Jones, Elizabeth	8/26/1936	21.17	7.47	0.00	0.00	28.64
Last Pmt: -20.58 On: 9/30/2010	(614)123-5555					
KLEINRA0 Klein, Randall	10/11/1953	5.80	0.00	0.00	0.00	5.80
Last Pmt: -23.18 On: 9/17/2010	(614)022-2693					
WONGJO10 Wong, Jo	9/6/1940	7.47	0.00	7.47	0.00	14.94
Last Pmt: -29.89 On: 9/14/2010	(614)029-7777					
WONGLIY0 Wong, Li Y	12/13/1938	4.14	0.00	0.00	0.00	4.14
Last Pmt: -16.54 On: 9/14/2010	(614)029-7777					
Report Aging Total		$38.58	$7.47	$7.47	$0.00	$53.52
Percent of Aging Total		72.1%	14.0%	14.0%	0.0%	100.0%

Figure 9-16   Patient Aging Applied Payment report

EXERCISE 9-5

Print a Patient Aging Applied Payment report for the period ending September 30, 2010.

Date: September 30, 2010

1. On the Reports menu, click Aging Reports and then Patient Aging Applied Payment.
2. Leave the Chart Number Range boxes blank.
3. Accept the entry in the first Date From Range box and change the date in the second box to 09/30/2010.
4. Leave the reamining fields blank.
5. Click the Preview Report button. The aging report is displayed.
6. Send the report to the printer.
7. Exit the Report Preview window.

filed with insurance carriers. The report lists claims that have been on file 0–30 days, 31–60 days, 61–90 days, 91–120 days, and more than 120 days (see Figure 9-17). This information is used to follow up on overdue payments from insurance carriers. Printing the aging report and following up on overdue claims speeds the collection

Family Care Center
Primary Insurance Aging
December 31, 2002

Date of Service	Procedure	- Past - 0 to 30	- Past - 31 to 60	- Past - 61 to 90	- Past - 91 to 120	- Past - 121 +	Total Balance
Aetna (AET00)						Erik (602)333-3333 ext: 123	

SIMTA000 Tanus J. Simpson   SS:
Birthdate: 4/4/1968   Policy: GG93-GXTA   Group: 99999

Claim: 1   Initial Billing Date: 12/3/2002   Last Billing Date: 12/3/2002

Date of Service	Procedure	0 to 30	31 to 60	61 to 90	91 to 120	121 +	Total Balance
12/3/2002	43220	$275.00	$0.00	$0.00	$0.00	$0.00	$275.00
12/3/2002	71040	$50.00	$0.00	$0.00	$0.00	$0.00	$50.00
12/3/2002	81000	$11.00	$0.00	$0.00	$0.00	$0.00	$11.00
12/3/2002	99213	$60.00	$0.00	$0.00	$0.00	$0.00	$60.00
		$396.00	$0.00	$0.00	$0.00	$0.00	$396.00
Insurance Totals:		$396.00	$0.00	$0.00	$0.00	$0.00	$396.00

Cigna (CIG00)						Bill S. Preston 234-5678	

BRIJA000 Jay Brimley   SS:
Birthdate: 1/23/1964   Policy: 98547377   Group: 12d

Claim: 3   Initial Billing Date: 3/25/2002   Last Billing Date: 3/25/2002

Date of Service	Procedure	0 to 30	31 to 60	61 to 90	91 to 120	121 +	Total Balance
3/25/2002	99214	$0.00	$0.00	$0.00	$0.00	$65.00	$65.00
3/25/2002	97260	$0.00	$0.00	$0.00	$0.00	$30.00	$30.00
		$0.00	$0.00	$0.00	$0.00	$95.00	$95.00
Insurance Totals:		$0.00	$0.00	$0.00	$0.00	$95.00	$95.00

Medicare (MED01)						Ted T. Logan (800)999-9999	

AGADW000 Dwight Again   SS:
Birthdate: 3/30/1932   Policy: 780340761   Group: 23c

Claim: 7   Initial Billing Date: 12/6/2002   Last Billing Date: 12/6/2002

Date of Service	Procedure	0 to 30	31 to 60	61 to 90	91 to 120	121 +	Total Balance
9/3/2002	73130	$45.00	$0.00	$0.00	$0.00	$0.00	$45.00
9/3/2002	99213	$60.00	$0.00	$0.00	$0.00	$0.00	$60.00
		$105.00	$0.00	$0.00	$0.00	$0.00	$105.00
Insurance Totals:		$105.00	$0.00	$0.00	$0.00	$0.00	$105.00

Report Aging Totals:		$501.00	$0.00	$0.00	$0.00	$95.00	$596.00
Percent of Aging Total:		84.06%	0.00%	0.00%	0.00%	15.94%	100.00%

Figure 9-17   Primary Insurance Aging report

process. The aging begins on the date of billing. Medisoft provides three insurance aging reports: primary, secondary, and tertiary.

Note: There is no hands-on exercise for Insurance Aging. Since claims have not actually been sent to insurance carriers, it is not possible to print an Insurance Aging report that contains meaningful data.

COLLECTION REPORTS

Medisoft provides a number of collection reports that can be used to identify and follow up on overdue patient or insurance accounts. The topic of collections is presented in Chapter 10.

Family Care Center
Patient Account Ledger
As of 11/30/2010

Entry	Date	POS	Description	Procedure	Document	Provider	Amount
BATTIAN0	Anthony Battistuta				(614)500-3619		
	Last Payment: 0.00						
425	10/28/2010	11		99212	1009280000	4	54.00
426	10/28/2010	11		82947	1009280000	4	25.00
	Patient Totals						79.00
BROOKLA0	Lawana Brooks				(614)027-4242		
	Last Payment: -20.00		On: 10/29/2010				
428	10/29/2010	11		99212	1010290000	4	54.00
429	10/29/2010	11		73600	1010290000	4	96.00
431	10/29/2010	11		EAPCPAY	1010290000	4	-20.00
	Patient Totals						130.00
FITZWJO0	John Fitzwilliams				(614)002-1111		
	Last Payment: -13.72		On: 10/4/2010				
471	9/7/2010	11		99211	0506020000	2	36.00
472	9/7/2010	11		84478	0506020000	2	29.00
592	10/4/2010		#214778924 ChampVA	CHVPAY	0506020000	2	-5.68
593	10/4/2010		Adjustment	CHVADJ	0506020000	2	-15.32
594	10/4/2010		#214778924 ChampVA	CHVPAY	0506020000	2	-8.04
595	10/4/2010		Adjustment	CHVADJ	0506020000	2	-20.96
380	9/7/2010	11		CHVCPAY	1009070000	2	-15.00
585	10/4/2010	11		99212	1010040000	2	54.00
586	10/4/2010	11		82270	1010040000	2	19.00
587	10/4/2010	11		CHVCPAY	1010040000	2	-15.00
	Patient Totals						58.00
GILESSH0	Sheila Giles				(614)303-0579		
	Last Payment: -130.40		On: 11/4/2010				
432	10/29/2010	11		99213	1010290000	5	72.00
433	10/29/2010	11		87430	1010290000	5	29.00
434	10/29/2010	11		71010	1010290000	5	91.00
612	11/4/2010		#001234 Blue Cross/Blue Shiel	BCBPAY	1010290000	5	-57.60
613	11/4/2010		#001234 Blue Cross/Blue Shiel	BCBPAY	1010290000	5	0.00
614	11/4/2010		#001234 Blue Cross/Blue Shiel	BCBPAY	1010290000	5	-72.80
	Patient Totals						61.60
HSUDIAN0	Diane Hsu				(614)022-0202		
	Last Payment: -20.00		On: 10/29/2010				
435	10/29/2010	11		99213	1010290000	4	72.00
436	10/29/2010	11		80048	1010290000	4	50.00
438	10/29/2010	11		EAPCPAY	1010290000	4	-20.00
	Patient Totals						102.00

Figure 9-18 Patient Account Ledger report

PATIENT LEDGER REPORTS

A **patient ledger** lists the financial activity in each patient's account, including charges, payments, and adjustments (see Figure 9-18). This information is especially useful if there is a question about a patient's account. A full set of patient ledgers details the status of every patient's account.

patient ledger a report that lists the financial activity in each patient's account, including charges, payments, and adjustments

Patient ledgers are printed by clicking Patient Ledger on the Reports menu. The Data Selection Questions dialog box is displayed, as it is with other reports. The dialog box in this case provides options to select by chart numbers, patient reference balances, dates, and providers. A patient ledger is generated only for data that meet the selection criteria. If any selection box is left blank, all values are included in the report.

EXERCISE 9-6

Print patient ledgers for July 2010 for patients whose last names begin with the letters *R* through *W*.

Date: July 31, 2010

1. On the Reports menu, click Patient Ledger. The Data Selections Questions dialog box is displayed.

2. Key *R* in the first box of the Chart Number Range box and then click on the first chart number that begins with an *R* (RAMOSMA0) to select it. Press Tab to move to the next box, and key *W*. Notice that the program stopped at the first patient with a last name beginning with *W*. To include all patients with last names beginning with *W*, key *WR* to select Lisa Wright, the last patient, and press Tab.

3. Change the entry in the first Date From Range box to 07/01/2010 and the entry in the second box to 07/31/2010.

4. Make certain that the Print one patient per page box is not checked.

5. If it is not already checked, be sure to check the Show Accounts Receivable Totals box.

6. Click the Preview Report button.

7. Send the report to the printer.

8. Exit the Report Preview window.

STANDARD PATIENT LISTS

Medisoft includes several convenient reports for identifying patients by diagnosis, procedure, or insurance carrier. These reports are accessed via the Standard Patient Lists submenu (see Figure 9-19).

The Patient by Diagnosis report lists diagnosis code, chart number, patient name, age, attending provider, facility, and date of last visit.

The Patient by Procedure report lists chart number, patient name, age, and date of last visit for each procedure code. Data in the report can be grouped by facility or by provider.

The Patient by Insurance Carrier report lists patients, sorted by provider or facility, and then their insurance carrier.

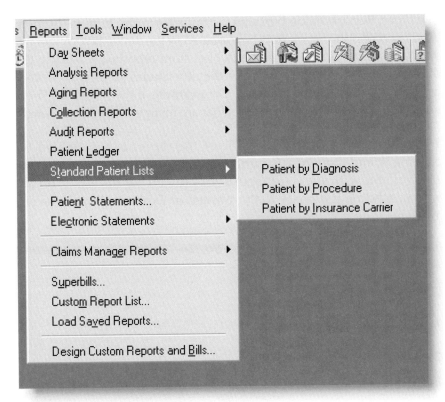

Figure 9-19   The Standard Patient Lists submenu

CUSTOM REPORTS

Medisoft has already created a number of custom reports using the built-in Report Designer. These reports include:

◆ Lists of addresses, billing codes, EDI receivers, patients, patient recalls, procedure codes, providers, and referring providers

◆ The CMS-1500 and Medicare CMS-1500 forms in a variety of printer formats

◆ Patient statements and walkout receipts

◆ Superbills (encounter forms)

When Custom Report List is clicked on the Reports menu, the Open Report dialog box, listing a variety of custom reports already created in Medisoft using the Report Designer, is displayed (see Figure 9-20). Additional custom reports can be created using the Report Designer. When a new custom report is created, it is added to the list of custom reports that is displayed on the screen.

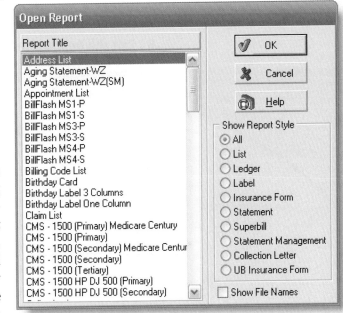

Figure 9-20   Open Report dialog box

The Open Report dialog box also contains ten radio buttons that are used to control the list of reports displayed in the dialog box. When the All radio button is clicked, all types of custom reports are listed in the dialog box. However, when one of the other radio buttons is clicked, only reports of that style are listed. For example, if the Insurance Form radio button is clicked, only reports that are insurance forms are listed.

SHORT CUT   To print a custom report, double-click the report title.

To print a custom report, the title of the report is highlighted by clicking it, and then the OK button is clicked. The same options that are available with standard reports for previewing the report on the screen, sending it directly to the printer, or exporting it to a file are available with custom reports.

EXERCISE 9-7

Print a list of all patients.

Date: July 31, 2010

1. On the Reports menu, click Custom Report List.
2. Select Patient List. Click the OK button.
3. Click the radio button to preview the report on the screen. Click the Start button.
4. Leave the Chart Number Range boxes blank to select all patients.
5. Click the OK button.
6. View the report on the screen. Notice the toolbar that appears in the window for a custom report is somewhat simplified compared to the toolbar that appears with other reports.
7. Send the report to the printer.
8. Exit the Report Preview window.

EXERCISE 9-8

Print a list of all procedure codes in the database.

Date: July 31, 2010

1. On the Reports menu, click Custom Report List.
2. In the Show Report Style section of the dialog box, click the List radio button so that only list styles are displayed.
3. Select Procedure Code List. Click the OK button.
4. Click the radio button to preview the report on the screen. Click the Start button.

5. Leave the Code 1 Range boxes blank to select all procedure codes. Click the OK button.

6. View the report on the screen.

7. Send the report to the printer.

8. Exit the Report Preview window.

USING REPORT DESIGNER

Medisoft's Report Designer provides maximum flexibility and control over data in the report and over how the data are displayed. Formatting styles include list, ledger, statement, and insurance. Reports can be created from scratch, or an existing report can be used as a starting point. The details of how to create new custom reports with the Report Designer are beyond the coverage of this book, but Exercise 9-9 offers practice working with the Report Designer to modify an existing report. The Report Designer is accessed by clicking Design Custom Reports and Bills on the Reports menu. This action causes the Report Designer window to be displayed (see Figure 9-21).

Figure 9-21 The Report Designer window

EXERCISE 9-9

Modify the Patient List report so that a work telephone number replaces a home telephone number in the report.

Date: July 31, 2010

1. On the Reports menu, click Design Custom Reports and Bills. The Report Designer window is displayed.

2. Click Open Report on the File menu. The Open Report dialog box is displayed.

3. Double-click Patient List in the list. The Patient List report is displayed (see Figure 9-22).

4. Double-click Phone, which appears between the two horizontal black lines near the top of the report, to select it. Then, double-click Phone again to edit it. The Text Properties dialog box is displayed (see Figure 9-23).

5. Enter **Work Phone** in the Text box that currently reads "Phone."

6. Since *Work Phone* contains more letters than *Phone,* it is necessary to lengthen the space allotted for the label on the report so all the letters can be displayed. This is done in the section of the dialog box labeled Size. Click in the Auto Size box to deselect that option. In the Width box, delete the existing entry by using the Backspace key, and enter **120**.

7. Click the OK button. Work Phone is displayed in the band where Phone used to be.

8. In the green band below the band in which Work Phone appears, click the Phone 1 box to select it. Then double-click the Phone 1 box again to edit its contents. The Data Field Properties dialog box is displayed (see Figure 9-24).

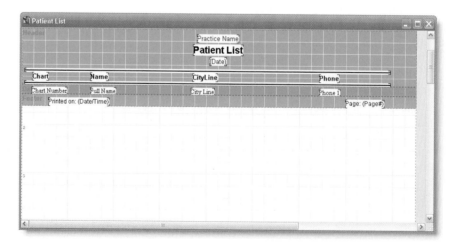

Figure 9-22   Patient List report open in Medisoft Report Designer

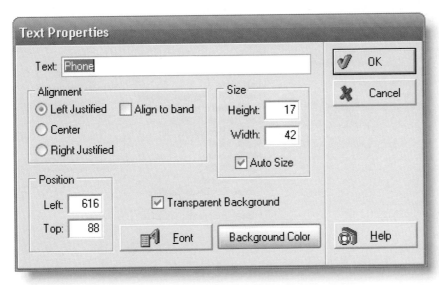

Figure 9-23 Text Properties dialog box

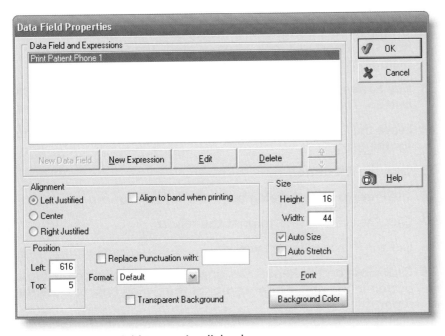

Figure 9-24 Data Field Properties dialog box

9. The current data box, Print Patient Phone 1, is active in the Data Field and Expressions box. Click the Edit button to change this box. The Select Data Field dialog box is displayed (see Figure 9-25).

10. In the Fields column, scroll down, highlight Work Phone, and click OK. The Data Field and Expressions box now lists Print Patient Work Phone.

11. To increase the space allotted in the report for this new value, click the Auto Size box to deselect it. Then go to the Width box, delete the existing entry, and key **120**. Click the OK button. Work Phone is displayed where Phone 1 used to be.

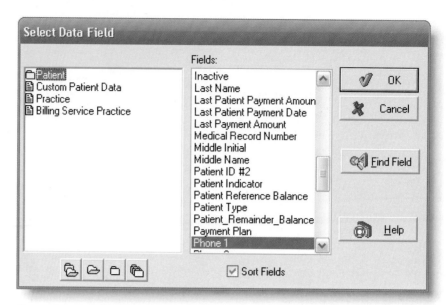

Figure 9-25   Select Data Field dialog box

12. On the Report Designer File menu, click Preview Report to see how the report will look when printed. The Save Report As . . . dialog box is displayed.

13. Key *Patient List—Work* in the Report Title box. Click the OK button. The Data Selection Questions dialog box is displayed.

14. Leave the Chart Number Range boxes blank to select all patients for the report.

15. Click the OK button.

16. The Preview Report dialog box is displayed, showing the report.

17. Click the Print button to print the report.

18. Exit the Preview Report window.

19. Click Close on the Report Designer File menu, or click the Close button in the upper-right corner of the dialog box, to close the report file.

20. Click Exit on the File menu, or click the Exit button on the toolbar, to leave Medisoft's Report Designer.

21. Select Custom Report List on the Reports menu. Scroll down and confirm that Patient List—Work appears in the list of custom reports. Click Cancel to close the Open Report dialog box.

ON YOUR OWN EXERCISE 8 Print a Patient Day Sheet

September 6, 2010

Print a Patient Day Sheet for September 6, 2010.

Electronic Medical Record Exchange

Viewing Data Transfer Reports

In addition to the many standard reports available in Medisoft, the Communications Manager program provides reports on inbound and outbound data transfers to and from an electronic medical record. Communications Manager is the program that makes it possible for Medisoft and an electronic medical record to exchange information.

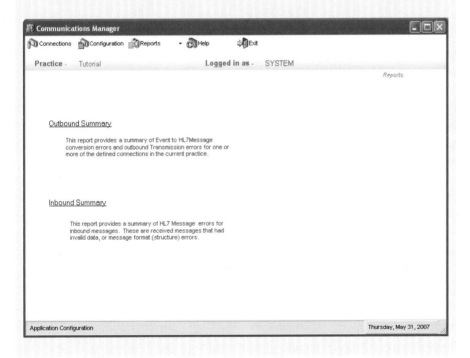

Name: _____ Date: _____

CHAPTER 9 WORKSHEET

After completing all the exercises in the chapter, answer the following questions in the spaces provided. You will need to refer to your printouts of the reports created in the exercises to complete this worksheet.

1. In the Patient Day Sheet created in Exercise 9-1, what is the total of the adjustments to Jonathan Bell's account?

    _____

2. In the Patient Day Sheet created in Exercise 9-1, what is the patient's balance on John Fitzwilliams's account?

    _____

3. In the Procedure Day Sheet created in Exercise 9-2, how many procedures were listed for the day of the report?

    _____

4. In the Payment Day Sheet created in Exercise 9-3, which provider had the highest total payments?

    _____

5. In the Practice Analysis report created in Exercise 9-4, what were the total insurance payments?

    _____

6. In the Patient Aging Applied Payment report created in Exercise 9-5, what amount of outstanding revenue is 61–90 days past due?

    _____

7. In the Patient Account Ledger created in Exercise 9-6, what is the amount of the Medicare payment on July 20, 2010?

    _____

8. According to the Patient Day Sheet created in On Your Own Exercise 8, how many procedures were performed on September 6, 2010?

    _____

9. According to the Practice Analysis report created in On Your Own Exercise 9, what is the amount of the check copayments?

    _____

10. According to the Practice Analysis report created in On Your Own Exercise 9, what is the amount of charges for procedure code 99212?

    _____

CHAPTER REVIEW

USING TERMINOLOGY

Match the terms on the left with the definitions on the right.

_____ **1.** aging report

_____ **2.** day sheet

_____ **3.** insurance aging report

_____ **4.** patient aging report

_____ **5.** patient day sheet

_____ **6.** patient ledger

_____ **7.** payment day sheet

_____ **8.** practice analysis report

_____ **9.** procedure day sheet

a. A summary of the activity of a patient on a given day.

b. A report that lists the amount of money owed the practice, organized by the length of time the money has been owed.

c. A report that provides information on practice activities for a twenty-four-hour period.

d. A report that lists the financial activity in each patient's account, including charges, payments, and adjustments.

e. A report that lists a patient's balance by age, the date and amount of the last payment, and the telephone number.

f. A report that lists payments received on a given day, organized by provider.

g. A report that analyzes the revenue of a practice for a specified period of time, usually a month or a year.

h. A report that lists the procedures performed on a given day, listed in numerical order.

i. A report that lists how long a payer has taken to respond to insurance claims.

CHECKING YOUR UNDERSTANDING

Answer the questions below in the space provided.

10. What is the difference between a patient day sheet and a procedure day sheet?

_____

_____

11. What is the name of the dialog box that provides options for filtering data included on a report?

_____

_____

12. What is the difference between a patient aging report and a patient aging applied report?

_____

_____

13. Which entries print in a report if the boxes in the Data Selection Questions dialog box are left blank?

_____

_____

APPLYING KNOWLEDGE

Answer the questions below in the space provided.

14. One of the providers in a practice asks for a report of yesterday's transactions. How would this report be created?

_____

_____

15. A patient is unsure whether she mailed a check last month for an outstanding balance on her account. How could you use Medisoft's reports feature to help answer her question?

_____

_____

Collections in the Medical Office

10

WHAT YOU NEED TO KNOW

To use this chapter, you need to know how to:

◆ Start Medisoft, use menus, and enter and edit text.

◆ Work with chart numbers and codes.

◆ Create an aging report.

LEARNING OUTCOMES

When you finish this chapter, you will be able to:

◆ Explain the importance of a financial policy in a medical practice.

◆ Identify the laws that regulate collections from patients.

◆ Describe the role of a collection agency in obtaining payment on overdue accounts.

◆ Discuss what happens to uncollectible accounts in the medical practice.

◆ Use a patient aging report to identify past due patient accounts.

◆ Create a collection report.

◆ Create collection letters.

◆ Create a Collection Tracer report.

KEY TERMS

collection agency
collection list
Collection Tracer report
payment plan
prompt payment laws
tickler
uncollectible accounts

THE IMPORTANCE OF COLLECTIONS IN THE MEDICAL PRACTICE

The average patient is now responsible for paying nearly 35 percent of medical bills, more than three times the amount paid by a patient in 1980, according to the Centers for Medicare and Medicaid Services (CMS). While most patients pay their bills on time, every practice has some patients who do not. Patients' reasons for not paying range from forgetfulness or inability to pay to dissatisfaction with the services or charges. The office staff may be asked to work with patients to resolve problems and collect payments.

At the same time, third-party payers often dispute claims. They may contend that patient care services were not medically necessary or that the method in which services were provided violated the payer-provider contract. When a carrier contests a claim or delays payment because more information is needed, providers frequently are not given notice in a timely manner. When further documentation is requested and the physician provides the information, an insurer or health plan can further delay payment by asking for additional information or clarification. Resubmitting rejected claims is a time-consuming process, resulting in increased practice expenses and more delay in payment.

THE PATIENT COLLECTION PROCESS

The patient collection process begins with a clear financial policy and effective communications with patients about their financial responsibilities. When patients understand the charges and the practice's financial policy in advance, collecting payments is not usually problematic. As a result, it is important to have a written financial policy that spells out patients' responsibilities.

The financial policy of a medical practice explains how the practice handles financial matters. When new patients register, they should be given copies of the financial policy along with the practice's HIPAA privacy policies and patient registration material. The policy should tell patients how the practice handles:

- Collecting copayments and past-due balances
- Setting up financial arrangements for unpaid balances
- Providing charity care or using a sliding scale for patients with low incomes
- Collecting payments for services not covered by insurance
- Collecting prepayment for services
- Accepting cash, checks, money orders, and credit cards

Figure 10-1 shows a sample financial policy of a medical practice.

Financial Policy of
Any Medical Practice
Any Town, USA

Thank you for choosing Any Medical Practice for your health care needs. The following information is being provided to assist you in understanding our financial policies and to address the questions most frequently asked by our patients.

Account Responsibility
You are responsible for all charges incurred on your account. It is also your responsibility to make sure all information on your account is current and accurate. Incorrect information can cause payment delays, which may result in late fees being applied to your account. Many people are under the impression that it is up to the physician and staff to make sure that all charges are paid or covered by insurance. This is not the case. Please remember that the insurance contract is between you and the insurance company, not the physician. It is your responsibility to know what your contract covers and pays and to communicate this to physicians and staff. Therefore, you are responsible for charges incurred regardless of insurance coverage.

Insurance Billing
If you have medical insurance, we will be happy to bill your insurance carrier for you. As a courtesy we will also bill the carrier of any secondary insurance coverage that you may have. Any Medical Practice contracts with many insurance companies, but due to the fact that these companies have many different plans available, it is impossible for us to know if your specific plan is included. You will need to check with your insurance company in advance. Please remember that your insurance may not cover or pay all charges incurred. Any unpaid balance after insurance is your responsibility.

Copays
All copays are due at time of service. A $5.00 billing fee is assessed if your copay is not paid at time of service. This fee will not be waived. It is your responsibility to know whether your insurance requires you to pay a copay.

No Insurance
If you have no insurance, payment in full is expected at time of service, unless payment arrangements have been made prior to your visit.

Late Fees
All patient balances are to be paid in full within 60 days. This refers to balances after your insurance has paid. If you are unable to pay your balance in full within 60 days, please contact the business office to set up a payment plan. A late fee of $20.00 per month will be assessed on patient balances over 60 days.

Cash Only
If your account has been turned over to collection, it will also be changed to a cash-only account. This means that all services will need to be paid in full at time of service. A letter will be sent to inform you if your account has been changed to a cash-only basis.

Dishonored Checks
A $25.00 service charge will be assessed on all dishonored checks.

Payment Methods
Any Medical Practice accepts cash, personal checks, and the following credit cards: Visa, MasterCard, American Express, and Discover. Payments can be made at any reception area. For your convenience, an ATM machine is located in the lobby of the building.

Figure 10-1   A sample medical practice financial policy

Despite the practice's efforts to communicate the financial policy to all patients, some individuals still do not pay in full and on time. Medical insurance specialists are often responsible for some aspect of the collection process. Each practice sets its own procedures. Large bills have priority over smaller ones. Usually, an automatic reminder notice and a second statement are mailed when a bill has not been paid within thirty days after it was issued. Some practices phone a patient whose account is thirty days overdue. If the bill is not then paid, a series of collection letters is generated at intervals, each more stringent in tone and more direct in approach. Table 10-1 provides an example of one practice's collection timeline; different approaches are used in other practices.

Laws Governing Patient Collections

Collections from insurance carriers are considered business collections. Collections from patients, however, are consumer collections and are regulated by federal and state laws. The Fair Debt Collection Practices Act of 1977 and the Telephone Consumer Protection Act of 1991 regulate debt collections, forbidding unfair practices. General guidelines include the following:

◆ Do not call a patient before 8 A.M. or after 9 P.M.

◆ Do not make threats or use profane language.

◆ Do not discuss the patient's debt with anyone except the person who is responsible for payment. If the patient has a lawyer, discuss the problem only with the lawyer, unless the lawyer gives permission to talk with the patient.

◆ Do not use any form of deception or violence to collect a debt. For example, do not impersonate a law officer to try to force a patient to pay.

If the practice's printed or displayed payment policy covers adding finance charges on late accounts, it is acceptable to do so. The amount of the finance charge must comply with federal and state law.

Table 10-1	Patient Collection Timeline
30 days	Bill patient
45 days	Call patient regarding bill
60 days	Letter 1
75 days	Letter 2 and call
80 days	Letter 3
90 days	Turn over to collections

Working with Collection Agencies

After a number of collection attempts that do not produce results, some practices use collection agencies to pursue large unpaid bills. A **collection agency** is an outside firm hired to collect on delinquent accounts. The agency that is selected should have a reputation for fair and ethical handling of collections.

When a patient's account is referred to an agency for collection, the medical insurance specialist no longer contacts the patient or sends statements. If a payment is received from a patient while the account is with the agency, the agency is notified. Collection agencies are often paid on the basis of the amount of money they collect.

collection agency an outside firm hired to collect on delinquent accounts

Using Payment Plans

For large bills or special situations, some practices may offer payment plans to patients. A **payment plan** is an agreement between a patient and a practice in which the patient agrees to make regular monthly payments over a specified period of time. If no finance charges are applied to unpaid balances, this type of arrangement is between the practice and the patient, and no legal regulations apply. If, however, the practice adds finance charges and the payments are to be made in more than four installments, the arrangement is subject to the Truth in Lending Act, which is part of the Consumer Credit Protection Act. In this case, the practice notifies the patient in writing about the total amount, the finance charges (stated as a percentage), when each payment is due and the amount, and the date the last payment is due. The agreement must be signed by the practice manager and the patient.

payment plan an agreement between a patient and a practice in which the patient agrees to make regular monthly payments over a specified period of time

Writing Off Uncollectible Accounts

When all collection attempts have been exhausted and the cost of continuing to pursue the debt is higher than the total amount owed, the collection process is ended. Medical practices have policies on how to handle bills they do not expect to collect. Usually, the amount owed is called an **uncollectible account** or a bad debt, and it is written off the practice's expected accounts receivable.

uncollectible account an account that does not respond to collection efforts and is written off the practice's expected accounts receivable

TIP In the Medicare and Medicaid programs, it is fraudulent to forgive or write off any payments that beneficiaries are responsible for, such as copayments or coinsurance, unless a rigid set of steps has been followed to verify the patient's financial situation. Similarly, it is fraudulent to discount services for other providers or their families, which was formerly a common practice.

LAWS GOVERNING TIMELY PAYMENT OF INSURANCE CLAIMS

prompt payment laws state laws that mandate a time period within which clean claims must be paid; if they are not, financial penalties are levied against the payer

Most states have enacted prompt payment laws to ensure that claims are paid in a timely manner. **Prompt payment laws** are state laws that mandate a time period within which clean claims must be paid and that call for financial penalties to be levied against late payers. (Clean claims are error-free claims that do not require additional documentation.) For example, under the New York Prompt Payment Law, when a managed care organization or insurance company fails to make payment on a clean claim within forty-five days of submission, the physician is entitled to receive interest on the late payment at the rate of 12 percent per year. In Texas, payers can be fined up to $1,000 per day for each claim that remains unpaid in violation of the prompt payment requirements.

If a clean claim is not paid within the allotted time frame, the payer should be notified in writing that payment has not been received according to applicable prompt payment laws. Practices should also request written explanations for all claim delays, partial payments, and denials. If satisfaction is not achieved, the applicable state or federal regulatory agency may be notified of the violation.

USING A PRACTICE MANAGEMENT PROGRAM FOR COLLECTION ACTIVITIES

Medical practices frequently use practice management software to monitor collection activities. While specific collection features vary from program to program, common features used for this purpose include aging reports, collection lists, collection letters, and collection reports.

The collection process begins with an analysis of the aging report, which shows the status of each account over time. Aging begins on the date the statement or claim was sent. For each account, an aging report shows the name of the patient, the last payment amount and date, and the amount of unpaid charges in each of these categories:

◆ Current: Up to thirty days

◆ Past: Thirty-one to sixty days

◆ Past: Sixty-one to ninety days

◆ Past: More than ninety-one days

Figure 10-2 shows a sample patient aging report created in Medisoft.

Family Care Center
Patient Aging Applied Payment
by Date From
From January 01, 2010 to September 30, 2010

Chart # Name	Birthdate	Current 0 - 30	Past 31 - 60	Past 61 - 90	Past 91 +	Total Balance
JONESEL0 Jones, Elizabeth	8/26/1936	72.00	21.17	7.47	0.00	100.64
Last Pmt: -20.58 On: 9/30/2010	(614)123-5555					
KLEINRA0 Klein, Randall	10/11/1953	0.00	5.80	0.00	0.00	5.80
Last Pmt: -23.18 On: 9/17/2010	(614)022-2693					
WONGJO10 Wong, Jo	9/6/1940	0.00	7.47	0.00	7.47	14.94
Last Pmt: -29.89 On: 9/14/2010	(614)029-7777					
WONGLIY0 Wong, Li Y	12/13/1938	0.00	4.14	0.00	0.00	4.14
Last Pmt: -16.54 On: 9/14/2010	(614)029-7777					
Report Aging Total		$72.00	$38.58	$7.47	$7.47	$125.52
Percent of Aging Total		57.4%	31.4%	5.6%	5.6%	100.0%

Figure 10-2   Sample Patient Aging Applied Payment report

EXERCISE 10-1

Review the Patient Aging Applied Payment report displayed in Figure 10-2. Using the information contained in the report, locate the patient account that is ninety-one or more days overdue. List the chart number, patient name, and account balance below.

Chart #	Name	Past 31–60	Past 61–90	Past 91+

USING THE COLLECTION LIST

Once overdue accounts have been identified, the next step is to add collection items to a collection list. The **collection list** is designed to track activities that need to be completed as part of the collection process. Ticklers or collection reminders are displayed as collection list items. A **tickler** is a reminder to follow-up on an account that is entered on the collection list.

In Medisoft, the selections for the Collection List feature are located on the Activities menu (see Figure 10-3).

The Collection List dialog box displays ticklers that have already been entered into the database (see Figure 10-4).

collection list a tool for tracking activities that need to be completed as part of the collection process

tickler a reminder to follow up on an account

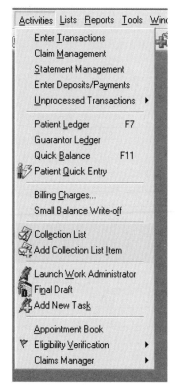

Figure 10-3 Collection List options on the Activities menu

Options for controlling what appears in the Collection List dialog box are at the top of the dialog box and include the following:

Date Items can be displayed for the current date, for a range of dates, or for all dates. By default, the current date (the Windows System Date) is used as the range of dates, and only those tickler items that are due on that date are displayed. To see all ticklers regardless of the date, click the Show All Ticklers box.

Show All Ticklers A check in this box results in the listing of all tickler items.

Show Deleted Only A check in this box displays only ticklers that have been deleted.

Exclude Deleted A check in this box indicates that deleted ticklers are not displayed.

The Collection List dialog box contains the following information about each tickler item:

Item This unique number identifying a tickler item is assigned automatically by the program.

Responsible Party This field contains the chart number (patient/guarantor) or insurance code (insurance carrier) that identifies the responsible party for this item. By clicking the plus sign (+) to the left of the entry, the field can be expanded to view more information about the responsible party.

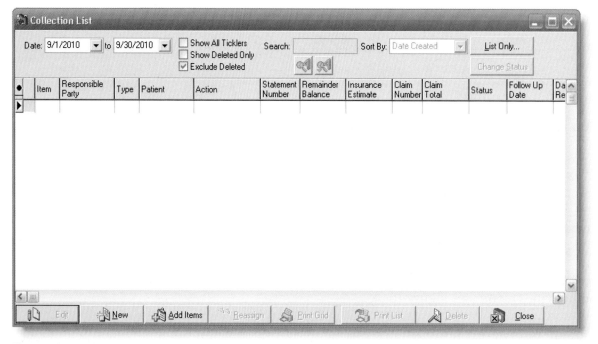

Figure 10-4 Collection List dialog box

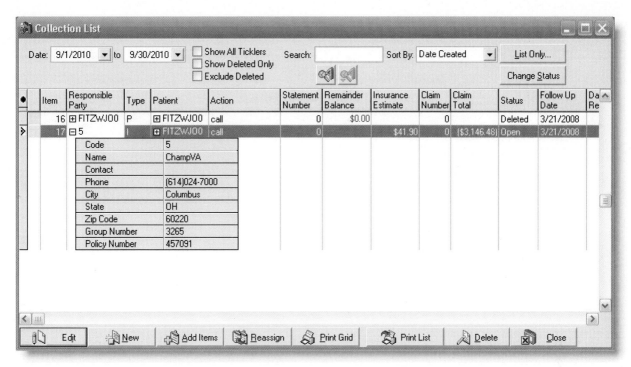

Figure 10-5 Additional information displayed when the responsible party is an insurance carrier

When the responsible party is an insurance carrier, the following additional information appears (see Figure 10-5):

◆ Code

◆ Name

◆ Contact

◆ Phone

◆ City

◆ State

◆ Zip Code

◆ Group Number

◆ Policy Number

When the responsible party is a guarantor, the following additional information is displayed (see Figure 10-6):

◆ Chart Number

◆ Name

◆ City

◆ Zip Code

◆ Phone 1

◆ Patient Reference Balance

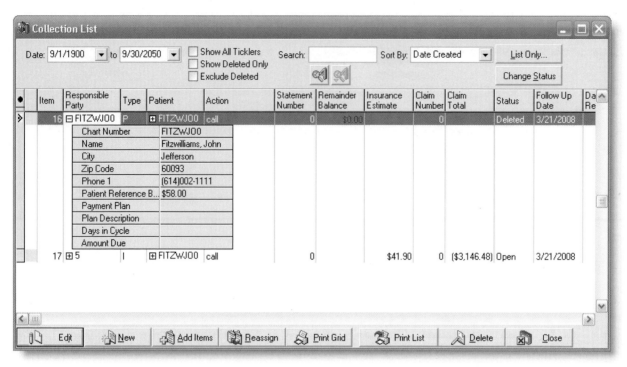

Figure 10-6   Additional information displayed when the responsible party is a guarantor

◆ Payment Plan

◆ Plan Description

◆ Days in Cycle

◆ Amount Due

Type   The type is either a *P* for *Patient* or an *I* for *Insurance*. If the type is P, the responsible party is a patient. If the type is I, the responsible party is the insurance carrier.

Patient   This field contains the patient chart number for this tickler. By clicking the plus sign (+), it can be expanded to get more information on the patient (see Figure 10-7).

The additional information displayed includes:

◆ Chart Number

◆ Last Name

◆ First Name

◆ Middle Initial

◆ Phone 1

◆ Zip Code

◆ Date of Birth

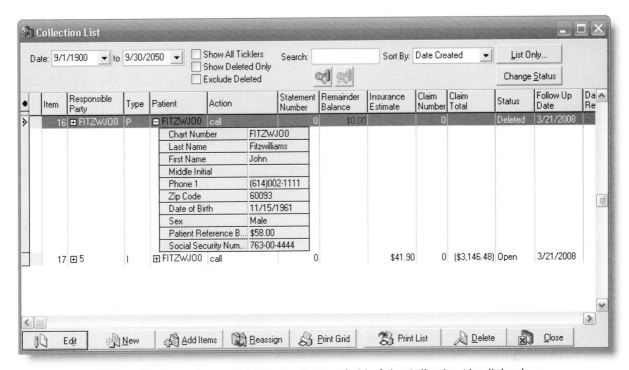

Figure 10-7   Additional information available in the Patient field of the Collection List dialog box

◆   Sex

◆   Patient Reference Balance

◆   Social Security Number

Other information in the Collection List dialog box includes the following:

Action   This field lists the action required. To see all of the text entered for this field, double-click in the field. This opens a window to view the complete text entry.

Statement Number   If the tickler is for a patient, the statement number is listed.

Remainder Balance   If the responsible type is Patient, the balance reported is the patient's balance as listed in Transaction Entry. If the responsible type is Insurance, the balance reported is an estimated balance for the patient's specified carrier. This is the balance at the time the tickler is created. This balance does not refresh when payments are made to the patient's account. To manually update the amounts, the tickler must be edited and saved again.

Insurance Estimate   This field displays an estimate of the amount of payment expected from the insurance carrier.

Claim Number   If the tickler is for an insurance carrier, the claim number is listed in this column.

Claim Total   If the tickler is for an insurance carrier, the total amount of charges on the claim is listed here.

Status   The entries in the field are Open, Resolved, or Deleted.

Follow Up Date   This is the date the tickler will appear on the collection list.

Date Resolved   This is the date that the status of the item was changed to Resolved. Resolution is determined by the user.

User ID   The User ID identifies the user who is responsible for following up on the item. In an actual practice, users are assigned login names and passwords in the Security Setup area of the program.

ENTERING A TICKLER ITEM

A new tickler item is created by pressing the New button in the Collection List dialog box. The Tickler Item dialog box is displayed in Figure 10-8.

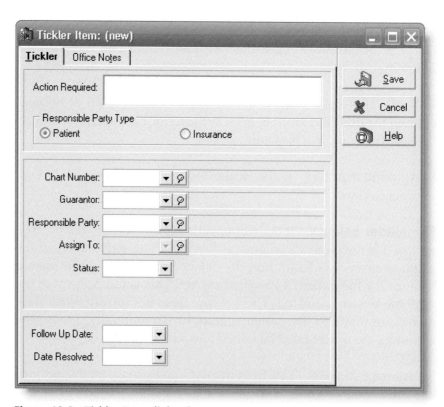

Figure 10-8   Tickler Item dialog box

The Tickler Item dialog box contains two tabs for information: Tickler and Office Notes.

Tickler Tab

The following information is entered in the Tickler tab:

Action Required   Action Required specifies the action that is to be taken to remedy the problem. Up to eighty characters of text can be entered.

Responsible Party Type   The button selected in this field indicates whether the patient or the insurance carrier is responsible for the account balance. This entry also controls the contents of the drop-down lists for the Responsible Party field below.

Chart Number   The patient's chart number is selected from the list.

Guarantor   The Guarantor field lists the account guarantor chart number for this tickler item.

Responsible Party   If the responsible party type is Patient, a chart number is selected from the drop-down list. If the responsible party type is Insurance, the code for an insurance carrier is selected.

Assign To   The Assign To box lists the name of the individual responsible for following up on the tickler item. These names are set up by selecting Security Setup on the File menu. *Note:* This feature is not demonstrated in this text/workbook, so the field is grayed out, and an entry cannot be made.

Status   The status of the tickler item is chosen from a drop-down list. The options are Open, Resolved, or Deleted.

Follow Up Date   This is the date the tickler will appear on the collection list if the Date range in the Collection List window is used. By default, Medisoft enters the current date—the Windows System Date—in this field.

Date Resolved   This field lists the date on which the status of the item was changed to Resolved. When the status is set to Resolved, the Date Resolved is set to the current date. Again, this is determined by the Windows System Date.

Office Notes Tab

The Office Notes tab consists of several buttons and a large area in which to enter notes. Notes that relate to the collection process of the selected tickler are entered in the large box.

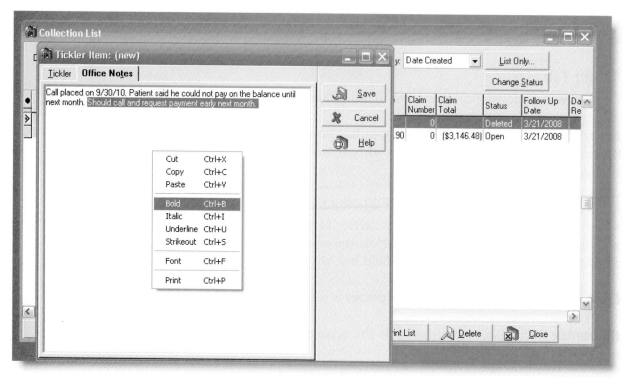

Figure 10-9 Office Notes tab of the Tickler Item dialog box with shortcut menu displayed

When the right mouse button is clicked within the typing area, a shortcut menu is displayed (see Figure 10-9). Using this menu, notes can be edited, formatted, and printed from within the Office Notes tab.

Once a new tickler has been saved, the program automatically assigns a unique identifier code to the item.

EXERCISE 10-2

Using the information in Exercise 10-1, create a tickler item for the patient whose account is more than ninety days overdue.

Date: November 5, 2010

1. Start Medisoft and restore the data from your last work session. Change the Medisoft Program Date to November 5, 2010.

2. Select Collection List on the Activities menu.

3. Change the entries in the Date fields to *10/01/2010* and *11/30/2010*. (*Note:* It is not necessary to enter the slashes when keying in the dates.)

4. Click the New button to display the Tickler Item dialog box.

5. In the Action Required box, enter *Telephone call about overdue balance. See notes.*

6. Select Patient as the Responsible Party Type.

7. Select the patient's chart number in the Chart Number field.

8. Select the guarantor in the Guarantor field.

9. Complete the Responsible Party field.

10. Leave the Assign to field blank. (In a real practice setting, this field would contain the name of the staff member who was assigned to follow up on this collection list item.)

11. Set the Status of the item to Open.

12. Change the entry in the Follow-up Date field to **November 12, 2010.**

13. Leave the Date Resolved field blank.

14. Click on the Office Notes tab, and enter the following text: **Patient said she could not pay the balance on the account until her November Social Security check was deposited. Call to follow-up.**

15. Click the Save button. The item is added to the Collection List.

16. Close the Collection List dialog box.

TIP When an account is added to the collection list, the current balance for the tickler is determined. Once recorded in the tickler, it is not updated when new transactions are entered in the program.

For patient-responsible ticklers, the balance is the balance shown in Transaction Entry. It could also include insurance balances. For insurance-responsible ticklers, the balance is the estimated amount due from the assigned insurance carrier.

CREATING COLLECTION LETTERS

A number of actions must be taken within Medisoft before collection letters can be sent. A patient-responsible tickler item for the patient's account must be entered in the collection list. Also, a Collection Letter report must be printed. This report is generated when the Patient Collection Letters option is selected on the Reports menu. The Patient Collection report lists patients with overdue accounts to whom statements have been mailed (see Figure 10-10 on page 278).

After the Patient Collection report is printed (or the Preview window is closed), the program displays a Confirm window that asks whether to print collection letters (see Figure 10-11 on page 278).

Patient Collection

11/5/2010

	Statement Number	Initial Bill Date	Last Bill Date	Last Patient Pay Date	Last Patient Pay Amount	Submission Count	Statement Type	Statement Total
JONESEL0- Jones, Elizabeth				Phone: (614)123-5555				
	8	9/30/2010	4/2/2008			3	Remainder	$28.64
								$28.64
KLEINRA0- Klein, Randall				Phone: (614)022-2693				
	9	9/30/2010	4/2/2008			3	Remainder	$5.80
								$5.80
SIMMOJI0- Simmons, Jill				Phone: (614)011-6767				
	11	4/2/2008	4/2/2008			1	Remainder	$21.00
								$21.00
WONGJO10- Wong, Jo				Phone: (614)029-7777				
	6	9/30/2010	9/30/2010			2	Remainder	$14.94
								$14.94

Figure 10-10   Patient Collection report

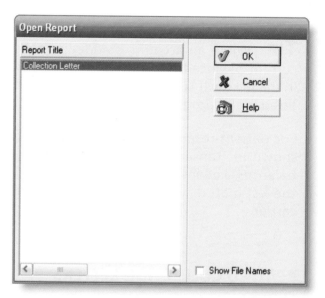

Figure 10-12   Open Report window for printing collection letters

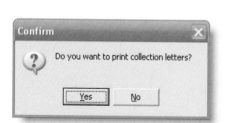

Figure 10-11   Confirm dialog box

If the Yes button is clicked, an Open Report dialog box appears (see Figure 10-12).

Once the OK button in the Open Report window is clicked, the program generates collection letters (see Figure 10-13).

After printing collection letters, an account alert appears in the Transaction Entry, Quick Ledger, and Appointment Entry windows

Family Care Center
285 Stephenson Boulevard
Stephenson, OH 60089
(614)555-0000

Jo Wong
736 East Street
Grandville, OH 60092

11/5/2010
Patient Account: Wong, Jo

Dear Jo Wong

Our records indicate that your account with us is overdue. The total unpaid amount is *$ 14.94

If you have already forwarded your payment, please disregard this letter; otherwise, please forward
your payment immediately.

Please contact us at (614)555-0000 if you have any questions or concerns about your account.

Sincerely,

Katherine Yan

WONGJO1

*Balance does not reflect any outstanding insurance payments

Figure 10-13 Patient collection letter

and remains until the patient no longer has an open tickler in the collection list. There are three account alert abbreviations:

- ◆ RB The patient has a remainder balance greater than the amount specified in the General tab in the Program Options window.

- ◆ DP The patient is delinquent on his or her payment plan.

- ◆ IC The patient account is in collections (for this message to appear, a collection letter must have been printed).

A sample account alert in the Transaction Entry window is displayed in Figure 10-14.

EXERCISE 10-3

Create collection letters.

Date: November 12, 2010

1. Select Collection Reports > Patient Collection Letters on the Reports menu. The Print Report Where? dialog box appears. Accept the default entry to preview the report on the screen, and click the Start button.

2. Make sure the three boxes at the bottom of the dialog box are checked: Exclude items that follow Payment Plan, Generate Collection Letters, and Add to Collection Tracer. Click Generate Collection Letters and Add to Collection Tracer. Do not change any other entries in the Data Selection Questions dialog box. Click the OK button. The Collection Letter report appears.

3. Click the Close button to exit the Preview window.

4. A Confirm dialog box is displayed, asking if collection letters should be printed. Click the Yes button. The Open Report window appears.

5. Select Collection letter if it is not already selected, and then click OK. Click the Start button to preview the letter.

6. The collection letter is displayed in the Preview window. Select the option to send the report directly to the printer. (*Note:* If the letter is not actually printed, the Account Alert message feature will not work.)

7. When you are finished printing the letter, click the Close button to close the Preview window.

8. Open the Transaction Entry dialog box, and select Jo Wong in the Chart field. Notice that the letters *RB IC* appear in red in the upper-left section of the window. This is an account alert message, indicating that the account has a remainder balance and is in collections. Close the Transaction Entry dialog box.

Note: The date shown in the collection letter is the current date—the Windows System Date. In an actual office setting, this date would be the actual date the letter was created.

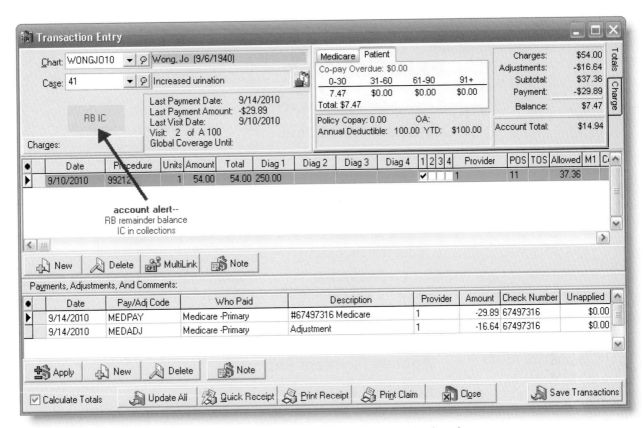

Figure 10-14   Transaction Entry dialog box with Account Alert message displayed

PRINTING A COLLECTION TRACER REPORT

A **Collection Tracer report** is used to keep track of collection letters that were sent. The report lists the tickler item number, the responsible party, the chart number, the account balance (as of the date the tickler was created), the date the collection letter was sent, and the reasons the account is in collections (see Figure 10-15).

Collection Tracer report   a tool for keeping track of collection letters that were sent

Family Care Center
Collection Tracer Report
11/1/2010

Item #	Responsible Party	Patient Chart	Balance	Date Letter Sent	Reasons
Jo Wong					
1	Jo Wong	WONGJO10	14.94	11/1/2010	The outstanding balance is greater than 0.01.

Total Letters Sent: 1

Figure 10-15   Collection Tracer report

EXERCISE 10-4

Create a Collection Tracer report.

Date: November 30, 2010

1. Select Collection Reports > Collection Tracer Report on the Reports menu.

2. In the Print Report Where? dialog box, click the Start button to preview the report on the screen.

3. Leave all boxes blank in the Data Selection Questions dialog box. Click the OK button.

4. The report appears in the Preview window. When you are finished viewing the report, close the Preview window.

ON YOUR OWN EXERCISE 10 Print a Patient Aging Applied Payment Report

November 30, 2010

Print a Patient Aging Applied Payment report for the period from 1/1/2010 to 11/30/2010. Review the status of Lisa Wright's account.

ON YOUR OWN EXERCISE 11 Add an Item to the Collection List

November 30, 2010

Add an item to the collection list for patient Lisa Wright. Notice that her account has an overdue balance. Enter a tickler for a telephone call about her account. Enter *12/7/2010* as the follow-up date.

ON YOUR OWN EXERCISE 12 Create a Collection Letter

December 14, 2010

Create a collection letter for Lisa Wright, since she did not respond to phone calls about her account.

Remember to create a backup of your work before exiting Medisoft! To help you keep track of your work, name the backup file after the chapter you are working on, for example, StudentID-c10.mbk.

CHAPTER 10 WORKSHEET

After completing all the exercises in the chapter, answer the following questions in the spaces provided.

1. In Exercise 10-1, what is the amount of the balance that is 91 or more days overdue?

   _____

2. In Exercise 10-2, who is listed in the Responsible Party field of the Tickler Item dialog box?

   _____

3. In Exercise 10-2, what is listed in the Status column of the Collection List dialog box?

   _____

4. In the Collection Letter report created in Exercise 10-3, what is listed in the Balance column?

   _____

5. After completing Exercise 10-3, what four letters are displayed under the Case field in the Transaction Entry dialog box for Jo Wong?

   _____

6. What is listed in the Reasons column of the Collection Tracer report created in Exercise 10-4?

   _____

7. In the report created in On Your Own Exercise 10, what percent of the aging total is 31–60 days late?

   _____

8. What is listed in the Guarantor field in the Tickler Item dialog box in On Your Own Exercise 11?

   _____

9. In On Your Own Exercise 11, what is listed as the Follow Up date for Lisa Wright?

   _____

10. In On Your Own Exercise 12, what is listed as the total unpaid amount in the letter to Lisa Wright?

    _____

CHAPTER REVIEW

USING TERMINOLOGY

Match the terms on the left with the definitions on the right.

_____ **1.** collection agency

_____ **2.** collection list

_____ **3.** Collection Tracer report

_____ **4.** payment plan

_____ **5.** prompt payment laws

_____ **6.** tickler

_____ **7.** uncollectible account

a. An agreement between a patient and a practice in which the patient agrees to make regular monthly payments over a specified period of time.

b. A reminder to follow up on an account.

c. An outside firm hired to collect on delinquent accounts.

d. An account that does not respond to collection efforts and is written off the practice's expected accounts receivable.

e. Legislation that mandates a time period within which clean claims must be paid; if they are not, financial penalties are levied against the payer.

f. A tool for tracking activities that need to be completed as part of the collection process.

g. A tool for tracking collection letters that were sent.

CHECKING YOUR UNDERSTANDING

Write "T" or "F" in the blank to indicate whether you think the statement is true or false.

8. Accounts that are overdue are treated equally; accounts with small balances are just as likely to be sent for collections as accounts with large balances. _____

9. Collection activities regarding patient accounts are considered business collections and are not regulated by federal or state law. _____

10. By law, payment plans cannot include finance charges. _____

11. Aging reports are used to determine which accounts are overdue. _____

12. An account is considered current if it is paid within thirty days. _____

13. A tickler item entered on the collection list includes a follow-up date for action. _____

Choose the best answer.

14. The entry in the Responsible Party field in the Collection List is either *P* for Patient or _____.

    a. *G* for Guarantor

    b. *C* for Child

    c. *I* for Insurance

15. General guidelines for telephone collection practices recommend not calling before 8:00 A.M. or after _____.

    a. 8:00 P.M.

    b. 9:00 P.M.

    c. 10:00 P.M.

16. An arrangement in which a patient agrees to make a regular monthly payment on an account for a specified period of time is known as a _____.

    a. financial plan

    b. payment plan

    c. payment policy

17. An account that must be written off the practice's expected accounts receivable is _____.

    a. an overdue account

    b. an uncollectible account

    c. a tickler account

APPLYING KNOWLEDGE

Answer the questions below in the space provided.

18. What is the purpose of a medical practice's financial policy?

_____

_____

19. What is the first step in the collection process?

_____

_____

20. How is an aging report used to identify accounts for collection?

_____

_____

21. What two steps need to occur before a collection letter can be printed in Medisoft?

_____

_____

AT THE COMPUTER

Answer the following question at the computer.

22. Create a Patient Aging Applied Payment report for the period ending December 31, 2010. Which overdue account has the largest outstanding balance (regardless of number of days past due)? How many account(s) are more than ninety days overdue?

_____

_____

Scheduling

11

WHAT YOU NEED TO KNOW

To use this chapter, you need to know how to:

◆ Start Medisoft, use menus, and enter and edit text.

◆ Work with chart numbers and codes.

◆ Locate patient information.

LEARNING OUTCOMES

When you finish this chapter, you will be able to:

◆ Start Office Hours.

◆ View the appointment schedule.

◆ Enter an appointment.

◆ Change or delete an appointment.

◆ Search for an appointment.

◆ Create a recall list.

◆ Enter a break in a provider's schedule.

◆ Print appointment schedules.

KEY TERMS

Office Hours break
Office Hours schedule

INTRODUCTION TO OFFICE HOURS

Appointment scheduling is one of the most important tasks in a medical office. Different medical procedures take different lengths of time, and each appointment must be the right length. On the one hand, a physician wants to be able to go from one appointment to another without unnecessary breaks. On the other hand, a patient should not be kept waiting more than a few minutes for a physician. Managing and juggling the schedule are usually the job of a medical office assistant working at the front desk. Medisoft provides a special program called Office Hours to handle appointment scheduling.

OVERVIEW OF THE OFFICE HOURS WINDOW

The Office Hours program has its own window (see Figure 11-1), including its own menu bar and toolbar. The Office Hours menu bar lists the menus available: File, Edit, View, Lists, Reports, Tools, and Help (see Figure 11-2). Under the menu bar is a toolbar with shortcut buttons. The functions of Office Hours are accessed by selecting a choice from one of the menus or by clicking a button on the toolbar.

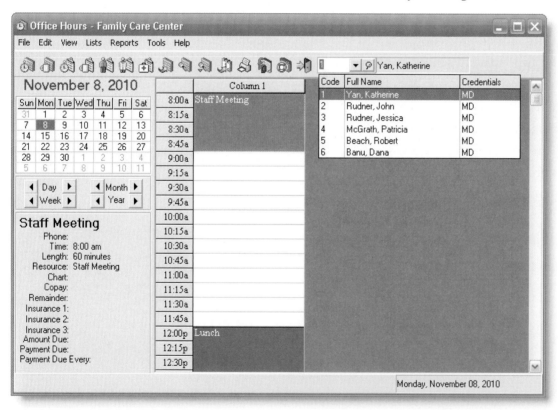

Figure 11-1　The Office Hours window

Figure 11-2　The Office Hours menu bar

Located just below the menu bar, the toolbar contains a series of buttons that represent the most common activities performed in Office Hours. These buttons are shortcuts for frequently used menu commands. The toolbar displays fifteen buttons (see Figure 11-3 and Table 11-1).

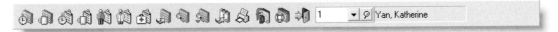

Figure 11-3   The Office Hours toolbar

Table 11-1	**Office Hours Toolbar Buttons**		
Button	**Button Name**	**Associated Function**	**Activity**
	Appointment Entry	New Appointment Entry dialog box	Enter appointments
	Break Entry	New Break Entry dialog box	Enter breaks
	Appointment List	Appointment List dialog box	Display list of appointments
	Break List	Break List dialog box	Display list of breaks
	Patient List	Patient List dialog box	Display list of patients
	Provider List	Provider List dialog box	Display list of providers
	Resource List	Resource List dialog box	Display list of resources
	Go to a Date	Go to a Date dialog box	Change calendar to a different date
	Search for Open Time Slot	Find Open Time dialog box	Locate first available time slot
	Search Again	Find Open Time dialog box	Locate next available time slot
	Go to Today		Return calendar to current date
	Print Appointment List		Print appointment list
	Edit Patient Notes in Final Draft	Final Draft word processor	Use Final Draft word processor
	Help	Office Hours Help	Display Office Hours Help contents
	Exit	Exit	Exit the Office Hours program

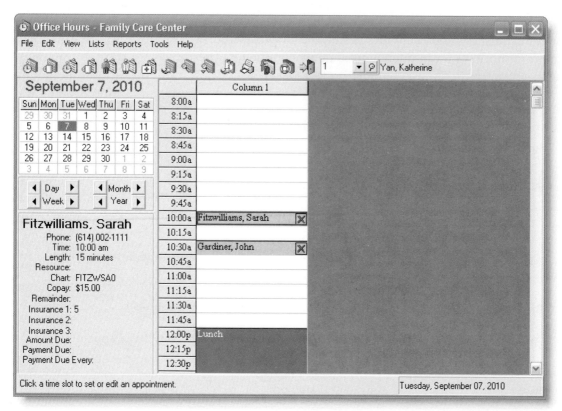

Figure 11-4 The left side of the Office Hours window displaying the date and a monthly calendar, and the right side displaying the selected provider's schedule for the day selected in the calendar

The left half of the Office Hours screen displays the current date and a calendar of the current month (see Figure 11-4). The current date is highlighted on the calendar. When a different date is clicked on the calendar, the calendar switches to the new date.

Office Hours schedule   a listing of time slots for a particular day for a specific provider

The **Office Hours schedule,** shown in the right half of the screen, is a listing of time slots for a particular day for a specific provider. The provider's name and number are displayed at the top to the right of the shortcut buttons. The provider can be easily changed by clicking the triangle button in the Provider box.

PROGRAM OPTIONS

When Office Hours is installed in a medical practice, it is set up to reflect the needs of that particular practice. Most offices that use Medisoft already have Office Hours set up and running. However, if Medisoft is just being installed, the options to set up the Office Hours program can be found in the Program Options dialog box, which is accessed by clicking Program Options on the Office Hours File menu.

ENTERING AND EXITING OFFICE HOURS

Office Hours can be started from within Medisoft or directly from Windows. To access Office Hours from within Medisoft, Appointment

Book is clicked on the Activities menu. Office Hours can also be started by clicking the corresponding shortcut button on the toolbar.

To start Office Hours without entering Medisoft first:

1. Click Start > All Programs.

2. Click Medisoft on the Programs submenu.

3. Click Office Hours on the Medisoft submenu.

The Office Hours program is closed by clicking Exit on the Office Hours File menu or by clicking the Exit button on its toolbar. If Office Hours was started from within Medisoft, exiting will return you to Medisoft. If Office Hours was started directly from Windows, clicking Exit will return you to the Windows desktop.

ENTERING APPOINTMENTS

Entering an appointment begins with selecting the provider for whom the appointment is being scheduled. The current provider is listed in the Provider box at the top right of the screen (see Figure 11-5). Clicking the arrow button displays a drop-down list of providers

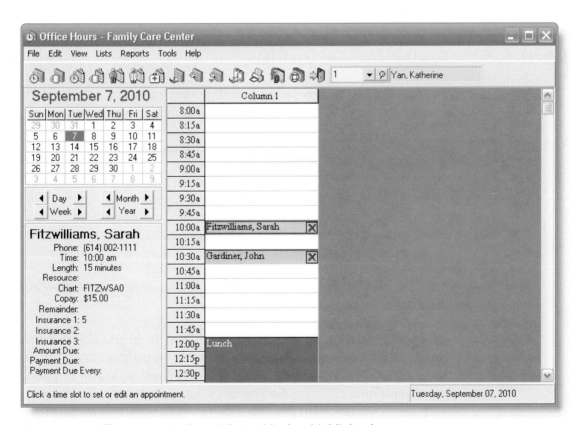

Figure 11-5 Office Hours window with Provider box highlighted

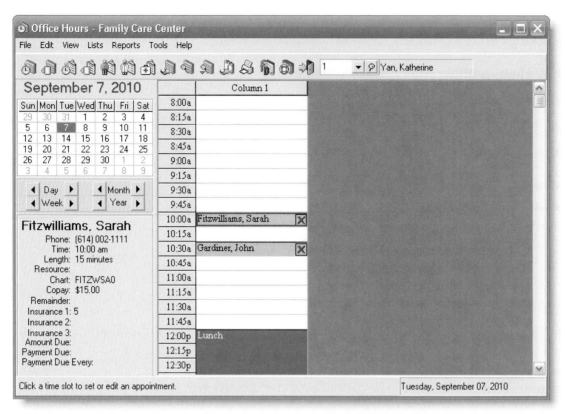

Figure 11-6 Office Hours window with Day, Week, Month, and Year arrow buttons highlighted

in the system. To choose a different provider, click the name of the provider on the drop-down list.

After the provider is selected, the date of the desired appointment must be chosen. Dates are changed by clicking the Day, Week, Month, and Year right and left arrow buttons located under the calendar (see Figure 11-6). After the provider and date have been selected, patient appointments can be entered.

Appointments are entered by clicking the Appointment Entry shortcut button or by double-clicking in a time slot on the schedule. When either action is taken, the New Appointment Entry dialog box is displayed (see Figure 11-7).

The New Appointment Entry dialog box contains the following fields:

Chart A patient's chart number is chosen from the Chart drop-down list. To select the desired patient, click on the patient's name in the drop-down list and press Tab. If you are setting up an appointment for a new patient who has not been assigned a chart number, skip the Chart box, and key the patient's name directly in the blank box to the right of the Chart box.

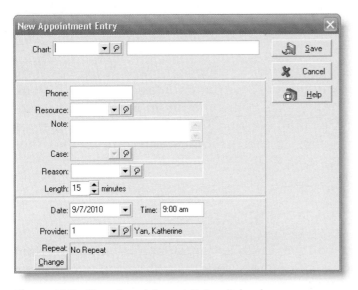

Figure 11-7 New Appointment Entry dialog box

Phone After a patient's chart is selected, that patient's phone number is automatically entered in the Phone box.

Resource This box is used if the practice assigns codes to resources, such as exam rooms or equipment.

Note Any special information about an appointment is entered in the Note box.

Case The case that pertains to the appointment is selected from the drop-down list of cases.

Reason Reason codes can be set up in the program to reflect the reason for an appointment.

Length The amount of time an appointment will take (in minutes) is entered in the Length box by keying the number of minutes or using the up and down arrows.

Date The Date box displays the date that is currently displayed on the calendar. If this is not the desired date, it may be changed by keying in a different date or by clicking the arrow button and selecting a date from the pop-up calendar that appears.

Time The Time box displays the appointment time that is currently selected on the schedule. If this is not the desired time, it may be changed by keying in a different time.

Provider The provider who will be treating the patient during this appointment is selected from the drop-down list of providers.

Repeat The Repeat box is used to enter appointments that recur on a regular basis.

After the boxes in the New Appointment Entry dialog box have been completed, clicking the Save button enters the information on the schedule. The patient's name appears in the time slot corresponding to the appointment time. In addition, information about the patient's insurance appears in the lower-left corner of the Office Hours window.

LOOKING FOR A FUTURE DATE

Often a patient will need a follow-up appointment at a certain time in the future. For example, suppose a physician would like a patient to return for a checkup in three weeks. The most efficient way to search for a future appointment in Office Hours is to use the Go to a Date shortcut button on the toolbar. (This feature can also be accessed on the Edit menu.)

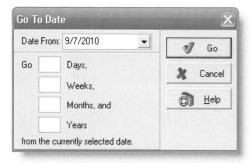

Figure 11-8   Go to Date dialog box

Clicking the Go to a Date shortcut button displays the Go to Date dialog box (see Figure 11-8). Within the dialog box, five boxes offer options for choosing a future date.

Date From This box indicates the current date in the appointment search.

Go __ Days This box is used to locate a date that is a specific number of days in the future. For example, if a patient needs an appointment ten days from the current day, *10* would be entered in this box.

Go __ Weeks This box is used when a patient needs an appointment a specific number of weeks in the future, such as six weeks from the current day.

Go __ Months This box is used when a patient needs an appointment a specific number of months in the future, such as three months from the current day.

Go __ Years Similar to the weeks and months options, this box is used when an appointment is needed in one year or several years in the future.

After a future date option has been selected, clicking the Go button closes the dialog box and begins the search. The system locates the future date and displays the calendar schedule for that date.

EXERCISE 11-1

Enter an appointment for Herbert Bell at 3:00 P.M. on Monday, November 15, 2010. The appointment is sixty minutes in length and is with Dr. John Rudner.

1. Start Medisoft and restore the data from your last work session.

2. Start Office Hours by clicking the Appointment Book shortcut button on the toolbar.

3. If John Rudner is not already selected, click "2, Rudner, John" on the drop-down list in the Provider box to select him.

4. Change the date on the calendar to Monday, November 15, 2010. Use the arrow keys to change the month and year, and then click the day on the calendar.

5. In the schedule, double-click the 3:00 P.M. time slot. (You may need to use the scroll bar to view 3:00 P.M.) The New Appointment Entry dialog box is displayed.

6. Click Herbert Bell from the list of names on the drop-down list in the Chart box, and press Tab. The system automatically fills in a number of boxes in the dialog box, such as the patient's name and phone number.

7. Accept the default entry in the Case box.

8. Notice that the Length box already contains an entry of fifteen minutes. This is the default appointment length set up in Medisoft. Since Herbert Bell's appointment is for an annual exam, this entry must be changed to sixty minutes. Key **60** in the Length box, or use the up arrow next to the Length box to change the appointment length to sixty minutes.

9. Verify the entries in the Date, Time, and Provider boxes, and then click the Save button. Medisoft saves the appointment, closes the dialog box, and displays the appointment on the schedule as well as in the lower-left corner of the Office Hours window. Herbert Bell's name is displayed in the 3:00 P.M. time slot on the schedule.

EXERCISE 11-2

Enter the following appointments with Dr. John Rudner.

1. The first appointment is Monday (November 15, 2010) at 4:00 P.M. for John Fitzwilliams, thirty minutes in length. Verify that "2 Rudner, John" is displayed in the Provider box.

2. In the schedule, double-click the 4:00 P.M. time-slot box.

3. Select John Fitzwilliams on the Chart drop-down list.

4. Press the Tab key. The program automatically completes several boxes in the dialog box.

5. Press the Tab key until the entry in the Length box is highlighted.

6. Key *30* in the Length box, or click the up arrow once to change the length to thirty minutes.

7. Click the Save button. Verify that the appointment for John Fitzwilliams appears on the schedule for November 15, 2010, at 4:00 P.M. for a length of thirty minutes.

8. Enter an appointment on Monday, November 15, 2010, at 4:30 P.M. for Leila Patterson, fifteen minutes in length.

9. Enter an appointment on Tuesday, November 16, 2010, at 12:15 P.M. for James Smith, thirty minutes in length.

10. To schedule an appointment for James Smith two weeks after November 16, 2010, at 12:15 P.M., fifteen minutes in length, click the Go To a Date shortcut button.

11. Key *2* in the Go _____ Weeks box. Click the Go button. The program closes the Go To Date box and displays the appointment schedule for November 30, 2010.

12. Enter James Smith's appointment.

EXERCISE 11-3

Enter these appointments with Dr. Jessica Rudner.

1. Click Dr. Jessica Rudner from the list of providers in the Provider drop-down list.

2. Enter an appointment for Friday, November 19, 2010, at 3:00 P.M. for Janine Bell, fifteen minutes in length.

3. Use the Go to a Date feature to schedule an appointment three weeks from November 19, 2010, at 1:15 P.M. for Sarina Bell, thirty minutes in length.

4. Schedule an appointment for Sarah Fitzwilliams one week from November 19, 2010, at 9:00 A.M., fifteen minutes in length.

5. Temporarily leave Office Hours by clicking the minimize button in the upper-right corner of the window.

EXERCISE 11-4

Enter an appointment on Thursday, November 11, 2010, at 9:00 A.M. for John Gardiner, thirty minutes in length. You do not know his provider, so this information must be looked up in Medisoft before you enter the appointment.

1. Go to the Patient List dialog box.

2. Select John Gardiner as the patient.

3. Click the Other Information tab to find his assigned provider.

4. Click the Office Hours button on the Windows task bar (bottom of screen). Notice that the Patient/Guarantor dialog box is still partially visible underneath the Office Hours window.

5. Select Gardiner's provider in the Provider box in Office Hours.

6. Enter the appointment. Remember to set the calendar to the correct date.

7. Minimize Office Hours.

8. In Medisoft, close the open dialog boxes.

SEARCHING FOR AVAILABLE APPOINTMENT TIME

Often it is necessary to search for available appointment space on a particular day of the week and at a specific time. For example, a patient needs a thirty-minute appointment and would like it to be during his lunch hour, which is from 12:00 P.M. to 1:00 P.M. He can get away from the office only on Mondays and Fridays. Office Hours makes it easy to locate an appointment slot that meets these requirements with the Search for Open Time Slot shortcut button.

EXERCISE 11-5

Maritza Ramos needs an appointment, but she has very limited times she can come in to the office. Search for the next available appointment slot with Dr. Yan on a Tuesday, 30 minutes in length, between 11:00 A.M. and 2:00 P.M., beginning November 11, 2010.

1. Click the Office Hours button on the Windows taskbar. Verify that Dr. Katherine Yan is displayed in the Provider box.

2. On the Edit menu, click Find Open Time, or click the Search for Open Time Slot shortcut button. The Find Open Time dialog box is displayed (see Figure 11-9).

3. Key *30* in the Length box. Press the Tab key.

4. Key *11* in the Start Time box. Press the Tab key.

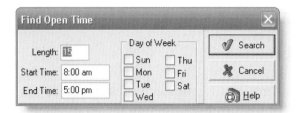

Figure 11-9   Find Open Time dialog box

5. Key **2** in the End Time box. Press the Tab key.

6. To search for an appointment on Tuesday, click the Tuesday box in the Day of Week area of the dialog box.

7. Click the Search button to begin looking for an appointment slot. Medisoft closes the dialog box and locates the first available time slot that meets these specifications. The time slot is outlined on the schedule.

8. Double-click the selected time slot. Click Maritza Ramos on the drop-down list in the Chart box.

9. Press the Tab key until the cursor is in the Length box.

10. Key **30,** and press the Tab key.

11. Click the Save button.

12. Verify that the appointment has been entered by looking at the schedule.

EXERCISE 11-6

Schedule Randall Klein for a thirty-minute appointment with Dr. John Rudner sometime after November 15, 2010. Mr. Klein is available only on Mondays between 3:00 P.M. and 5:00 P.M.

1. Click the desired provider in the Provider box.

2. Change the calendar to November 15, 2010.

3. Click Find Open Time on the Edit menu to display the Find Open Time dialog box.

4. In the Length box, key **30.** Press the Tab key to move the cursor to the Start Time box.

5. Key **3** in the Start Time box. Press Tab. Click on "am" to highlight it, and then key **p** to change "am" to "pm." Press Tab to move to the End Time box.

6. Key **5** in the End Time box. Press Tab.

7. In the Day of Week boxes, select Monday. If necessary, deselect any other days that are selected.

8. Click the Search button. The first available slot that meets the requirements is outlined on the schedule.

9. Double-click in the time slot to open the New Appointment Entry dialog box.

10. Click Randall Klein in the drop-down list in the Chart box. Press tab several times to move the cursor to the Length box.

11. Key *30* in the Length box, and press the Tab key.

12. Click the Save button. The dialog box closes, and Randall Klein's appointment appears on the schedule.

ENTERING APPOINTMENTS FOR NEW PATIENTS

When a new patient phones the office for an appointment, the appointment can be scheduled in Office Hours before the patient information is entered in Medisoft. However, while the prospective patient is still on the phone, most offices obtain basic data and enter it in the appropriate Medisoft dialog boxes (Patient/Guarantor and Case).

EXERCISE 11-7

Schedule Lisa Green, a new patient, for a forty-five-minute appointment with Dr. John Rudner on November 15, 2010, at 1:15 P.M.

1. Verify that November 15, 2010, is displayed on the schedule and that Dr. John Rudner is selected as the provider.

2. Double-click the 1:15 P.M. time slot.

3. In the box to the right of the Chart box, key *Green, Lisa.* Press the Tab key to move the cursor to the Phone box.

4. Key *6145553604* in the Phone box, and press Tab until the cursor is in the Length box.

5. Key *45* in the Length box.

6. Click the Save button. The appointment is displayed on the November 15, 2010, schedule.

BOOKING REPEATED APPOINTMENTS

Some patients require appointments on a repeated basis, such as every Thursday for eight weeks. Repeated appointments are also set up in the New Appointment Entry dialog box. The Repeat feature is located at the bottom of the dialog box. When the Change button is clicked, the Repeat Change dialog box is displayed. The Repeat Change dialog box provides a number of choices for setting up repeating appointments (see Figure 11-10).

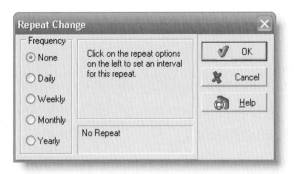

Figure 11-10   Repeat Change dialog box with the default settings (None button selected)

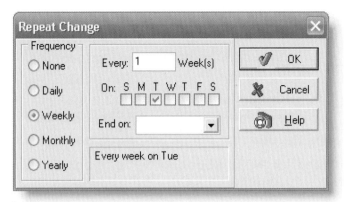

Figure 11-11   Repeat Change dialog box when an option other than None is selected

The left side of the dialog box contains information about the frequency of the appointments. The default is set to None. Other options include Daily, Weekly, Monthly, and Yearly. When an option other than None is selected, the center section of the dialog box changes and displays additional options for setting up the appointments (see Figure 11-11).

In the center section, an option is provided to indicate how often the appointments should be scheduled, such as once every week. Below that there is an option to indicate the day of the week on which the appointments should be scheduled. Finally, there is a box to indicate when the repeating appointments should stop. When all the information has been entered, clicking the OK button closes the Repeat Change dialog box, and the New Appointment Entry dialog box is once again visible. Clicking the Save button enters the repeating appointments on the schedule.

EXERCISE 11-8

Schedule Li Y. Wong for a fifteen-minute appointment once a week for six weeks with Dr. Katherine Yan. Mrs. Wong has requested that the appointments be at the same time every week, preferably in the early morning, beginning on Wednesday, November 17, 2010.

1. Click the desired provider on the Provider drop-down list.

2. Change the schedule to November 17, 2010.

3. Double-click in the 8:00 A.M. time slot. The New Appointment Entry dialog box is displayed.

4. Select Li Y. Wong from the Chart drop-down list. Press the Tab key.

5. Confirm that the entry in the Length box is fifteen minutes.

6. Click the Change button to schedule the repeating appointments.

7. In the Frequency column, select Weekly.

8. Accept the default entry of 1 in the Every ___ Week(s) box.

9. Accept the default entry of W to accept Wednesday as the day of the week.

10. Click the arrow for the drop-down list in the End on box. A calendar pops up. Count six weeks from November 17, 2010. When you find the sixth Wednesday (counting November 17 as the first week), click in the calendar box for that day. The date 12/22/2010 appears in the End on box.

11. Click the OK button. Notice that "Every week on Wed" is displayed in the Repeat area of the New Appointment Entry dialog box.

12. Click the Save button to enter the appointments.

13. Go to December 22, 2010, to verify that Mrs. Wong is scheduled for an appointment at 8:00 A.M.

14. Go to December 29, 2010, and confirm that Mrs. Wong is not scheduled. This is the seventh week, and her repeating appointments were scheduled for six weeks, so no appointment should appear on December 29, 2010.

CHANGING OR DELETING APPOINTMENTS

It is often necessary to change or cancel a patient's appointment. Changing an appointment is accomplished with the Cut and Paste commands on the Office Hours Edit menu.

The following steps are used to reschedule an appointment:

1. Locate the appointment that needs to be changed. Make sure the appointment slot is visible on the schedule.

2. Click on the existing time-slot box. A black border surrounds the slot to indicate that it is selected.

3. Click Cut on the Edit menu. The appointment disappears from the schedule.

4. Click the date on the calendar when the appointment is to be rescheduled.

5. Click the desired time-slot box on the schedule. The slot becomes active.

6. Click Paste on the Edit menu. The patient's name appears in the new time-slot box.

The following steps are used to cancel an appointment without rescheduling:

1. Locate the appointment on the schedule.

2. Click the time-slot box to select the appointment.

3. Click Cut on the Edit menu. The appointment disappears from the schedule.

> **TIP** Instead of using the Cut and Paste commands to change or delete an appointment, select the appointment, and press the right mouse button. A shortcut menu appears with several options, including Cut, Copy, and Delete.

EXERCISE 11-9

Change Janine Bell's and John Gardiner's appointments.

1. Click Jessica Rudner on the Provider box drop-down list.

2. Go to Friday, November 19, 2010, on the calendar.

3. Locate Janine Bell's 3:00 P.M. appointment on the schedule. Click the 3:00 P.M. time-slot box.

4. Click Cut on the Edit menu. Janine Bell's appointment is removed from the 3:00 P.M. time-slot box. (You may also use the right-mouse-click shortcut.)

5. Click the 4:00 P.M. time-slot box.

6. Click Paste on the Edit menu. Janine Bell's name is displayed in the 4:00 P.M. time-slot box.

7. Click Katherine Yan on the Provider drop-down list.

8. Go to Thursday, November 11, 2010, on the calendar.

9. Locate John Gardiner's 9:00 A.M. appointment. Remove his appointment from the 9:00 A.M. time slot.

10. Go to Friday, November 19, 2010, on the calendar.

11. Enter John Gardiner's appointment in the 9:15 A.M. time slot.

12. Exit Office Hours.

CREATING A RECALL LIST

Medical offices frequently must keep track of patients who need to return for future appointments. Some offices schedule future appointments when the patient is leaving the office. For example, if a patient has just seen a physician and needs to return for a follow-up appointment in six weeks, the appointment is usually made before the patient leaves the office. However, when the appointment is needed farther in the future, such as one year later, it is not always practical to set up the appointment. It is difficult for the patient and the physician to know their schedules a year in advance. For this reason, many offices keep lists of patients who need to be contacted for future appointments.

In Medisoft, a recall list can be created and maintained by clicking Patient Recall on the Lists menu. Patients can also be added to the recall list by clicking the Patient Recall Entry shortcut button on the toolbar. When Patient Recall is selected from the Lists menu, the Patient Recall List dialog box is displayed (see Figure 11-12). This dialog box organizes the recall information in a column format. The scroll bar is used to display the last three columns on the right.

Date of Recall   Lists the date on which the recall is scheduled.

Name   Displays the patient's name.

Phone   Lists the patient's phone number, making it easy to call patients for appointments without having to look up phone numbers in another dialog box.

Extension   Lists the patient's phone extension.

Status   Indicates the patient's recall status: Call, Call Again, Appointment Set, No Appointment.

Provider   Displays the provider code for the patient's provider.

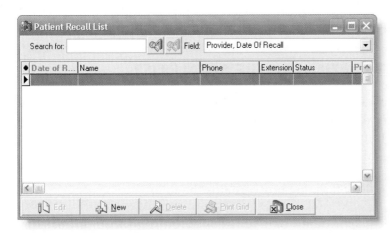

Figure 11-12   Patient Recall List dialog box

Message Displays the entry made in the Message box of the Patient Recall dialog box.

Chart Number Displays the patient's chart number.

Procedure Code Lists the procedure code for the procedure for which the patient is being recalled.

The Patient Recall List dialog box contains the following boxes:

Search For The Search For box is used to locate a specific patient on the recall list. Entering the first few letters or numbers in the Search For box displays the selection that is the closest match to the search criteria.

Field The choices in the Field box determine the order in which patients are listed in the dialog box. There are three sorting options:

1. Provider, Date of Recall

2. Date of Recall, Provider, Chart Number

3. Chart Number, Date of Recall

The Patient Recall List dialog box also contains these buttons: Edit, New, Delete, Print Grid, and Close.

Edit Clicking the Edit button displays the Patient Recall dialog box for the patient whose entry is highlighted. The information on the patient can then be edited by making different selections in the boxes.

New Clicking the New button displays an empty Patient Recall dialog box in which data on a new recall patient can be entered.

Delete Clicking the Delete button deletes data on the patient whose entry is highlighted from the patient recall list.

Print Grid The Print Button is used to print data in the window.

Close The Close button is used to exit the Patient Recall List dialog box.

ADDING A PATIENT TO THE RECALL LIST

Patients are added to the recall list by clicking the New button in the Patient Recall List dialog box or by clicking the Patient Recall Entry shortcut button. When either of these actions is performed, the Patient Recall dialog box is displayed (see Figure 11-13).

The Patient Recall dialog box contains the following boxes:

Recall Date The date a patient needs to return to see a physician is entered in the Recall Date box.

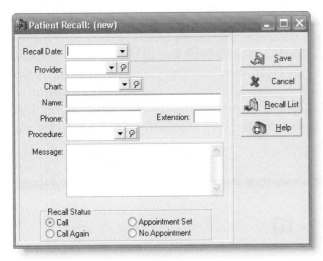

Figure 11-13   Patient Recall (new) dialog box

Provider   A patient's provider is selected from the drop-down list.

Chart   A patient's chart number is selected from the drop-down list, or the first few letters of a patient's chart number are entered in the Chart box.

Name, Phone, Extension   After a chart number is entered, the system automatically completes the Name, Phone, and Extension boxes.

Procedure   If the procedure for which a patient is returning is known, it is entered in the Procedure box in one of two ways. The procedure code can be selected from the drop-down list, or the first few numbers can be entered so that the drop-down list will display the entry that most closely matches the entered numbers. This is especially valuable in practices that use hundreds of procedure codes because it eliminates the need to scroll through the codes to locate the desired one.

Message   The Message box is used to record any special notes, reminders, or instructions about a patient and his or her appointment.

Recall Status   The choices in the Recall Status box are used to indicate the action that needs to be taken. They include:

Call   The Call button is used when a patient needs to be telephoned about a future appointment.

Call Again   The Call Again button is used when a patient has been called once, but contact was not made and an additional call is necessary.

Appointment Set   The Appointment Set button is used when a patient has an appointment already scheduled.

No Appointment   The No Appointment button is used when a patient has been contacted for an appointment but has declined for some reason.

After the information has been entered in the dialog box, clicking the Save button saves the data and adds the patient to the recall list. In addition to the Save button, the Patient Recall dialog box contains Cancel, Recall List, and Help buttons. The Cancel button exits the dialog box without saving the data entered. The Recall List button in the Patient Recall dialog box is used to display the Patient Recall List dialog box. The Help button displays Medisoft's online help for the Patient Recall dialog box.

EXERCISE 11-10

John Fitzwilliams needs to receive a phone call one year from November 15, 2010, to set up an appointment for an annual physical. Add John Fitzwilliams to the recall list.

1. Click the Patient Recall Entry shortcut button. The Patient Recall dialog box is displayed.

2. In the Recall Date box, enter November 15, 2011. Press Tab.

3. Determine which physician is John Fitzwilliams's provider. (Look in the Patient/Guarantor dialog box for this information.)

4. Click John Fitzwilliams's provider on the drop-down list in the Provider box. Press Tab.

5. Enter John Fitzwilliams's chart number in the Chart box by keying the first few letters of his last name. Notice that the system automatically completes the Name and Phone box. (The Extension box would also be completed if there were an extension.)

6. Enter the procedure code in the Procedure box by keying **99396** (Preventive est., 40–64 years).

7. Verify that the Call radio button in the Recall Status box is selected.

8. Click the Save button to save the entry.

9. Click Patient Recall on the Lists menu.

10. Verify that the entry for John Fitzwilliams has been added to the recall list.

11. Close the Patient Recall List dialog box.

CREATING BREAKS

Office Hours break a block of time when a physician is unavailable for appointments with patients

Office Hours provides features for inserting standard breaks in providers' schedules. The **Office Hours break** is a block of time when a physician is unavailable for appointments with patients. Some examples of breaks include Lunch, Meeting, Personal, Emergency, Break, Vacation, Seminar, Holiday, Trip, and Surgery. In Office

Hours, breaks can be created one at a time or on a recurring basis for all providers. One-time breaks, such as those for vacations, are set up for individual providers. Other breaks, such as staff meetings, can be entered once for multiple providers.

Often breaks need to be inserted into a provider's schedule when he or she is not available for appointments with patients. For example, if a physician will be in surgery on Thursday from 9 A.M. until 12:00 P.M., that time period must be marked as unavailable on his or her schedule.

To set up a break for a current provider (that is, the provider listed in the Office Hours Provider box), click the Break Entry shortcut button. This action causes the New Break Entry dialog box to appear (see Figure 11-14).

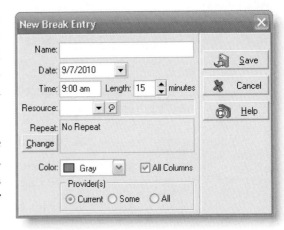

Figure 11-14   New Break Entry dialog box

The dialog box contains the following options:

Name   The name field is used to store a name or description of the break.

Date   The date field displays the current date on the Office Hours calendar. If this is not the correct date for the break entry, a different date can be entered.

Time   The starting time of the break is entered in this box.

Length   This box indicates the length of the break in minutes (from 0 to 720).

Resource   The drop-down list entries in the Resource box display the different types of breaks already set up in Office Hours.

Change   The Change button next to the Repeat box is used to enter breaks that recur at a regular interval.

Color   By selecting a different color from the drop-down list, the color of the break time slot in the schedule can be changed.

Provider(s)   The Provider(s) buttons are used to indicate whether a break is to be set for the current provider (the provider selected in the Provider box in Office Hours), some providers, or all providers. If some is selected, a Provider Selection dialog box will be displayed when the Save button is clicked. The appropriate providers can then be selected.

When all the information has been entered, clicking the Save button closes the dialog box and enters the break(s) in Medisoft.

EXERCISE 11-11

Dr. Jessica Rudner will be attending a seminar from 10:00 A.M. to 12:00 P.M. on Monday, Tuesday, and Wednesday, December 13–15, 2010. Enter this as a break on her schedule.

1. Start Office Hours.

2. Select Jessica Rudner from the Provider drop-down list.

3. Change the date on the calendar to December 13, 2010.

4. Click in the 10:00 A.M. time slot.

5. Click the Break Entry shortcut button. The New Break Entry dialog box appears.

6. Enter *HIPAA Update Seminar* in the Name box.

7. Confirm that the date and time are correct.

8. Click the up arrow in the Length box to change the length of time to 120 minutes.

9. Select Seminar Break in the Resource box.

10. Press the Change button (to repeat the break for two additional days). The Repeat Change dialog box is displayed.

11. If it is not already selected, click the Daily button in the Frequency column.

12. Accept the default entry of 1 in the Every __ Day(s) box, since the break occurs every day for a period of three days.

13. Key *12152010* in the End On box.

14. Click the OK button. You are returned to the New Break Entry dialog box.

15. Click the Save button to enter the break in Office Hours. Notice that the time slot from 10:00 A.M. to 12:00 P.M. on December 13, 2010, has been filled in on the calendar.

16. Change the calendar to December 14 and 15, 2010, to verify that the break has been entered correctly.

PREVIEWING AND PRINTING SCHEDULES

In most medical offices, providers' schedules are printed on a daily basis. To view a list of all appointments for a provider for a given day, the Appointment List option on the Office Hours Reports menu is used. The report can be previewed on the screen or sent

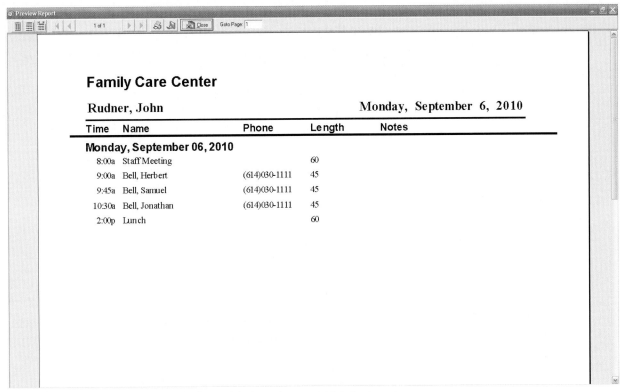

1 of 1   Close   Goto Page: 1

Family Care Center

Rudner, John   Monday, September 6, 2010

Time	Name	Phone	Length	Notes
Monday, September 06, 2010				
8:00a	Staff Meeting		60	
9:00a	Bell, Herbert	(614)030-1111	45	
9:45a	Bell, Samuel	(614)030-1111	45	
10:30a	Bell, Jonathan	(614)030-1111	45	
2:00p	Lunch		60	

Figure 11-15   Preview Report window with Appointment List displayed

directly to the printer. If the preview option is selected, the appointment list is displayed in a preview window (see Figure 11-15). Various buttons are used to view the schedule at different sizes, to move from page to page, to print the schedule, and to save the schedule as a file. Clicking the Close button closes the preview window.

The schedule can also be printed without using the Preview option by clicking the Print Appointment List shortcut button. (Office Hours prints the schedule for the provider who is listed in the Provider box. To print the schedule of a different provider, change the entry in the Provider box before printing the schedule.)

EXERCISE 11-12

Print Dr. John Rudner's schedule for November 15, 2010.

1. Select Dr. John Rudner as the provider.

2. Go to Monday, November 15, 2010, on the calendar.

3. Click Appointment List on the Office Hours Reports menu. The Report Setup dialog box appears.

4. Under Print Selection, click the button that sends the report directly to the printer.

5. Click the Start button. The Data Selection dialog box is displayed.

6. Enter *11152010* in both Dates boxes.

7. Select John Rudner in both Providers boxes.

8. Click the OK button. The Print dialog box appears.

9. Click OK to print the report.

ON YOUR OWN EXERCISE 13 Enter an Appointment

December 6, 2010

Book a 15-minute appointment for Lisa Wright as soon as possible. She is experiencing dizziness and will have to get someone to drive her in for an appointment. Because of this, the appointment will need to be at 3:00 P.M. or later.

ON YOUR OWN EXERCISE 14 Change an Appointment

November 22, 2010

James Smith calls to say that he will be out of town and cannot make his appointment on November 30. He is available after 12:00 P.M. beginning on December 6. Reschedule his appointment.

ON YOUR OWN EXERCISE 15 Print a Physician's Schedule

December 6, 2010

Print today's appointment list for Dr. Jessica Rudner.

Remember to create a backup of your work before exiting Medisoft! To help you keep track of your work, name the backup file after the chapter you are working on, for example, StudentID-c11.mbk.

Electronic Medical Record Exchange

Transferring Appointment Information

The first time Medisoft exchanges information with an electronic medical record, all appointments and patient demographics are transferred. After that first transmission, only new or edited appointments and demographics are transmitted. The illustration below shows patient appointments in Office Hours, the Medisoft scheduling program.

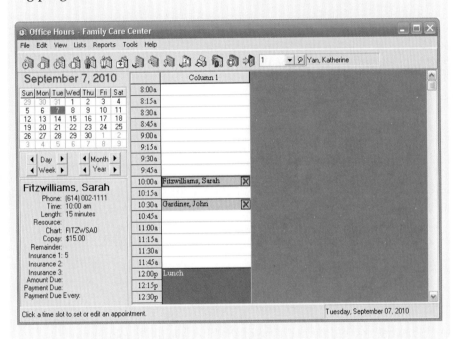

Name: _____   Date: _____

CHAPTER 11 WORKSHEET

After completing all the exercises in the chapter, answer the following questions in the spaces provided.

1. In Exercise 11-1, what is listed on the appointment schedule immediately before Herbert Bell's appointment?

   _____

2. In Exercise 11-2, what is listed on the appointment schedule immediately after John Fitzwilliams's appointment on November 15, 2010?

   _____

3. In Exercise 11-2, how long is James Smith's appointment on November 16, 2010?

   _____

4. In Exercise 11-3, are there any other patient appointments on the day of Janine Bell's appointment?

   _____

5. In Exercise 11-4, who is John Gardiner's provider?

   _____

6. In Exercise 11-5, what is the date and time of the next available appointment slot for Maritza Ramos to see Dr. Yan?

   _____

7. In Exercise 11-6, what is the date and time of Randall Klein's appointment?

   _____

8. In Exercise 11-8, what is the date of Li Wong's last fifteen-minute appointment with Dr. Yan?

   _____

9. In Exercise 11-11, what is listed in the 10:00 A.M. time slot for Dr. Jessica Rudner on December 15, 2010?

   _____

10. In Exercise 11-12, who has the last appointment with Dr. John Rudner on November 15, 2010?

    _____

CHAPTER REVIEW

USING TERMINOLOGY

Define the terms below as they apply to Office Hours.

1. Office Hours schedule

_____

_____

2. Office Hours break

_____

_____

CHECKING YOUR UNDERSTANDING

Answer the questions below in the space provided.

3. What are the different ways of starting Office Hours?

_____

_____

4. How do you display the schedule for a specific date?

_____

_____

5. If the Office Hours calendar shows October 6, how do you move to November 6?

_____

_____

6. How do you display the schedule for a specific provider?

_____

_____

7. How do you schedule a new appointment in Office Hours?

_____

_____

8. How is an appointment deleted?

_____

_____

9. How is an appointment moved from one time slot to another?

_____

_____

10. Suppose your office has set up Office Hours so that the default appointment length is fifteen minutes. If you need to make a one-hour appointment for a patient, in what box do you change fifteen to sixty?

_____

_____

APPLYING KNOWLEDGE

Answer the questions below in the space provided.

11. After you entered a personal break for Dr. Katherine Yan for February 24, she tells you that she gave you the wrong date. The break should be February 25. How do you correct the schedule?

_____

_____

12. A patient calls to request an appointment on a specific day next week. You determine that the appointment is for a routine checkup, not an emergency. What steps should you follow to schedule the appointment?

_____

_____

314 PART 2 ◆ MEDISOFT ADVANCED TRAINING
Copyright © 2009 The McGraw-Hill Companies

AT THE COMPUTER

Answer the following questions at the computer.

13. Today is Friday, September 3, 2010. Dr. Katherine Yan asks you to find out when Sarah Fitzwilliams is coming in for her next two appointments. Locate the appointments in Office Hours. *Hint:* Use the Appointment List option on the Office Hours Lists menu, or click the Appointment List button on the Office Hours toolbar.

_____

_____

14. Today is November 15, 2010. Samuel Bell needs to be scheduled as soon as possible for a thirty-minute appointment between 10:00 A.M. and 12:00 P.M. with Dr. John Rudner. When is the next available time slot that meets these requirements? How did you locate the open slot?

_____

_____

PART 3

APPLYING YOUR KNOWLEDGE

Chapter 12
Handling Patient Records and Transactions

Chapter 13
Setting Up Appointments

Chapter 14
Printing Lists and Reports

Chapter 15
Putting It All Together

Handling Patient Records and Transactions

WHAT YOU NEED TO KNOW

To complete the exercises in this chapter, you need to know how to:

◆ Locate patient information.

◆ Change the Medisoft Program Date.

◆ Assign a new chart number and enter information on a new patient.

◆ Create a new case for a patient.

◆ Change information on an established patient.

◆ Enter procedures, charges, and diagnoses.

◆ Record payments from patients and insurance carriers.

◆ Print walkout receipts.

All office personnel at the Family Care Center (FCC) know how to input patient information in the Patient/Guarantor dialog box and in the Case dialog box. Whenever possible, information for both dialog boxes is entered into the computer as soon as patients complete the handwritten information sheet and return it to the receptionist. On busy days, however, or when the office is understaffed because one of the medical assistants is sick or on vacation, input operations may be delayed.

EXERCISE 12-1: INPUTTING PATIENT INFORMATION

For this exercise, you need Source Documents 13–19.

It is Monday, November 15, 2010. You are a records/billing clerk at the Family Care Center. On your desk is a small pile of information sheets and encounter forms from Friday afternoon, November 12. You decide to input all patient information first, and then go back to record the transactions. First, you arrange the papers alphabetically:

> Battistuta
>
> Brooks
>
> Hsu
>
> Syzmanski

Then you begin. (Remember to change the Medisoft Program Date to November 12, 2010.)

PATIENT 1: ANTHONY BATTISTUTA

Record the address change that is written on Mr. Battistuta's encounter form (Source Document 13).

1. Start Medisoft, and restore the data from your last work session.

2. Click Patients/Guarantors and Cases on the Lists menu. The Patient List dialog box is displayed.

3. Select Anthony Battistuta from the list of patients.

4. Click the Edit Patient button. The Patient/Guarantor dialog box is displayed, with the Name, Address tab active.

5. Enter the new address.

6. Click the Save button.

PATIENT 2: LAWANA BROOKS

You can see from the encounter form (Source Document 14) that Ms. Brooks is an established patient. There are no changes to be made in the Patient/Guarantor dialog box. The work you need to do must take place in the Case dialog box. Ms. Brooks has had an accident at work, so a new case must be created.

1. After saving the changes for Mr. Battistuta in the Patient/Guarantor dialog box, the Patient List dialog box is redisplayed.

2. In the list of patients, click the listing for Brooks to select her as the patient. In the list of cases, click the ankle sprain case. You will not enter new information in the ankle sprain case; instead, you will copy information from the ankle sprain case to create a new case.

3. Click the Copy Case button to copy the information from the existing case into a new case. A duplicate case is displayed.

4. Using Source Documents 14 and 15, edit the information in the case to reflect the information relevant to the new case by changing the information in the Medisoft boxes listed below. If a box is not listed, either the information in that box does not need to be changed or the box is to remain blank.

Personal Tab

> Description

Diagnosis Tab

> Principal Diagnosis
>
> Default Diagnosis 2
>
> Default Diagnosis 3

Condition Tab

> Injury/Illness/LMP Date
>
> Illness Indicator
>
> First Consultation Date (when a message about the date entry appears, click the No button)
>
> Employment Related
>
> Emergency
>
> Accident Related to
>
> Nature of

5. Save your work.

TIP When entering information on different tabs within a dialog box, it is not necessary to click the Save button after completing work on each tab. However, the Save button must be clicked once all the tabs are complete and before exiting the dialog box.

PATIENT 3: EDWIN HSU

The information you need to make the necessary changes for Edwin Hsu is on Source Documents 16 and 17. Changes need to be made in Edwin Hsu's Patient/Guarantor and Case dialog boxes.

1. If the Patient List dialog box is not still displayed, open it now. Select Edwin Hsu from the list of patients, and click the Edit button.

2. Move to the Street box, and enter the new address.

3. Move to the home phone box, and enter the new phone number.

4. Save the information you just entered.

5. Create a new case for Edwin Hsu by copying his existing case.

6. Using Source Documents 16 and 17, edit the information in the copied case to reflect the information relevant to the new case. Change information in the following boxes:

Personal Tab

> Description

Diagnosis Tab

> Principal Diagnosis

7. Click the Save button to save the new case.

PATIENT 4: HANNAH SYZMANSKI

Use Source Documents 18 and 19 to enter information on a new patient, Hannah Syzmanski. Hannah is the daughter of Michael and Debra Syzmanski, who are Dr. Dana Banu's patients. Hannah's pediatrician, Dr. Harold Gearhart, has referred her to the Family Care Center. This is noted on Source Document 19.

1. Go to the Patient List dialog box, click the Patient radio button to make the Patient section of the dialog box active, and then click the New Patient button.

2. Key *SYZMAHAØ* in the Chart Number box.

3. Complete the boxes for name, address, phone, birth date, sex, and Social Security number.

4. Complete the following boxes in the Other Information tab:

> Type
>
> Assigned Provider
>
> Flag (East Ohio PPO)
>
> Signature on File
>
> Signature Date

5. Save your work. (If a message about the signature date appears, click the No button, click OK, and then save your work.)

6. Click the Case radio button to make the Case portion of the Patient List dialog box active.

7. Click the New Case button to open a new Case dialog box.

8. Complete the following tabs in the Case dialog box:

Personal Tab

> Description
>
> Guarantor
>
> Marital Status
>
> Student Status

Account Tab

> Referring Provider

Diagnosis Tab

> Principal Diagnosis
>
> Allergies and Notes

Policy 1 Tab

> When you attempt to complete the Policy 1 tab, you notice that Hannah has not filled in her insurance information. Since she is covered under her father's policy, it is easy to locate the information required to complete the Policy 1 tab.
>
> First save your work on Hannah's case. As before, open the Case dialog box for the acne case for Michael Syzmanski. This time go to the Policy 1 tab. Use the information on that tab to fill in the missing insurance data for Hannah Syzmanski.
>
> When completing the Policy 1 tab for Hannah, remember to list Michael Syzmanski in the Policy Holder 1 box and to click Child in the Relationship to Insured field. Also be sure that all of the Insurance Coverage Percents by Service Classification boxes at the bottom are set to 100.

9. Save your work.

EXERCISE 12-2: AN EMERGENCY VISIT

You will need Source Document 20 for this exercise.

It is still Monday morning, November 15, 2010. Carlos Lopez has just seen Dr. McGrath on an emergency basis. Mr. Lopez was experiencing chest tightness. Dr. McGrath has determined that he was suffering from heart palpitations. You need to enter the procedure charges, accept Mr. Lopez's payment, and print a walkout receipt. Make sure all transaction information is properly recorded in the database.

1. Change the Medisoft Program Date to November 15, 2010.

2. From the Patient List dialog box, create a new case for Carlos Lopez by copying the information in the case that already exists.

3. Using Source Document 20, complete the following boxes:

Personal Tab

    Description

Diagnosis Tab

    Default Diagnosis 1

Condition Tab

    Injury/Illness/LMP Date

    Illness Indicator

    First Consultation Date

    Emergency

4. Save your work. Close the Patient List dialog box.

5. Click Enter Transactions on the Activities menu.

6. Select Mr. Lopez in the Chart box.

7. Select Heart Palpitations in the Case box.

8. Click the New button in the Charges section to create a new transaction.

9. Verify that the entry in the Date box is 11/15/2010.

10. Enter the procedures marked on the encounter form. A reminder appears stating that the case requires a copayment. Click OK and continue.

11. Enter Lopez's payment. Remember to enter a check number in the Check Number box. Then click the Apply button, and apply the payment.

12. Click the Save Transactions button to save your work. When the Date of Service Validation boxes appear, click Yes to save the transactions. *Note:* The box will appear once for each transaction entered that has a date in the future.

13. Click the Quick Receipt button to print a walkout statement.

14. Close the Transaction Entry dialog box.

EXERCISE 12-3: INPUTTING TRANSACTION DATA

For this exercise, you need Source Documents 13, 14, 16, and 19.

You are now ready to record the transactions from Friday's four encounter forms. Before you begin, set the Medisoft Program Date to November 12, 2010.

ANTHONY BATTISTUTA

1. Click Enter Transactions on the Activities menu.

2. Select Anthony Battistuta in the Chart box.

3. Verify that Diabetes is displayed to the right of the Case box.

4. Record the procedures, one at a time.

5. Save your work.

LAWANA BROOKS

Follow essentially the same procedures to enter the transaction data. Remember to save your work.

EDWIN HSU

Follow essentially the same procedures to enter the transaction data. Then enter Hsu's payment, apply the payment to the charges, and save your work.

HANNAH SYZMANSKI

Follow essentially the same procedures to enter the transaction data. You need to record the date and procedure and Syzmanski's payment. Apply the payment to the charges, and save your work.

EXERCISE 12-4: ENTERING A NEW PATIENT AND TRANSACTIONS

For this exercise, you need Source Documents 21 and 22.

The date is November 12, 2010. Enter patient information and all transactions for Christopher Palmer, a new patient of Dr. Beach. (*Note:* When completing the Policy 1 tab in the Case dialog box, enter 100 in all of the Insurance Coverage by Service Classification boxes.)

EXERCISE 12-5: ENTERING AND APPLYING AN INSURANCE CARRIER PAYMENT

For this exercise, you need Source Document 23.

The date is November 12, 2010. A remittance advice and electronic funds transfer (EFT) have just been received from East Ohio PPO. Enter the deposit in Medisoft, and apply the payment to the appropriate patient accounts.

1. Open the Deposit List dialog box.

2. If necessary, change the date in the Deposit Date box to November 12, 2010.

3. Enter the deposit.

4. Apply the payment to the patient charges. Be sure to click the Save Payments/Adjustments button after each patient. Notice that as you enter and save payments, the amount listed in the Unapplied box decreases.

5. When you are finished, click the Detail button in the Deposit List dialog box to verify that the amount in the Unapplied column for each patient is 0.00.

6. Payments entered in the Deposit List dialog box are automatically linked to data in the Transaction Entry dialog box. Open the Transaction Entry dialog box, and confirm that the insurance company payments and adjustments appear in the transaction list at the bottom of the window for each patient in this exercise. Close the Transaction Entry dialog box.

Remember to create a backup of your work before exiting Medisoft! To help you keep track of your work, name the backup file after the chapter you are working on, for example, StudentID-c12.mbk.

Setting Up Appointments

13

WHAT YOU NEED TO KNOW

To complete the exercises in this chapter, you need to know how to:

◆ Start Office Hours.

◆ Move around in the schedule.

◆ Enter appointments.

◆ Change appointment information.

◆ Move or copy an appointment.

◆ Schedule a recall appointment.

◆ Create a new case record for a patient.

◆ Change a transaction record.

The Family Care Center uses Office Hours as the primary tool for recording appointments. For the simulations in this chapter, assume that you are the front-desk receptionist and are responsible for most of the center's scheduling tasks. Remember, you can access Office Hours at any time, no matter what you are working on. For example, suppose you are typing a letter for one of the doctors and a patient calls to make an appointment. All you have to do is click the Start button on the task bar, select Programs—Medisoft and then Office Hours, enter the appointment, exit Office Hours, and return to your word-processing program. Office Hours can also be accessed from within Medisoft, either by clicking the shortcut button or by clicking Appointment Book on the Activities menu.

EXERCISE 13-1: SCHEDULING APPOINTMENTS

It is Monday, November 15, 2010. In Office Hours, schedule the following patient appointments on December 10, 2010:

Patient	Provider	Time	Length
Nancy Stern	P. McGrath	9:30	30 minutes
Sheila Giles	R. Beach	10:00	45 minutes
Raji Patel	D. Banu	2:45	30 minutes

1. Start Medisoft, and restore the data from your last work session.
2. Set the Medisoft Program Date to November 15, 2010. Open Office Hours.
3. Go to December 10, 2010.
4. Select each patient's provider from the Provider drop-down list, and enter the appointments.

EXERCISE 13-2: MAKING AN APPOINTMENT CHANGE

Carlos Lopez has just called to say that he lost his appointment card and cannot remember the time of his December 1 appointment. He thinks he may have a scheduling conflict. If the appointment is in the morning, he wants it changed to 2:00 the same day. If the 2:00 slot is not available, he needs to make the appointment for the next day at the earliest possible time.

1. In Office Hours, go to December 1, 2010.
2. Find out who Lopez's doctor is by calling up the Patient/Guarantor dialog box in Medisoft. Select the Other Information tab, and

check the Assigned Provider box. Then select Lopez's provider from the Provider drop-down list in Office Hours.

3. Locate Mr. Lopez's appointment.

4. Check to see whether 2:00 P.M., the time he wants the appointment changed to, is available.

5. Since 2:00 is not available, move to December 2 on the calendar, and see if 8:00 A.M. is available.

6. Go back to December 1. Move Mr. Lopez's appointment from December 1 to December 2. (If you do not remember how to move an appointment, see Chapter 11.)

EXERCISE 13-3: JUGGLING SCHEDULES

Mrs. Jackson's sister is on the phone. She will be taking care of the Jackson twins, Darnell and Tyrone, on Saturday, December 11, 2010, and she needs to make appointments for both of them for physicals and tetanus shots sometime after 9:00 A.M. That is the only day they can come in, so she hopes you can accommodate her. She does not remember the name of their doctor.

1. Find out who the boys' doctor is by looking up the information in Medisoft.

2. Go into Office Hours, and check the provider's schedule for December 11. The doctor is booked solid from 8:00 A.M. until she leaves at 1:00 P.M.

3. Check the schedules of Dr. McGrath and Dr. Beach. Since Dr. McGrath is unavailable, book Darnell in the 10:30 A.M. time slot and Tyrone in the 10:45 A.M. slot with Dr. Beach.

EXERCISE 13-4: ADDING PATIENTS TO THE RECALL LIST

Darnell and Tyrone Jackson need to be called back for follow-up appointments in six months. Add both names to the Recall list for six months from December 11, 2010.

1. Click Patient Recall on the Lists menu in Medisoft. The Patient Recall List dialog box is displayed.

2. Click the New button.

3. Enter June 11, 2011, in the Recall Date box.

4. Select Dr. Dana Banu in the Provider box.

5. Select Darnell Jackson's chart number from the drop-down list in the Chart box. Press the Tab key.

6. In the Message box, key *Six month follow-up appointment needed.*

7. Verify that the Call radio button in the Recall Status box is selected.

8. Click the Save button to save the entry.

9. Repeat the steps to add Tyrone Jackson to the Patient Recall List.

10. Close the Patient Recall List dialog box.

EXERCISE 13-5: DIANE HSU AND MICHAEL SYZMANSKI

For this exercise, you will need Source Documents 24 and 25.

It is Monday, November 15, 2010. Diane Hsu and Michael Syzmanski are leaving the office after their appointments. Use the information on Source Documents 24 and 25 to perform the following tasks.

1. Create new cases for both patients by copying existing cases.

   For Hsu, complete the boxes listed below in the Personal and Diagnosis tabs:

Personal Tab

   Description

Diagnosis Tab

   Principal Diagnosis

   For Syzmanski, complete the following boxes in the Personal and Diagnosis tabs:

Personal Tab

   Description

Diagnosis Tab

   Principal Diagnosis

2. Record the charges in the Transaction Entry dialog box.

3. Record the payments, and apply the payments to the charges.

4. Make the appointment indicated on Mrs. Hsu's encounter form, using Office Hours. Do not exit Medisoft.

EXERCISE 13-6: CHANGING A TRANSACTION RECORD

Just as you finish making Mrs. Hsu's appointment, Dr. Robert Beach comes to the desk to say that he thinks he forgot to add the strep test he performed on Christopher Palmer on November 12, 2010, to the encounter form. He asks you to check and to add the charge if necessary.

1. Go to the Transaction Entry dialog box. Check through the entries to find out whether the charge was entered. (It was not.)

2. Enter the new charge. (*Hint:* Remember to change the default date entry in the Date box to November 12, 2010.)

Remember to create a backup of your work before exiting Medisoft! To help you keep track of your work, name the backup file after the chapter you are working on, for example, StudentID-c13.mbk.

Printing Lists and Reports

14

WHAT YOU NEED TO KNOW

To complete the exercises in this chapter, you need to know how to:

- ◆ Create a patient ledger.
- ◆ Create a day sheet report.
- ◆ Understand what aging means in an accounting sense.
- ◆ Create a patient aging report.
- ◆ Enter transactions.
- ◆ Print an appointment list.
- ◆ Print a patient ledger report.
- ◆ Add an item to the Work List.

Because Medisoft is an accounting package, its most powerful features involve computerized manipulation of account data for patients. Medisoft uses information in the system to produce reports on any facet of patients' or insurers' accounts and to generate bills for patients and for insurance companies. For example, as long as the office personnel in the Family Care Center have entered transactions correctly and have performed basic accounting procedures, Medisoft can be used to print current reports on the center's finances. You can print a report showing details of a day's transactions for any one of the center's physicians or for all physicians. You can print a report of late accounts for a particular patient or for all patients, for one insurance company or for all insurance companies.

Before starting the exercises in this chapter, you should understand some basic aspects of medical office accounting procedures.

Every medical office must keep a daily record of charges for and payments made for and by every patient of every doctor. For charges, the record usually includes the name of the patient, the type of service provided, and the amount of the charge. For payments, a record usually includes the name of the patient whose account is being credited and the payment amount. Whereas day sheets record information on charges and payments for a single day, ledgers show all current information up to and including the date shown on the ledger.

EXERCISE 14-1: FINDING A PATIENT'S BALANCE

It is still Monday, November 15, 2010. Anthony Battistuta calls. He would like to know the amount of the charges from November 12 that he is responsible for, assuming that Medicare pays its portion of the total charges. How can you find the amount he is responsible for?

1. Start Medisoft, set the Program Date to November 15, 2010, and restore the data from your last work session.

2. On the Activities menu, click Enter Transactions.

3. In the Chart box, select Anthony Battistuta's chart number.

4. Verify that the Diabetes case is active in the Case box.

5. Look at the Allowed column in the Charges section for the three procedures on 11/12/2010. Add up the amounts in the Allowed column to determine how much Medicare is likely to pay. Since Medicare pays 80 percent of the allowed amount and the patient is responsible for the remaining 20 percent, calculate how much the patient is likely to owe for the November 12th visit.

EXERCISE 14-2: PRINTING A SCHEDULE

Print the appointment schedule for Dr. Dana Banu for Saturday, December 11, 2010.

1. Open Office Hours.

2. Click Appointment List on the Office Hours Reports menu.

3. Select the option to print the report on the printer.

4. Click the Start button. The Data Selection dialog box appears.

5. Enter *12112010* in both Dates boxes.

6. Enter *6* in both Providers boxes.

7. Click the OK button.

8. When the Print dialog box is displayed, click the OK button.

9. Exit Office Hours.

EXERCISE 14-3: PRINTING DAY SHEET REPORTS

Patient day sheets and procedure day sheets can be viewed and/or printed using options on the Reports menu.

Medisoft Program Date: November 12, 2010

CREATING A PATIENT DAY SHEET REPORT

1. On the Reports menu, click Day Sheets and then Patient Day Sheet.

2. Leave the Chart Number Range boxes blank in order to include all patients.

3. Change the entry in the first Date Created Range box to January 1, 2008, and change the entry in the second box to January 1, 2018.

4. Change the entries in both Date From Range boxes to November 12, 2010.

5. If it is not already selected, click the Show Accounts Receivable Totals box.

6. Leave all other boxes blank.

7. Click the Preview Report button.

8. The patient day sheet report is displayed on the screen.

9. Print the report, and then close the Preview Report window.

CREATING A PROCEDURE DAY SHEET REPORT

1. On the Reports menu, click Day Sheets and then Procedure Day Sheet.

2. Leave the Procedure Code Range boxes blank.

3. Change the entry in the first Date Created Range box to January 1, 2008, and change the entry in the second box to January 1, 2018.

4. Change the entries in both Date From Range boxes to November 12, 2010.

5. If it is not already selected, click the Show Accounts Receivable Totals box.

6. Leave all other boxes blank.

7. Click the Preview Report button.

8. The procedure day sheet report is displayed on the screen.

9. Print the report, and then close the Preview Report window.

EXERCISE 14-4: CREATING A PATIENT AGING APPLIED PAYMENT REPORT

Print a patient aging report as a first step in the billing process. The aging report shows which accounts are overdue and how long they have been overdue.

Medisoft Program Date: November 30, 2010

1. On the Reports menu, click Aging Reports and then Patient Aging Applied Payment.

2. Accept the default entry in the first Date From Range box (1/1/1900), and change the entries in the second box to November 30, 2010.

3. Leave all other boxes blank.

4. Click the Preview Report button.

5. The patient aging applied payment report is displayed on the screen.

6. Print the report, and then close the Report Preview window.

EXERCISE 14-5: ADDING ITEMS TO THE COLLECTION LIST

Study the Patient Aging Applied Payment report created in Exercise 14-4. Determine which patients have outstanding balances of greater then $5.00 that are more than sixty days past due.

Add these patient accounts to the Collection List. (*Note:* Do not include Jo Wong's account, since you added it to the list in Chapter 10.)

The following information is common to all tickler entries:

> Action Required: Telephone call about overdue balance

> Status: Active

> Follow-up Date: December 14, 2010

Medisoft Program Date: November 30, 2010

1. Select Collection List on the Activities menu.
2. Click the New button.
3. Complete the following fields in the Tickler tab:

> Action Required

> Responsible Party Type

> Chart Number

> Guarantor

> Responsible Party

> Status

> Follow-up Date

4. Click the Save button.
5. Close the Collection List dialog box.

EXERCISE 14-6: CREATING A PRACTICE ANALYSIS REPORT

Print a practice analysis report for the month of November 2010.

Medisoft Program Date: November 30, 2010

1. On the Reports menu, click Analysis Reports and then Practice Analysis.

2. Change the entry in the first Date Created Range box to January 1, 2008, and change the entry in the second box to January 1, 2018.

3. Change the entry in the first Date From Range box to November 1, 2010, and change the entry in the second box to November 30, 2010.

4. If it is not already selected, click the Show Accounts Receivable Totals Page box.

5. Leave all other boxes blank.

6. Click the Preview Report button.

7. The practice analysis report is displayed on the screen.

8. Print the report, and then close the Preview Report window.

EXERCISE 14-7: STEWART ROBERTSON

You need Source Documents 26 and 27 for this exercise, which has two parts.

PART ONE : DECEMBER 10, 2010

A new patient of Dr. Beach, Stewart Robertson, has stopped by to schedule an appointment and to fill out a patient information form. He wants an appointment for a routine physical in December, specifically for the third Saturday of the month, as early as possible.

Medisoft Program Date: December 10, 2010

1. Using Source Document 26, enter the patient information for Mr. Robertson. Complete the Patient/Guarantor dialog box and the Case dialog box. You need to create a new case. Since Stewart's insurance is a capitated plan, remember to check the Capitated Plan box in the Policy 1 tab of the Case folder. Also enter 100 in all of the Insurance Coverage Percents by Service Classification boxes.

2. In Office Hours, schedule Robertson for his appointment (sixty minutes).

PART TWO: DECEMBER 18, 2010

Stewart Robinson completes his office visit with Dr. Beach.

Medisoft Program Date: December 18, 2010

1. Using Source Document 27, enter Robertson's diagnosis in Medisoft.

2. Enter the charges and payments for Stewart Robertson's visit.

EXERCISE 14-8: MICHAEL SYZMANSKI

You need Source Document 28 for this exercise.

Medisoft Program Date: December 18, 2010

1. Read the following account of Michael Syzmanski's visit to the Family Care Center on December 18, 2010:

   While driving to his daughter Hannah's soccer game, Syzmanski had a minor automobile accident in Jefferson and has a cut on his eyelid. He has come in to see Dr. Banu on an emergency basis. Dr. Banu is unavailable, so he is treated by Dr. McGrath. She determines that there has been no serious damage. After an examination using a local anesthetic, Dr. McGrath stitches the cut and tells Syzmanski to come back in a week. The procedure is simple suture.

2. In Medisoft, enter all the information pertaining to this visit using Source Document 28. *Hint:* Remember to change the default entry in the Provider column in the Transaction Entry dialog box.

3. Close the Transaction Entry dialog box.

Remember to create a backup of your work before exiting Medisoft! To help you keep track of your work, name the backup file after the chapter you are working on, for example, StudentID-c14.mbk.

Putting It All Together

15

WHAT YOU NEED TO KNOW

To complete the exercises in this chapter, you need to know how to:

◆ Schedule appointments.

◆ Create cases.

◆ Enter charges for procedures.

◆ Enter copayments from patients.

◆ Create claims.

◆ Enter payments from insurance carriers.

◆ Create patient statements.

◆ Print reports.

◆ Add items to the Collection List.

◆ Create collection letters.

In this chapter, you need to use almost all the skills you have practiced throughout the exercises in the book. If you have any problems, refer back to the chapters in the book that cover the material.

EXERCISE 15-1: SCHEDULING APPOINTMENTS

1. Start Medisoft, and restore the data from your last work session.

2. Enter January 5, 2011, as the program date in Medisoft.

3. Schedule appointments for January 5, 2011, for the following patients. Make sure they are scheduled for the right doctors.

Jackson, Luther	30 minutes	9:00 A.M.
Hsu, Edwin	15 minutes	9:15 A.M.
Simmons, Jill	15 minutes	10:15 A.M.
Stern, Nancy	1 hour	9:30 A.M.
Syzmanski, Debra	30 minutes	9:30 A.M.
Giles, Sheila	15 minutes	9:00 A.M.
Battistuta, Pauline	30 minutes	10:30 A.M.

4. Switch the appointment times for Giles and Simmons.

5. Cancel the appointment for Edwin Hsu.

6. Print the appointment lists for January 5, 2011, for Dr. Banu, Dr. Beach, and Dr. McGrath.

EXERCISE 15-2: CREATING CASES

Create new cases for all patients with appointments on January 5, 2011, using the information found on Source Documents 29–34.

EXERCISE 15-3: ENTERING TRANSACTIONS

Using Source Documents 29–34, record the charge and payment transactions for all of the patients who had appointments.

EXERCISE 15-4: CREATING CLAIMS

Create insurance claims for all transactions that have not already been placed on claims. (*Hint:* Leave the Transaction Dates boxes blank in the Create Claims dialog box.) Change the status of the newly created claims from Ready to Send to Sent.

EXERCISE 15-5: ENTERING INSURANCE PAYMENTS

Change the Medisoft Program Date to December 31, 2010. Enter the insurance payments listed on Source Documents 35–39, and apply the payments to patient charges. For capitated payments, remember to identify patients covered by this plan who had visited the practice during the month of November 2010, using the List Only button in the Claim Management window, then enter a zero insurance deposit to adjust capitated patient accounts to a zero balance.

EXERCISE 15-6: CREATING PATIENT STATEMENTS

Create remainder statements as of 12/31/2010 for patients whose last names begin with the letters *J* through *Z*. Print any statements that were created.

EXERCISE 15-7: PRINTING REPORTS

1. Print a patient day sheet for 01/05/2011.

2. Print a Patient Aging Applied Payment report as of 12/31/2010.

3. Print a Practice Analysis report for the period of 1/1/2010 to 12/31/2010.

EXERCISE 15-8: ADDING ITEMS TO THE COLLECTION LIST

1. Study the Patient Aging Applied Payment report created in Exercise 15-7. Determine which patients have account balances of greater than $5.00 whose accounts are more than sixty days late.

2. Change the dates in the Collection List Date boxes to 1/1/2010 and 12/31/2010. Add these items to the Collection List on 12/31/2010. Note that you do not need to add anyone who is already on the Collection List. The patients should be called to alert them to the overdue accounts. A follow-up should be scheduled for two weeks from today.

EXERCISE 15-9: CREATING COLLECTION LETTERS

Change the Medisoft Program Date to January 14, 2011. Create collection letters for the patients added to the Collection List in Exercise 15-8. In the Data Selection Questions dialog box for the Collection Letter report, enter January 14, 2011 in both Follow Up Date Range boxes. Also make sure that all three boxes at the bottom of the dialog box, including Generate Collection Letters, are checked.

Remember to create a backup of your work before exiting Medisoft! To help you keep track of your work, name the backup file after the chapter you are working on, for example, StudentID-c15.mbk.

SOURCE DOCUMENTS

FAMILY CARE CENTER
285 Stephenson Boulevard
Stephenson, OH 60089-4000
614-555-0000

PATIENT INFORMATION FORM

Patient				
Last Name Tanaka	First Name Hiro	MI	Sex __ M X F	Date of Birth 2 / 20 / 1975
Address 80 Cedar Lane	City Stephenson	State OH		Zip 60089
Home Ph # (614) 555-7373 Cell Ph # (614) 555-0162		Marital Status Single		Student Status
SS# 812-73-6000	Email htanaka@abc.com		Allergies: penicillin	
Employment Status Full-time	Employer Name McCray Manufacturing Inc.	Work Ph # (614) 555-1001	Primary Insurance ID# 812736000 Group HJ31	
Employer Address 1311 Kings Highway	City Stephenson	State OH	Zip 60089	
Referred By Dr. Bertram Brown		Ph # of Referral (614) 567-7896		

Responsible Party (Complete this section if the person responsible for the bill is not the patient)

Last Name	First Name	MI	Sex __ M __ F	Date of Birth / /
Address	City	State Zip	SS#	
Relation to Patient __ Spouse __ Parent __ Other	Employer Name		Work Phone # ( )	
Spouse, or Parent (if minor):			Home Phone # ( )	

Insurance (If you have multiple coverage, supply information from both carriers)

Primary Carrier Name OhioCare HMO	Secondary Carrier Name
Name of the Insured (Name on ID Card) Hiro Tanaka	Name of the Insured (Name on ID Card)
Patient's relationship to the insured X Self __ Spouse __ Child	Patient's relationship to the insured __ Self __ Spouse __ Child
Insured ID # 812736000	Insured ID #
Group # or Company Name Group HJ31	Group # or Company Name
Insurance Address 147 Central Ave., Halevile, OH 60890	Insurance Address
Phone #614-555-0101	Copay $ 20	Phone #	Copay $
	Deductible $		Deductible $

Other Information

Is patient's condition related to:	Reason for visit:Accident - back pain
__ Employment X Auto Accident (if yes, state in which accident occurred: OH) __ Other Accident	

Date of Accident: 9 /26 /2010   Date of First Symptom of Illness: 9 /26 /2010

Financial Agreement and Authorization for Treatment

I authorize treatment and agree to pay all fees and charges for the person named above. I agree to pay all charges shown by statements, promptly upon their presentation, unless credit arrangements are agreed upon in writing.

I authorize payment directly to FAMILY CARE CENTER of insurance benefits otherwise payable to me. I hereby authorize the release of any medical information necessary in order to process a claim for payment in my behalf.

Signed: Hiro Tanaka

Date: 10/4/2010

FAMILY CARE CENTER
285 Stephenson Boulevard
Stephenson, OH 60089-4000
614-555-0000

PATIENT INFORMATION FORM

Patient				
Last Name Wright	First Name Lisa	MI	Sex __ M _X_ F	Date of Birth 3 / 15/ 1970
Address 39 Woodlake Rd.	City Stephenson	State OH	Zip 60089	

Home Ph # (614) 555-7059 Cell Ph # (614) 505-1397   Marital Status Divorced   Student Status

SS# 333-46-7904	Email lwright@abc.com	Allergies: none
Employment Status Full-time	Employer Name Wheeler, Sampson, & Hull	Work Ph # (614) 086-9000	Primary Insurance ID# 0032697 Group A4
Employer Address 100 Central Ave.	City Stephenson	State OH	Zip 60089
Referred By Dr. Marion Davis		Ph # of Referral (614) 444-3200	

Responsible Party (Complete this section if the person responsible for the bill is not the patient)

Last Name	First Name	MI	Sex __ M __ F	Date of Birth / /
Address	City	State Zip	SS#	
Relation to Patient __ Spouse __ Parent __ Other	Employer Name	Work Phone # ( )	
Spouse, or Parent (if minor):		Home Phone # ( )	

Insurance (If you have multiple coverage, supply information from both carriers)

Primary Carrier Name Blue Cross Blue Shield	Secondary Carrier Name
Name of the Insured (Name on ID Card) Lisa Wright	Name of the Insured (Name on ID Card)
Patient's relationship to the insured _X_ Self __ Spouse __ Child	Patient's relationship to the insured __ Self __ Spouse __ Child
Insured ID # 0032697	Insured ID #
Group # or Company Name Group A4	Group # or Company Name
Insurance Address 340 Boulevard, Columbus, OH 60220	Insurance Address
Phone # 614-024-9000 Copay $ Deductible $ $500 (met)	Phone # Copay $ Deductible $

Other Information

Is patient's condition related to: Reason for visit: cough

__ Employment   __ Auto Accident (if yes, state in which accident occurred: ___)   __ Other Accident

Date of Accident: /   /   Date of First Symptom of Illness: /   /

Financial Agreement and Authorization for Treatment

I authorize treatment and agree to pay all fees and charges for the person named above. I agree to pay all charges shown by statements, promptly upon their presentation, unless credit arrangements are agreed upon in writing.

I authorize payment directly to FAMILY CARE CENTER of insurance benefits otherwise payable to me. I hereby authorize the release of any medical information necessary in order to process a claim for payment in my behalf.

Signed: Lisa Wright   Date: 10/4/2010

ENCOUNTER FORM

10/4/2010		3:00 pm	
DATE		TIME	
Hiro Tanaka		TANAKHI0	
PATIENT NAME		CHART #	

OFFICE VISITS - SYMPTOMATIC

NEW

99201	OF--New Patient Minimal	
99202	OF--New Patient Low	X
99203	OF--New Patient Detailed	
99204	OF--New Patient Moderate	
99205	OF--New Patient High	

ESTABLISHED

99211	OF--Established Patient Minimal	
99212	OF--Established Patient Low	
99213	OF--Established Patient Detailed	
99214	OF--Established Patient Moderate	
99215	OF--Established Patient High	

PREVENTIVE VISITS

NEW

99381	Under 1 Year	
99382	1 - 4 Years	
99383	5 - 11 Years	
99384	12 - 17 Years	
99385	18 - 39 Years	
99386	40 - 64 Years	
99387	65 Years & Up	

ESTABLISHED

99391	Under 1 Year	
99392	1 - 4 Years	
99393	5 - 11 Years	
99394	12 - 17 Years	
99395	18 - 39 Years	
99396	40 - 64 Years	
99397	65 Years & Up	

PROCEDURES

12011	Simple suture--face--local anes.	
29125	App. of short arm splint; static	
29425	App. of short leg cast, walking	
50390	Aspiration of renal cyst by needle	
71010	Chest x-ray, single view, frontal	

PROCEDURES

71020	Chest x-ray, two views, frontal & lateral	
71030	Chest x-ray, complete, four views	
73070	Elbow x-ray, AP & lateral views	
73090	Forearm x-ray, AP & lateral views	
73100	Wrist x-ray, AP & lateral views	
73510	Hip x-ray, complete, two views	
73600	Ankle x-ray, AP & lateral views	

LABORATORY

80019	19 clinical chemistry tests	
80048	Basic metabolic panel	
80061	Lipid panel	
82270	Blood screening, occult; feces	
82947	Glucose screening--quantitative	
82951	Glucose tolerance test, three specimens	
83718	HDL cholesterol	
84478	Triglycerides test	
85007	Manual differential WBC	
85018	Hemoglobin	
85651	Erythrocyte sedimentation rate--non-auto	
86580	TB Mantoux test	
87072	Culture by commercial kit, nonurine...	
87076	Culture, anaerobic isolate	
87077	Bacterial culture, aerobic isolate	
87086	Urine culture and colony count	
87430	Strep test	
87880	Direct streptococcus screen	

INJECTIONS

90471	Immunization administration	
90703	Tetanus injection	
90772	Injection	
92516	Facial nerve function studies	
93000	Electrocardiogram--ECG with interpretation	
93015	Treadmill stress test, with physician...	
96900	Ultraviolet light treatment	
99070	Supplies and materials provided	

FAMILY CARE CENTER
286 Stephenson Blvd.
Stephenson, OH 60089
614-555-0000

☐ DANA BANU, M.D.
☐ ROBERT BEACH, M.D.
☐ PATRICIA MCGRATH, M.D.

☐ JESSICA RUDNER, M.D.
☐ JOHN RUDNER, M.D.
☒ KATHERINE YAN, M.D.

NOTES

REFERRING PHYSICIAN	NPI	AUTHORIZATION #
Bertram Brown, MD	1234567890	

DIAGNOSIS
724.2

PAYMENT AMOUNT
$20, check #123

FAMILY CARE CENTER
285 Stephenson Boulevard
Stephenson, OH 60089
614-555-0000

KATHERINE YAN, M.D.
PHYSICIAN'S NOTES

PATIENT NAME	Hiro Tanaka
CHART NUMBER	TANAKHI0
DATE	10/4/10
CASE	Accident - Back Pain

NOTES

Condition related to auto accident in Stephenson, Ohio that occurred on 9/26/10.

Patient was hospitalized from 9/26/10 to 9/27/10.

Patient was totally disabled from 9/26/10 to 9/27/10.

Patient was partially disabled from 9/28/10 to 10/4/10.

Patient was unable to work from 9/26/10 to 10/4/10.

ENCOUNTER FORM

10/4/2010		9:45 am	
DATE		TIME	
Elizabeth Jones		**JONESEL0**	
PATIENT NAME		CHART #	

OFFICE VISITS - SYMPTOMATIC		
NEW		
99201	OF--New Patient Minimal	
99202	OF--New Patient Low	
99203	OF--New Patient Detailed	
99204	OF--New Patient Moderate	
99205	OF--New Patient High	
ESTABLISHED		
99211	OF--Established Patient Minimal	
99212	OF--Established Patient Low	
99213	OF--Established Patient Detailed	X
99214	OF--Established Patient Moderate	
99215	OF--Established Patient High	
PREVENTIVE VISITS		
NEW		
99381	Under 1 Year	
99382	1 - 4 Years	
99383	5 - 11 Years	
99384	12 - 17 Years	
99385	18 - 39 Years	
99386	40 - 64 Years	
99387	65 Years & Up	
ESTABLISHED		
99391	Under 1 Year	
99392	1 - 4 Years	
99393	5 - 11 Years	
99394	12 - 17 Years	
99395	18 - 39 Years	
99396	40 - 64 Years	
99397	65 Years & Up	
PROCEDURES		
12011	Simple suture--face--local anes.	
29125	App. of short arm splint; static	
29425	App. of short leg cast, walking	
50390	Aspiration of renal cyst by needle	
71010	Chest x-ray, single view, frontal	

PROCEDURES		
71020	Chest x-ray, two views, frontal & lateral	
71030	Chest x-ray, complete, four views	
73070	Elbow x-ray, AP & lateral views	
73090	Forearm x-ray, AP & lateral views	
73100	Wrist x-ray, AP & lateral views	
73510	Hip x-ray, complete, two views	
73600	Ankle x-ray, AP & lateral views	
LABORATORY		
80019	19 clinical chemistry tests	
80048	Basic metabolic panel	
80061	Lipid panel	
82270	Blood screening, occult; feces	
82947	Glucose screening--quantitative	
82951	Glucose tolerance test, three specimens	
83718	HDL cholesterol	
84478	Triglycerides test	
85007	Manual differential WBC	
85018	Hemoglobin	
85651	Erythrocyte sedimentation rate--non-auto	
86580	TB Mantoux test	
87072	Culture by commercial kit, nonurine...	
87076	Culture, anaerobic isolate	
87077	Bacterial culture, aerobic isolate	
87086	Urine culture and colony count	
87430	Strep test	
87880	Direct streptococcus screen	
INJECTIONS		
90471	Immunization administration	
90703	Tetanus injection	
90772	Injection	
92516	Facial nerve function studies	
93000	Electrocardiogram--ECG with interpretation	
93015	Treadmill stress test, with physician...	
96900	Ultraviolet light treatment	
99070	Supplies and materials provided	

FAMILY CARE CENTER
286 Stephenson Blvd.
Stephenson, OH 60089
614-555-0000

- ☐ DANA BANU, M.D.
- ☐ ROBERT BEACH, M.D.
- ☐ PATRICIA MCGRATH, M.D.
- ☐ JESSICA RUDNER, M.D.
- ☐ JOHN RUDNER, M.D.
- ☒ KATHERINE YAN, M.D.

NOTES

REFERRING PHYSICIAN	NPI	AUTHORIZATION #

DIAGNOSIS
250.00

PAYMENT AMOUNT

ENCOUNTER FORM

10/4/2010	11:00 am
DATE	TIME
John Fitzwilliams	FITZWJO0
PATIENT NAME	CHART #

OFFICE VISITS - SYMPTOMATIC

NEW

99201	OF--New Patient Minimal	
99202	OF--New Patient Low	
99203	OF--New Patient Detailed	
99204	OF--New Patient Moderate	
99205	OF--New Patient High	

ESTABLISHED

99211	OF--Established Patient Minimal	
99212	OF--Established Patient Low	X
99213	OF--Established Patient Detailed	
99214	OF--Established Patient Moderate	
99215	OF--Established Patient High	

PREVENTIVE VISITS

NEW

99381	Under 1 Year	
99382	1 - 4 Years	
99383	5 - 11 Years	
99384	12 - 17 Years	
99385	18 - 39 Years	
99386	40 - 64 Years	
99387	65 Years & Up	

ESTABLISHED

99391	Under 1 Year	
99392	1 - 4 Years	
99393	5 - 11 Years	
99394	12 - 17 Years	
99395	18 - 39 Years	
99396	40 - 64 Years	
99397	65 Years & Up	

PROCEDURES

12011	Simple suture--face--local anes.	
29125	App. of short arm splint; static	
29425	App. of short leg cast, walking	
50390	Aspiration of renal cyst by needle	
71010	Chest x-ray, single view, frontal	

PROCEDURES

71020	Chest x-ray, two views, frontal & lateral	
71030	Chest x-ray, complete, four views	
73070	Elbow x-ray, AP & lateral views	
73090	Forearm x-ray, AP & lateral views	
73100	Wrist x-ray, AP & lateral views	
73510	Hip x-ray, complete, two views	
73600	Ankle x-ray, AP & lateral views	

LABORATORY

80019	19 clinical chemistry tests	
80048	Basic metabolic panel	
80061	Lipid panel	
82270	Blood screening, occult; feces	X
82947	Glucose screening--quantitative	
82951	Glucose tolerance test, three specimens	
83718	HDL cholesterol	
84478	Triglycerides test	
85007	Manual differential WBC	
85018	Hemoglobin	
85651	Erythrocyte sedimentation rate--non-auto	
86580	TB Mantoux test	
87072	Culture by commercial kit, nonurine...	
87076	Culture, anaerobic isolate	
87077	Bacterial culture, aerobic isolate	
87086	Urine culture and colony count	
87430	Strep test	
87880	Direct streptococcus screen	

INJECTIONS

90471	Immunization administration	
90703	Tetanus injection	
90772	Injection	
92516	Facial nerve function studies	
93000	Electrocardiogram--ECG with interpretation	
93015	Treadmill stress test, with physician...	
96900	Ultraviolet light treatment	
99070	Supplies and materials provided	

FAMILY CARE CENTER
286 Stephenson Blvd.
Stephenson, OH 60089
614-555-0000

☐ DANA BANU, M.D.
☐ ROBERT BEACH, M.D.
☐ PATRICIA MCGRATH, M.D.

☐ JESSICA RUDNER, M.D.
☒ JOHN RUDNER, M.D.
☐ KATHERINE YAN, M.D.

NOTES

REFERRING PHYSICIAN	NPI	AUTHORIZATION #

DIAGNOSIS
531.30

PAYMENT AMOUNT
$15 copay, check #456

ENCOUNTER FORM

10/4/2010
DATE

1:00 pm
TIME

Lisa Wright
PATIENT NAME

WRIGHLI0
CHART #

OFFICE VISITS - SYMPTOMATIC		
NEW		
99201	OF--New Patient Minimal	
99202	OF--New Patient Low	
99203	OF--New Patient Detailed	X
99204	OF--New Patient Moderate	
99205	OF--New Patient High	
ESTABLISHED		
99211	OF--Established Patient Minimal	
99212	OF--Established Patient Low	
99213	OF--Established Patient Detailed	
99214	OF--Established Patient Moderate	
99215	OF--Established Patient High	
PREVENTIVE VISITS		
NEW		
99381	Under 1 Year	
99382	1 - 4 Years	
99383	5 - 11 Years	
99384	12 - 17 Years	
99385	18 - 39 Years	
99386	40 - 64 Years	
99387	65 Years & Up	
ESTABLISHED		
99391	Under 1 Year	
99392	1 - 4 Years	
99393	5 - 11 Years	
99394	12 - 17 Years	
99395	18 - 39 Years	
99396	40 - 64 Years	
99397	65 Years & Up	
PROCEDURES		
12011	Simple suture--face--local anes.	
29125	App. of short arm splint; static	
29425	App. of short leg cast, walking	
50390	Aspiration of renal cyst by needle	
71010	Chest x-ray, single view, frontal	

PROCEDURES		
71020	Chest x-ray, two views, frontal & lateral	X
71030	Chest x-ray, complete, four views	
73070	Elbow x-ray, AP & lateral views	
73090	Forearm x-ray, AP & lateral views	
73100	Wrist x-ray, AP & lateral views	
73510	Hip x-ray, complete, two views	
73600	Ankle x-ray, AP & lateral views	
LABORATORY		
80019	19 clinical chemistry tests	
80048	Basic metabolic panel	
80061	Lipid panel	
82270	Blood screening, occult; feces	
82947	Glucose screening--quantitative	
82951	Glucose tolerance test, three specimens	
83718	HDL cholesterol	
84478	Triglycerides test	
85007	Manual differential WBC	
85018	Hemoglobin	
85651	Erythrocyte sedimentation rate--non-auto	
86580	TB Mantoux test	
87072	Culture by commercial kit, nonurine...	
87076	Culture, anaerobic isolate	
87077	Bacterial culture, aerobic isolate	
87086	Urine culture and colony count	
87430	Strep test	
87880	Direct streptococcus screen	
INJECTIONS		
90471	Immunization administration	
90703	Tetanus injection	
90772	Injection	
92516	Facial nerve function studies	
93000	Electrocardiogram--ECG with interpretation	
93015	Treadmill stress test, with physician...	
96900	Ultraviolet light treatment	
99070	Supplies and materials provided	

FAMILY CARE CENTER
286 Stephenson Blvd.
Stephenson, OH 60089
614-555-0000

☐ DANA BANU, M.D.
☐ ROBERT BEACH, M.D.
☐ PATRICIA MCGRATH, M.D.

☒ JESSICA RUDNER, M.D.
☐ JOHN RUDNER, M.D.
☐ KATHERINE YAN, M.D.

NOTES

REFERRING PHYSICIAN

NPI

AUTHORIZATION #

DIAGNOSIS
490

PAYMENT AMOUNT

CHAMPVA
240 CENTER ST.
COLUMBUS, OH 60220

PROVIDER REMITTANCE
THIS IS NOT A BILL
A PAYMENT SUMMARY AND AN EXPLANATION OF
CODES ARE AT THE END OF THIS STATEMENT

FAMILY CARE CENTER
285 STEPHENSON BLVD.
STEPHENSON, OH 60089-4000

PAGE: 1 OF 1
DATE: 10/04/2010
ID NUMBER: 214778924

PROVIDER: JOHN RUDNER, M.D.

PATIENT: FITZWILLIAMS JOHN   CLAIM: 123456789

FROM DATE	THRU DATE	PROC CODE	UNITS	AMOUNT BILLED	AMOUNT ALLOWED	DEDUCT	COPAY/ COINS	PROV PAID	REASON CODE
09/07/10	09/07/10	99211	1	36.00	20.68	.00	15.00	5.68	
09/07/10	09/07/10	84478	1	29.00	8.04	.00	.00	8.04	
	CLAIM TOTALS			64.00	28.72	.00	15.00	13.72	

PROVIDER: KATHERINE YAN, M.D.

PATIENT: FITZWILLIAMS SARAH   CLAIM: 234567891

FROM DATE	THRU DATE	PROC CODE	UNITS	AMOUNT BILLED	AMOUNT ALLOWED	DEDUCT	COPAY/ COINS	PROV PAID	REASON CODE
09/07/10	09/07/10	90471	1	15.00	15.00	.00	15.00	.00	
09/07/10	09/07/10	90703	1	29.00	14.30	.00	.00	14.30	
	CLAIM TOTALS			44.00	29.30	.00	15.00	14.30	

******************** CHECK #214778924 IN THE AMOUNT OF $28.02 IS ATTACHED ********************

PAYMENT SUMMARY		TOTAL ALL CLAIMS	
TOTAL AMOUNT PAID	28.02	AMOUNT CHARGED	108.00
PRIOR CREDIT BALANCE	.00	AMOUNT ALLOWED	58.02
CURRENT CREDIT DEFERRED	.00	DEDUCTIBLE	.00
PRIOR CREDIT APPLIED	.00	COPAY	30.00
NEW CREDIT BALANCE	.00	OTHER REDUCTION	.00
NET DISBURSED	28.02		

STATUS CODES:
A - APPROVED   AJ - ADJUSTMENT   IP - IN PROCESS   R - REJECTED   V - VOID

EAST OHIO PPO
10 CENTRAL AVENUE
HALEVILLE, OH 60890

PROVIDER REMITTANCE
THIS IS NOT A BILL
A PAYMENT SUMMARY AND AN EXPLANATION OF
CODES ARE AT THE END OF THIS STATEMENT

FAMILY CARE CENTER
285 STEPHENSON BLVD.
STEPHENSON, OH 60089-4000

PAGE: 1 OF 2
DATE: 10/04/2010
ID NUMBER: 00146972

PROVIDER: ROBERT BEACH, M.D.

PATIENT: ARLEN SUSAN   CLAIM: 123456789

FROM DATE	THRU DATE	PROC CODE	UNITS	AMOUNT BILLED	AMOUNT ALLOWED	DEDUCT	COPAY/ COINS	PROV PAID	REASON CODE
09/06/10	09/06/10	99212	1	54.00	48.60	.00	20.00	28.60	
	CLAIM TOTALS			54.00	48.60	.00	20.00	28.60	

PROVIDER: JOHN RUDNER, M.D.

PATIENT: BELL HERBERT   CLAIM: 234567891

FROM DATE	THRU DATE	PROC CODE	UNITS	AMOUNT BILLED	AMOUNT ALLOWED	DEDUCT	COPAY/ COINS	PROV PAID	REASON CODE
09/06/10	09/06/10	99211	1	36.00	32.40	.00	20.00	12.40	
	CLAIM TOTALS			36.00	32.40	.00	20.00	12.40	

PATIENT: BELL SAMUEL   CLAIM: 34567891

FROM DATE	THRU DATE	PROC CODE	UNITS	AMOUNT BILLED	AMOUNT ALLOWED	DEDUCT	COPAY/ COINS	PROV PAID	REASON CODE
09/06/10	09/06/10	99212	1	54.00	48.60	.00	20.00	28.60	
	CLAIM TOTALS			54.00	48.60	.00	20.00	28.60	

PROVIDER: KATHERINE YAN, M.D.

PATIENT: BELL JANINE   CLAIM: 45678912

FROM DATE	THRU DATE	PROC CODE	UNITS	AMOUNT BILLED	AMOUNT ALLOWED	DEDUCT	COPAY/ COINS	PROV PAID	REASON CODE
09/06/10	09/06/10	99213	1	72.00	64.80	.00	20.00	44.80	
09/06/10	09/06/10	73510	1	124.00	111.60	.00	.00	111.60	
	CLAIM TOTALS			196.00	176.40	.00	20.00	156.40	

PATIENT: BELL JONATHAN   CLAIM: 56789123

FROM DATE	THRU DATE	PROC CODE	UNITS	AMOUNT BILLED	AMOUNT ALLOWED	DEDUCT	COPAY/ COINS	PROV PAID	REASON CODE
09/06/10	09/06/10	99394	1	222.00	199.80	.00	20.00	179.80	
	CLAIM TOTALS			222.00	199.80	.00	20.00	179.80	

STATUS CODES:
A - APPROVED   AJ - ADJUSTMENT   IP - IN PROCESS   R - REJECTED   V - VOID

EAST OHIO PPO
10 CENTRAL AVENUE
HALEVILLE, OH 60890

PROVIDER REMITTANCE
THIS IS NOT A BILL
A PAYMENT SUMMARY AND AN EXPLANATION OF
CODES ARE AT THE END OF THIS STATEMENT

FAMILY CARE CENTER
285 STEPHENSON BLVD.
STEPHENSON, OH 60089-4000

PAGE:	2 OF 2
DATE:	10/04/2010
ID NUMBER:	00146972

PROVIDER: KATHERINE YAN, M.D.

PATIENT: BELL SARINA   CLAIM: 56789123

FROM DATE	THRU DATE	PROC CODE	UNITS	AMOUNT BILLED	AMOUNT ALLOWED	DEDUCT	COPAY/ COINS	PROV PAID	REASON CODE
09/06/10	09/06/10	99213	1	72.00	64.80	.00	20.00	44.80	
	CLAIM TOTALS			72.00	64.80	.00	20.00	44.80	

PAYMENT SUMMARY		TOTAL ALL CLAIMS		EFT INFORMATION	
TOTAL AMOUNT PAID	450.60	AMOUNT CHARGED	634.00	NUMBER	00146972
PRIOR CREDIT BALANCE	.00	AMOUNT ALLOWED	570.60	DATE	10/04/10
CURRENT CREDIT DEFERRED	.00	DEDUCTIBLE	.00	AMOUNT	450.60
PRIOR CREDIT APPLIED	.00	COPAY	120.00		
NEW CREDIT BALANCE	.00	OTHER REDUCTION	.00		
NET DISBURSED	450.60	AMOUNT APPROVED	450.60		

STATUS CODES:
A - APPROVED   AJ - ADJUSTMENT   IP - IN PROCESS   R - REJECTED   V - VOID

BLUE CROSS/BLUE SHIELD
340 BOULEVARD
COLUMBUS, OH 60220

PROVIDER REMITTANCE
THIS IS NOT A BILL
A PAYMENT SUMMARY AND AN EXPLANATION OF
CODES ARE AT THE END OF THIS STATEMENT

FAMILY CARE CENTER
285 STEPHENSON BLVD.
STEPHENSON, OH 60089-4000

PAGE:	1 OF 1
DATE:	11/04/2010
ID NUMBER:	001234

PROVIDER: ROBERT BEACH, M.D.

PATIENT: GILES SHEILA   CLAIM: 123456789

FROM DATE	THRU DATE	PROC CODE	UNITS	AMOUNT BILLED	AMOUNT ALLOWED	DEDUCT	COPAY/ COINS	PROV PAID	REASON CODE
10/29/10	10/29/10	99213	1	72.00	72.00	.00	.00	57.60	
10/29/10	10/29/10	71010	1	91.00	91.00	.00	.00	72.80	
10/29/10	10/29/10	87430	1	29.00	.00	.00	.00	.00	R
	CLAIM TOTALS			192.00	163.00	.00	.00	130.40	

R* OUTSIDE LAB WORK NOT BILLABLE BY PROVIDER

PATIENT: SIMMONS JILL   CLAIM: 234567891

FROM DATE	THRU DATE	PROC CODE	UNITS	AMOUNT BILLED	AMOUNT ALLOWED	DEDUCT	COPAY/ COINS	PROV PAID	REASON CODE
10/29/10	10/29/10	99212	1	54.00	54.00	.00	.00	43.20	
10/29/10	10/29/10	87086	1	51.00	51.00	.00	.00	40.80	
	CLAIM TOTALS			105.00	105.00	.00	.00	84.00	

PAYMENT SUMMARY		TOTAL ALL CLAIMS		EFT INFORMATION	
TOTAL AMOUNT PAID	214.40	AMOUNT CHARGED	297.00	NUMBER	001234
PRIOR CREDIT BALANCE	.00	AMOUNT ALLOWED	268.00	DATE	11/04/10
CURRENT CREDIT DEFERRED	.00	DEDUCTIBLE	.00	AMOUNT	214.40
PRIOR CREDIT APPLIED	.00	COINSURANCE	.00		
NEW CREDIT BALANCE	.00	OTHER REDUCTION	.00		
NET DISBURSED	214.40	AMOUNT APPROVED	214.40		

STATUS CODES:
A - APPROVED   AJ - ADJUSTMENT   IP - IN PROCESS   R - REJECTED   V - VOID

OHIOCARE HMO
147 CENTRAL AVENUE
HALEVILLE, OH 60890

FAMILY CARE CENTER
285 STEPHENSON BLVD.
STEPHENSON, OH 60089-4000

PAGE: 1 OF 1
DATE: 10/31/2010
ID NUMBER: 001006003

OHIOCARE HMO CAPITATION STATEMENT
MONTH OF OCTOBER 2010

PROVIDERS
BANU DANA
BEACH ROBERT
MCGRATH PATRICIA
RUDNER JESSICA
RUDNER JOHN
YAN KATHERINE

MEMBER NUMBER	MEMBER NAME	CONTRACT NUMBER	CONTRACT STATUS
0003602149	FAMILY CARE CENTER	YG34906	APPROVED

AMOUNT OF PAYMENT $2,500.00
EFT STATUS: SENT 10/31/10 8:46AM
TRANSACTION #343434

BLUE CROSS/BLUE SHIELD
340 BOULEVARD
COLUMBUS, OH 60220

PROVIDER REMITTANCE
THIS IS NOT A BILL
A PAYMENT SUMMARY AND AN EXPLANATION OF
CODES ARE AT THE END OF THIS STATEMENT

FAMILY CARE CENTER
285 STEPHENSON BLVD.
STEPHENSON, OH 60089-4000

PAGE: 1 OF 1
DATE: 10/29/2010
ID NUMBER: 2000000

PROVIDER: JESSICA RUDNER, M.D.

PATIENT: WRIGHT LISA   CLAIM: 345678901

FROM DATE	THRU DATE	PROC CODE	UNITS	AMOUNT BILLED	AMOUNT ALLOWED	DEDUCT	COPAY/ COINS	PROV PAID	REASON CODE
10/04/10	10/04/10	99203	1	120.00	120.00	.00	.00	96.00	
10/04/10	10/04/10	71020	1	112.00	112.00	.00	.00	89.60	
	CLAIM TOTALS			232.00	232.00	.00	.00	185.60	

PAYMENT SUMMARY		TOTAL ALL CLAIMS		EFT INFORMATION	
TOTAL AMOUNT PAID	185.60	AMOUNT CHARGED	232.00	NUMBER	2000000
PRIOR CREDIT BALANCE	.00	AMOUNT ALLOWED	232.00	DATE	10/29/10
CURRENT CREDIT DEFERRED	.00	DEDUCTIBLE	.00	AMOUNT	185.60
PRIOR CREDIT APPLIED	.00	COINSURANCE	.00		
NEW CREDIT BALANCE	.00	OTHER REDUCTION	.00		
NET DISBURSED	185.60	AMOUNT APPROVED	185.60		

STATUS CODES:
A - APPROVED   AJ - ADJUSTMENT   IP - IN PROCESS   R - REJECTED   V - VOID

ENCOUNTER FORM

11/12/2010
DATE

9:00 am
TIME

Anthony Battistuta
PATIENT NAME

BATTIAN0
CHART #

OFFICE VISITS - SYMPTOMATIC		
NEW		
99201	OF--New Patient Minimal	
99202	OF--New Patient Low	
99203	OF--New Patient Detailed	
99204	OF--New Patient Moderate	
99205	OF--New Patient High	
ESTABLISHED		
99211	OF--Established Patient Minimal	
99212	OF--Established Patient Low	X
99213	OF--Established Patient Detailed	
99214	OF--Established Patient Moderate	
99215	OF--Established Patient High	
PREVENTIVE VISITS		
NEW		
99381	Under 1 Year	
99382	1 - 4 Years	
99383	5 - 11 Years	
99384	12 - 17 Years	
99385	18 - 39 Years	
99386	40 - 64 Years	
99387	65 Years & Up	
ESTABLISHED		
99391	Under 1 Year	
99392	1 - 4 Years	
99393	5 - 11 Years	
99394	12 - 17 Years	
99395	18 - 39 Years	
99396	40 - 64 Years	
99397	65 Years & Up	
PROCEDURES		
12011	Simple suture--face--local anes.	
29125	App. of short arm splint; static	
29425	App. of short leg cast, walking	
50390	Aspiration of renal cyst by needle	
71010	Chest x-ray, single view, frontal	

PROCEDURES		
71020	Chest x-ray, two views, frontal & lateral	
71030	Chest x-ray, complete, four views	
73070	Elbow x-ray, AP & lateral views	
73090	Forearm x-ray, AP & lateral views	
73100	Wrist x-ray, AP & lateral views	
73510	Hip x-ray, complete, two views	
73600	Ankle x-ray, AP & lateral views	
LABORATORY		
80019	19 clinical chemistry tests	
80048	Basic metabolic panel	
80061	Lipid panel	
82270	Blood screening, occult; feces	
82947	Glucose screening--quantitative	
82951	Glucose tolerance test, three specimens	X
83718	HDL cholesterol	
84478	Triglycerides test	
85007	Manual differential WBC	
85018	Hemoglobin	
85651	Erythrocyte sedimentation rate--non-auto	
86580	TB Mantoux test	
87072	Culture by commercial kit, nonurine...	
87076	Culture, anerobic isolate	
87077	Bacterial culture, aerobic isolate	
87086	Urine culture and colony count	X
87430	Strep test	
87880	Direct streptococcus screen	
INJECTIONS		
90471	Immunization administration	
90703	Tetanus injection	
90772	Injection	
92516	Facial nerve function studies	
93000	Electrocardiogram--ECG with interpretation	
93015	Treadmill stress test, with physician...	
96900	Ultraviolet light treatment	
99070	Supplies and materials provided	

FAMILY CARE CENTER
286 Stephenson Blvd.
Stephenson, OH 60089
614-555-0000

☐ DANA BANU, M.D.
☐ ROBERT BEACH, M.D.
☒ PATRICIA MCGRATH, M.D.

☐ JESSICA RUDNER, M.D.
☐ JOHN RUDNER, M.D.
☐ KATHERINE YAN, M.D.

NOTES

**New address:
36 Grant Blvd.
Grandville, OH
60092**

REFERRING PHYSICIAN

NPI

AUTHORIZATION #

DIAGNOSIS
Diabetes mellitus, type II

PAYMENT AMOUNT

ENCOUNTER FORM

11/12/2010	**10:00 am**
DATE	TIME
Lawana Brooks	**BROOKLA0**
PATIENT NAME	CHART #

OFFICE VISITS - SYMPTOMATIC		
NEW		
99201	OF--New Patient Minimal	
99202	OF--New Patient Low	
99203	OF--New Patient Detailed	
99204	OF--New Patient Moderate	
99205	OF--New Patient High	
ESTABLISHED		
99211	OF--Established Patient Minimal	
99212	OF--Established Patient Low	X
99213	OF--Established Patient Detailed	
99214	OF--Established Patient Moderate	
99215	OF--Established Patient High	
PREVENTIVE VISITS		
NEW		
99381	Under 1 Year	
99382	1 - 4 Years	
99383	5 - 11 Years	
99384	12 - 17 Years	
99385	18 - 39 Years	
99386	40 - 64 Years	
99387	65 Years & Up	
ESTABLISHED		
99391	Under 1 Year	
99392	1 - 4 Years	
99393	5 - 11 Years	
99394	12 - 17 Years	
99395	18 - 39 Years	
99396	40 - 64 Years	
99397	65 Years & Up	
PROCEDURES		
12011	Simple suture--face--local anes.	
29125	App. of short arm splint; static	X
29425	App. of short leg cast, walking	
50390	Aspiration of renal cyst by needle	
71010	Chest x-ray, single view, frontal	

PROCEDURES		
71020	Chest x-ray, two views, frontal & lateral	
71030	Chest x-ray, complete, four views	
73070	Elbow x-ray, AP & lateral views	
73090	Forearm x-ray, AP & lateral views	X
73100	Wrist x-ray, AP & lateral views	
73510	Hip x-ray, complete, two views	
73600	Ankle x-ray, AP & lateral views	
LABORATORY		
80019	19 clinical chemistry tests	
80048	Basic metabolic panel	
80061	Lipid panel	
82270	Blood screening, occult; feces	
82947	Glucose screening--quantitative	
82951	Glucose tolerance test, three specimens	
83718	HDL cholesterol	
84478	Triglycerides test	
85007	Manual differential WBC	
85018	Hemoglobin	
85651	Erythrocyte sedimentation rate--non-auto	
86580	TB Mantoux test	
87072	Culture by commercial kit, nonurine...	
87076	Culture, anaerobic isolate	
87077	Bacterial culture, aerobic isolate	
87086	Urine culture and colony count	
87430	Strep test	
87880	Direct streptococcus screen	
INJECTIONS		
90471	Immunization administration	
90703	Tetanus injection	
90772	Injection	
92516	Facial nerve function studies	
93000	Electrocardiogram--ECG with interpretation	
93015	Treadmill stress test, with physician...	
96900	Ultraviolet light treatment	
99070	Supplies and materials provided	

FAMILY CARE CENTER
286 Stephenson Blvd.
Stephenson, OH 60089
614-555-0000

- ☐ DANA BANU, M.D.
- ☐ ROBERT BEACH, M.D.
- ☒ PATRICIA MCGRATH, M.D.
- ☐ JESSICA RUDNER, M.D.
- ☐ JOHN RUDNER, M.D.
- ☐ KATHERINE YAN, M.D.

REFERRING PHYSICIAN	NPI	AUTHORIZATION #

DIAGNOSIS
841.0   E885.9   E849.3

PAYMENT AMOUNT

NOTES

Accidental fall at work

Workers' comp, no copayment collected from patient

FAMILY CARE CENTER
285 Stephenson Boulevard
Stephenson, OH 60089
614-555-0000

CASE NOTES

PATIENT NAME	Lawana Brooks
CHART NUMBER	BROOKLA0
DATE	11/12/10
CASE	Fall at work - Workers' Compensation

NOTES

Emergency visit for injuries sustained due to a fall at work on 11/12/10.

This is classified as a work injury - non-collision.

ENCOUNTER FORM

11/12/2010	**11:15 am**
DATE	TIME
Edwin Hsu	**HSUEDWI0**
PATIENT NAME	CHART #

OFFICE VISITS - SYMPTOMATIC
NEW

99201	OF--New Patient Minimal	
99202	OF--New Patient Low	
99203	OF--New Patient Detailed	
99204	OF--New Patient Moderate	
99205	OF--New Patient High	

ESTABLISHED

99211	OF--Established Patient Minimal	X
99212	OF--Established Patient Low	
99213	OF--Established Patient Detailed	
99214	OF--Established Patient Moderate	
99215	OF--Established Patient High	

PREVENTIVE VISITS
NEW

99381	Under 1 Year	
99382	1 - 4 Years	
99383	5 - 11 Years	
99384	12 - 17 Years	
99385	18 - 39 Years	
99386	40 - 64 Years	
99387	65 Years & Up	

ESTABLISHED

99391	Under 1 Year	
99392	1 - 4 Years	
99393	5 - 11 Years	
99394	12 - 17 Years	
99395	18 - 39 Years	
99396	40 - 64 Years	
99397	65 Years & Up	

PROCEDURES

12011	Simple suture--face--local anes.	
29125	App. of short arm splint; static	
29425	App. of short leg cast, walking	
50390	Aspiration of renal cyst by needle	
71010	Chest x-ray, single view, frontal	

PROCEDURES

71020	Chest x-ray, two views, frontal & lateral	
71030	Chest x-ray, complete, four views	
73070	Elbow x-ray, AP & lateral views	
73090	Forearm x-ray, AP & lateral views	
73100	Wrist x-ray, AP & lateral views	
73510	Hip x-ray, complete, two views	
73600	Ankle x-ray, AP & lateral views	

LABORATORY

80019	19 clinical chemistry tests	
80048	Basic metabolic panel	
80061	Lipid panel	
82270	Blood screening, occult; feces	
82947	Glucose screening--quantitative	
82951	Glucose tolerance test, three specimens	
83718	HDL cholesterol	
84478	Triglycerides test	
85007	Manual differential WBC	
85018	Hemoglobin	
85651	Erythrocyte sedimentation rate--non-auto	
86580	TB Mantoux test	
87072	Culture by commercial kit, nonurine...	
87076	Culture, anerobic isolate	
87077	Bacterial culture, aerobic isolate	
87086	Urine culture and colony count	
87430	Strep test	
87880	Direct streptococcus screen	

INJECTIONS

90471	Immunization administration	
90703	Tetanus injection	
90772	Injection	
92516	Facial nerve function studies	
93000	Electrocardiogram--ECG with interpretation	
93015	Treadmill stress test, with physician...	
96900	Ultraviolet light treatment	
99070	Supplies and materials provided	

FAMILY CARE CENTER
286 Stephenson Blvd.
Stephenson, OH 60089
614-555-0000

☐ DANA BANU, M.D.
☐ ROBERT BEACH, M.D.
☒ PATRICIA MCGRATH, M.D.
☐ JESSICA RUDNER, M.D.
☐ JOHN RUDNER, M.D.
☐ KATHERINE YAN, M.D.

NOTES

REFERRING PHYSICIAN	NPI	AUTHORIZATION #

DIAGNOSIS
461.9 Acute sinusitis

PAYMENT AMOUNT
$20 copay, check #1066

FAMILY CARE CENTER
285 Stephenson Boulevard
Stephenson, OH 60089
614-555-0000

**CASE NOTES
PAGE 1 OF 1**

PATIENT NAME	Edwin Hsu
CHART NUMBER	HSUEDWI0
DATE	11/12/10
CASE	Acute sinusitis

NOTES

Patient has moved--new address is:
56 Reynolds St.
Stephenson, OH 60089

Telephone: 614-034-6729

FAMILY CARE CENTER
285 Stephenson Boulevard
Stephenson, OH 60089-4000
614-555-0000

PATIENT INFORMATION FORM

Patient				
Last Name Syzmanski	First Name Hannah	MI	Sex __ M X F	Date of Birth 2 / 26/ 2000
Address 3 Broadbrook Lane	City Stephenson		State OH	Zip 60089
Home Ph # (614) 086-4444 Cell Ph # ( )		Marital Status Single		Student Status Full-time
SS# Email 907-66-0003			Allergies Bee stings	
Employment Status	Employer Name	Work Ph # ( )	Primary Insurance ID#	
Employer Address	City		State	Zip
Referred By		Ph # of Referral ( )		

Responsible Party (Complete this section if the person responsible for the bill is not the patient)

Last Name Syzmanski	First Name Michael	MI	Sex X M __ F	Date of Birth 6 / 5 / 1970
Address 3 Broadbrook Lane	City Stephenson	State OH	Zip 60089	SS# 022-45-6789
Relation to Patient __ Spouse X Parent __ Other	Employer Name Nichol's Hardware		Work Phone # ( )	
Spouse, or Parent (if minor):			Home Phone # (614) 086-4444	

Insurance (If you have multiple coverage, supply information from both carriers)

Primary Carrier Name	Secondary Carrier Name
Name of the Insured (Name on ID Card)	Name of the Insured (Name on ID Card)
Patient's relationship to the insured __ Self __ Spouse __ Child	Patient's relationship to the insured __ Self __ Spouse __ Child
Insured ID #	Insured ID #
Group # or Company Name	Group # or Company Name
Insurance Address	Insurance Address

Phone #   Copay $
                    Deductible $
	Phone # Copay $
	                    Deductible $

Other Information

Is patient's condition related to:	Reason for visit: general check up
__ Employment __ Auto Accident (if yes, state in which accident occurred: ___) __ Other Accident	

Date of Accident: /   /   Date of First Symptom of Illness: /   /

Financial Agreement and Authorization for Treatment

I authorize treatment and agree to pay all fees and charges for the person named above. I agree to pay all charges shown by statements, promptly upon their presentation, unless credit arrangements are agreed upon in writing.

I authorize payment directly to FAMILY CARE CENTER of insurance benefits otherwise payable to me. I hereby authorize the release of any medical information necessary in order to process a claim for payment in my behalf.

Signed: Michael Syzmanski   Date: 11/12/2010

ENCOUNTER FORM

11/12/2010
DATE

Hannah Syzmanski
PATIENT NAME

10:00 am
TIME

SYZMAHA0
CHART #

OFFICE VISITS - SYMPTOMATIC		
NEW		
99201	OF--New Patient Minimal	
99202	OF--New Patient Low	
99203	OF--New Patient Detailed	
99204	OF--New Patient Moderate	
99205	OF--New Patient High	
ESTABLISHED		
99211	OF--Established Patient Minimal	
99212	OF--Established Patient Low	
99213	OF--Established Patient Detailed	
99214	OF--Established Patient Moderate	
99215	OF--Established Patient High	
PREVENTIVE VISITS		
NEW		
99381	Under 1 Year	
99382	1 - 4 Years	
99383	5 - 11 Years	X
99384	12 - 17 Years	
99385	18 - 39 Years	
99386	40 - 64 Years	
99387	65 Years & Up	
ESTABLISHED		
99391	Under 1 Year	
99392	1 - 4 Years	
99393	5 - 11 Years	
99394	12 - 17 Years	
99395	18 - 39 Years	
99396	40 - 64 Years	
99397	65 Years & Up	
PROCEDURES		
12011	Simple suture--face--local anes.	
29125	App. of short arm splint; static	
29425	App. of short leg cast, walking	
50390	Aspiration of renal cyst by needle	
71010	Chest x-ray, single view, frontal	

PROCEDURES		
71020	Chest x-ray, two views, frontal & lateral	
71030	Chest x-ray, complete, four views	
73070	Elbow x-ray, AP & lateral views	
73090	Forearm x-ray, AP & lateral views	
73100	Wrist x-ray, AP & lateral views	
73510	Hip x-ray, complete, two views	
73600	Ankle x-ray, AP & lateral views	
LABORATORY		
80019	19 clinical chemistry tests	
80048	Basic metabolic panel	
80061	Lipid panel	
82270	Blood screening, occult; feces	
82947	Glucose screening--quantitative	
82951	Glucose tolerance test, three specimens	
83718	HDL cholesterol	
84478	Triglycerides test	
85007	Manual differential WBC	
85018	Hemoglobin	
85651	Erythrocyte sedimentation rate--non-auto	
86580	TB Mantoux test	
87072	Culture by commercial kit, nonurine...	
87076	Culture, anerobic isolate	
87077	Bacterial culture, aerobic isolate	
87086	Urine culture and colony count	
87430	Strep test	
87880	Direct streptococcus screen	
INJECTIONS		
90471	Immunization administration	
90703	Tetanus injection	
90772	Injection	
92516	Facial nerve function studies	
93000	Electrocardiogram--ECG with interpretation	
93015	Treadmill stress test, with physician...	
96900	Ultraviolet light treatment	
99070	Supplies and materials provided	

FAMILY CARE CENTER
286 Stephenson Blvd.
Stephenson, OH 60089
614-555-0000

☒ DANA BANU, M.D.
☐ ROBERT BEACH, M.D.
☐ PATRICIA MCGRATH, M.D.
☐ JESSICA RUDNER, M.D.
☐ JOHN RUDNER, M.D.
☐ KATHERINE YAN, M.D.

NOTES

REFERRING PHYSICIAN
Harold Gearhart, M.D.

NPI

AUTHORIZATION #

DIAGNOSIS
v20.2

PAYMENT AMOUNT
$20 copay, check #3019

ENCOUNTER FORM

11/15/2010
DATE

9:00 am
TIME

Carlos Lopez
PATIENT NAME

LOPEZCA0
CHART #

OFFICE VISITS - SYMPTOMATIC		
NEW		
99201	OF--New Patient Minimal	
99202	OF--New Patient Low	
99203	OF--New Patient Detailed	
99204	OF--New Patient Moderate	
99205	OF--New Patient High	
ESTABLISHED		
99211	OF--Established Patient Minimal	
99212	OF--Established Patient Low	X
99213	OF--Established Patient Detailed	
99214	OF--Established Patient Moderate	
99215	OF--Established Patient High	
PREVENTIVE VISITS		
NEW		
99381	Under 1 Year	
99382	1 - 4 Years	
99383	5 - 11 Years	
99384	12 - 17 Years	
99385	18 - 39 Years	
99386	40 - 64 Years	
99387	65 Years & Up	
ESTABLISHED		
99391	Under 1 Year	
99392	1 - 4 Years	
99393	5 - 11 Years	
99394	12 - 17 Years	
99395	18 - 39 Years	
99396	40 - 64 Years	
99397	65 Years & Up	
PROCEDURES		
12011	Simple suture--face--local anes.	
29125	App. of short arm splint; static	
29425	App. of short leg cast, walking	
50390	Aspiration of renal cyst by needle	
71010	Chest x-ray, single view, frontal	

PROCEDURES		
71020	Chest x-ray, two views, frontal & lateral	
71030	Chest x-ray, complete, four views	
73070	Elbow x-ray, AP & lateral views	
73090	Forearm x-ray, AP & lateral views	
73100	Wrist x-ray, AP & lateral views	
73510	Hip x-ray, complete, two views	
73600	Ankle x-ray, AP & lateral views	
LABORATORY		
80019	19 clinical chemistry tests	
80048	Basic metabolic panel	
80061	Lipid panel	
82270	Blood screening, occult; feces	
82947	Glucose screening--quantitative	
82951	Glucose tolerance test, three specimens	
83718	HDL cholesterol	
84478	Triglycerides test	
85007	Manual differential WBC	
85018	Hemoglobin	
85651	Erythrocyte sedimentation rate--non-auto	
86580	TB Mantoux test	
87072	Culture by commercial kit, nonurine...	
87076	Culture, anaerobic isolate	
87077	Bacterial culture, aerobic isolate	
87086	Urine culture and colony count	
87430	Strep test	
87880	Direct streptococcus screen	
INJECTIONS		
90471	Immunization administration	
90703	Tetanus injection	
90772	Injection	
92516	Facial nerve function studies	
93000	Electrocardiogram--ECG with interpretation	
93015	Treadmill stress test, with physician...	
96900	Ultraviolet light treatment	
99070	Supplies and materials provided	

FAMILY CARE CENTER
286 Stephenson Blvd.
Stephenson, OH 60089
614-555-0000

☐ DANA BANU, M.D.
☐ ROBERT BEACH, M.D.
☒ PATRICIA MCGRATH, M.D.

☐ JESSICA RUDNER, M.D.
☐ JOHN RUDNER, M.D.
☐ KATHERINE YAN, M.D.

NOTES

REFERRING PHYSICIAN

NPI

AUTHORIZATION #

DIAGNOSIS
v65.5

PAYMENT AMOUNT
$20 copay, check #1001

FAMILY CARE CENTER
285 Stephenson Boulevard
Stephenson, OH 60089-4000
614-555-0000

PATIENT INFORMATION FORM

Patient				

Last Name	First Name	MI	Sex	Date of Birth
Palmer	Christopher		X M __ F	1 / 5 / 1954

Address	City	State	Zip
17 Red Oak Lane	Jefferson	OH	60093

Home Ph # (614) 077-2249   Cell Ph # (614) 077-2250   Marital Status Single   Student Status

SS#	Email	Allergies
607-50-7620	cpalmer@abc.com	

Employment Status	Employer Name	Work Ph #	Primary Insurance ID#
Not employed		( )	607507620

Employer Address	City	State	Zip

Referred By	Ph # of Referral (614) 444-3200
Dr. Marion Davis	

Responsible Party (Complete this section if the person responsible for the bill is not the patient)

Last Name	First Name	MI	Sex	Date of Birth
			__ M __ F	/ /

Address	City	State	Zip	SS#

Relation to Patient	Employer Name	Work Phone #
__ Spouse __ Parent __ Other		( )

Spouse, or Parent (if minor):	Home Phone # ( )

Insurance (If you have multiple coverage, supply information from both carriers)

Primary Carrier Name	Secondary Carrier Name
Medicaid	
Name of the Insured (Name on ID Card)	Name of the Insured (Name on ID Card)
Christopher Palmer	
Patient's relationship to the insured	Patient's relationship to the insured
X Self __ Spouse __ Child	__ Self __ Spouse __ Child
Insured ID #	Insured ID #
607507620	
Group # or Company Name	Group # or Company Name
Insurance Address	Insurance Address
248 West Main St., Cleveland, OH 60120	

Phone # 614-599-6000	Copay $ 10	Phone #	Copay $
	Deductible $		Deductible $

Other Information

Is patient's condition related to: Reason for visit: **difficulty breathing**

__ Employment   __ Auto Accident (if yes, state in which accident occurred: ___)   __ Other Accident

Date of Accident: / /   Date of First Symptom of Illness: / /

Financial Agreement and Authorization for Treatment

I authorize treatment and agree to pay all fees and charges for the person named above. I agree to pay all charges shown by statements, promptly upon their presentation, unless credit arrangements are agreed upon in writing.

I authorize payment directly to FAMILY CARE CENTER of insurance benefits otherwise payable to me. I hereby authorize the release of any medical information necessary in order to process a claim for payment in my behalf.

Signed: Christopher Palmer   Date: 11/12/2010

ENCOUNTER FORM

11/12/2010	10:00 am
DATE	TIME
Christopher Palmer	PALMECH0
PATIENT NAME	CHART #

OFFICE VISITS - SYMPTOMATIC		
NEW		
99201	OF--New Patient Minimal	X
99202	OF--New Patient Low	
99203	OF--New Patient Detailed	
99204	OF--New Patient Moderate	
99205	OF--New Patient High	
ESTABLISHED		
99211	OF--Established Patient Minimal	
99212	OF--Established Patient Low	
99213	OF--Established Patient Detailed	
99214	OF--Established Patient Moderate	
99215	OF--Established Patient High	
PREVENTIVE VISITS		
NEW		
99381	Under 1 Year	
99382	1 - 4 Years	
99383	5 - 11 Years	
99384	12 - 17 Years	
99385	18 - 39 Years	
99386	40 - 64 Years	
99387	65 Years & Up	
ESTABLISHED		
99391	Under 1 Year	
99392	1 - 4 Years	
99393	5 - 11 Years	
99394	12 - 17 Years	
99395	18 - 39 Years	
99396	40 - 64 Years	
99397	65 Years & Up	
PROCEDURES		
12011	Simple suture--face--local anes.	
29125	App. of short arm splint; static	
29425	App. of short leg cast, walking	
50390	Aspiration of renal cyst by needle	
71010	Chest x-ray, single view, frontal	

PROCEDURES		
71020	Chest x-ray, two views, frontal & lateral	
71030	Chest x-ray, complete, four views	
73070	Elbow x-ray, AP & lateral views	
73090	Forearm x-ray, AP & lateral views	
73100	Wrist x-ray, AP & lateral views	
73510	Hip x-ray, complete, two views	
73600	Ankle x-ray, AP & lateral views	
LABORATORY		
80019	19 clinical chemistry tests	
80048	Basic metabolic panel	
80061	Lipid panel	
82270	Blood screening, occult; feces	
82947	Glucose screening--quantitative	
82951	Glucose tolerance test, three specimens	
83718	HDL cholesterol	
84478	Triglycerides test	
85007	Manual differential WBC	
85018	Hemoglobin	
85651	Erythrocyte sedimentation rate--non-auto	
86580	TB Mantoux test	
87072	Culture by commercial kit, nonurine...	
87076	Culture, anaerobic isolate	
87077	Bacterial culture, aerobic isolate	
87086	Urine culture and colony count	
87430	Strep test	
87880	Direct streptococcus screen	
INJECTIONS		
90471	Immunization administration	
90703	Tetanus injection	
90772	Injection	
92516	Facial nerve function studies	
93000	Electrocardiogram--ECG with interpretation	
93015	Treadmill stress test, with physician...	
96900	Ultraviolet light treatment	
99070	Supplies and materials provided	

FAMILY CARE CENTER
286 Stephenson Blvd.
Stephenson, OH 60089
614-555-0000

- ☐ DANA BANU, M.D.
- ☒ ROBERT BEACH, M.D.
- ☐ PATRICIA MCGRATH, M.D.
- ☐ JESSICA RUDNER, M.D.
- ☐ JOHN RUDNER, M.D.
- ☐ KATHERINE YAN, M.D.

NOTES

REFERRING PHYSICIAN	NPI	AUTHORIZATION #
Dr. Marion Davis		

DIAGNOSIS
485 Bronchopneumonia

PAYMENT AMOUNT
$10 copay, cash

EAST OHIO PPO
10 CENTRAL AVENUE
HALEVILLE, OH 60890

PROVIDER REMITTANCE

FAMILY CARE CENTER
285 STEPHENSON BLVD.
STEPHENSON, OH 60089

PAGE: 1 OF 1
DATE: 11/12/2010
ID NUMBER: 4679323

PROVIDER: PATRICIA MCGRATH, M.D.

PATIENT: BROOKS LAWANA   CLAIM: 234567890

FROM DATE	THRU DATE	PROC CODE	UNITS	AMOUNT BILLED	AMOUNT ALLOWED	DEDUCT	COPAY/ COINS	PROV PAID	REASON CODE
10/29/10	10/29/10	99212	1	54.00	48.60	.00	20.00	28.60	
10/29/10	10/29/10	73600	1	96.00	86.40	.00	.00	86.40	
	CLAIM TOTALS			150.00	135.00	.00	20.00	115.00	

PATIENT: HSU DIANE   CLAIM: 345678901

FROM DATE	THRU DATE	PROC CODE	UNITS	AMOUNT BILLED	AMOUNT ALLOWED	DEDUCT	COPAY/ COINS	PROV PAID	REASON CODE
10/29/10	10/29/10	99213	1	72.00	64.80	.00	20.00	44.80	
10/29/10	10/29/10	80048	1	50.00	45.00	.00	.00	45.00	
	CLAIM TOTALS			122.00	109.80	.00	20.00	89.80	

PROVIDER: DANA BANU, M.D.

PATIENT: PATEL RAJI   CLAIM: 567890123

FROM DATE	THRU DATE	PROC CODE	UNITS	AMOUNT BILLED	AMOUNT ALLOWED	DEDUCT	COPAY/ COINS	PROV PAID	REASON CODE
10/29/10	10/29/10	99212	1	54.00	48.60	.00	20.00	28.60	
	CLAIM TOTALS			54.00	48.60	.00	20.00	28.60	

PATIENT: SYZMANSKI MICHAEL   CLAIM: 678901234

FROM DATE	THRU DATE	PROC CODE	UNITS	AMOUNT BILLED	AMOUNT ALLOWED	DEDUCT	COPAY/ COINS	PROV PAID	REASON CODE
10/29/10	10/29/10	99212	1	54.00	48.60	.00	20.00	28.60	
	CLAIM TOTALS			54.00	48.60	.00	20.00	28.60	

PAYMENT SUMMARY

TOTAL AMOUNT PAID	262.00
PRIOR CREDIT BALANCE	.00
CURRENT CREDIT DEFERRED	.00
PRIOR CREDIT APPLIED	.00
NEW CREDIT BALANCE	.00
NET DISBURSED	262.00

TOTAL ALL CLAIMS

AMOUNT CHARGED	380.00
AMOUNT ALLOWED	342.00
DEDUCTIBLE	.00
COPAY	.00
COINSURANCE	80.00

EFT INFORMATION

NUMBER	4679323
DATE	11/12/10
AMOUNT	262.00

STATUS CODES:
A - APPROVED   AJ - ADJUSTMENT   IP - IN PROCESS   R - REJECTED   V - VOID

ENCOUNTER FORM

11/15/2010	**11:30 am**
DATE	TIME
Diane Hsu	**HSUDIAN0**
PATIENT NAME	CHART #

OFFICE VISITS - SYMPTOMATIC		
NEW		
99201	OF--New Patient Minimal	
99202	OF--New Patient Low	
99203	OF--New Patient Detailed	
99204	OF--New Patient Moderate	
99205	OF--New Patient High	
ESTABLISHED		
99211	OF--Established Patient Minimal	
99212	OF--Established Patient Low	X
99213	OF--Established Patient Detailed	
99214	OF--Established Patient Moderate	
99215	OF--Established Patient High	
PREVENTIVE VISITS		
NEW		
99381	Under 1 Year	
99382	1 - 4 Years	
99383	5 - 11 Years	
99384	12 - 17 Years	
99385	18 - 39 Years	
99386	40 - 64 Years	
99387	65 Years & Up	
ESTABLISHED		
99391	Under 1 Year	
99392	1 - 4 Years	
99393	5 - 11 Years	
99394	12 - 17 Years	
99395	18 - 39 Years	
99396	40 - 64 Years	
99397	65 Years & Up	
PROCEDURES		
12011	Simple suture--face--local anes.	
29125	App. of short arm splint; static	
29425	App. of short leg cast, walking	
50390	Aspiration of renal cyst by needle	
71010	Chest x-ray, single view, frontal	

PROCEDURES		
71020	Chest x-ray, two views, frontal & lateral	
71030	Chest x-ray, complete, four views	
73070	Elbow x-ray, AP & lateral views	
73090	Forearm x-ray, AP & lateral views	
73100	Wrist x-ray, AP & lateral views	
73510	Hip x-ray, complete, two views	
73600	Ankle x-ray, AP & lateral views	
LABORATORY		
80019	19 clinical chemistry tests	
80048	Basic metabolic panel	
80061	Lipid panel	
82270	Blood screening, occult; feces	
82947	Glucose screening--quantitative	
82951	Glucose tolerance test, three specimens	
83718	HDL cholesterol	
84478	Triglycerides test	
85007	Manual differential WBC	
85018	Hemoglobin	
85651	Erythrocyte sedimentation rate--non-auto	
86580	TB Mantoux test	
87072	Culture by commercial kit, nonurine...	
87076	Culture, anaerobic isolate	
87077	Bacterial culture, aerobic isolate	
87086	Urine culture and colony count	
87430	Strep test	X
87880	Direct streptococcus screen	
INJECTIONS		
90471	Immunization administration	
90703	Tetanus injection	
90772	Injection	
92516	Facial nerve function studies	
93000	Electrocardiogram--ECG with interpretation	
93015	Treadmill stress test, with physician...	
96900	Ultraviolet light treatment	
99070	Supplies and materials provided	

FAMILY CARE CENTER
286 Stephenson Blvd.
Stephenson, OH 60089
614-555-0000

☐ DANA BANU, M.D.
☐ ROBERT BEACH, M.D.
☒ PATRICIA MCGRATH, M.D.

☐ JESSICA RUDNER, M.D.
☐ JOHN RUDNER, M.D.
☐ KATHERINE YAN, M.D.

NOTES

Next appt. 1 week from today, 2:00 pm, 15 minutes

REFERRING PHYSICIAN	NPI	AUTHORIZATION #

DIAGNOSIS
487.1 Influenza

PAYMENT AMOUNT
$20 copay, check 3419

ENCOUNTER FORM

11/15/2010	2:30 pm
DATE	TIME
Michael Syzmanski	SYZMAMI0
PATIENT NAME	CHART #

OFFICE VISITS - SYMPTOMATIC

NEW

99201	OF--New Patient Minimal	
99202	OF--New Patient Low	
99203	OF--New Patient Detailed	
99204	OF--New Patient Moderate	
99205	OF--New Patient High	

ESTABLISHED

99211	OF--Established Patient Minimal	
99212	OF--Established Patient Low	
99213	OF--Established Patient Detailed	
99214	OF--Established Patient Moderate	
99215	OF--Established Patient High	X

PREVENTIVE VISITS

NEW

99381	Under 1 Year	
99382	1 - 4 Years	
99383	5 - 11 Years	
99384	12 - 17 Years	
99385	18 - 39 Years	
99386	40 - 64 Years	
99387	65 Years & Up	

ESTABLISHED

99391	Under 1 Year	
99392	1 - 4 Years	
99393	5 - 11 Years	
99394	12 - 17 Years	
99395	18 - 39 Years	
99396	40 - 64 Years	
99397	65 Years & Up	

PROCEDURES

12011	Simple suture--face--local anes.	
29125	App. of short arm splint; static	
29425	App. of short leg cast, walking	
50390	Aspiration of renal cyst by needle	
71010	Chest x-ray, single view, frontal	

PROCEDURES

71020	Chest x-ray, two views, frontal & lateral	
71030	Chest x-ray, complete, four views	
73070	Elbow x-ray, AP & lateral views	
73090	Forearm x-ray, AP & lateral views	
73100	Wrist x-ray, AP & lateral views	
73510	Hip x-ray, complete, two views	
73600	Ankle x-ray, AP & lateral views	

LABORATORY

80019	19 clinical chemistry tests	
80048	Basic metabolic panel	
80061	Lipid panel	
82270	Blood screening, occult; feces	X
82947	Glucose screening--quantitative	
82951	Glucose tolerance test, three specimens	
83718	HDL cholesterol	
84478	Triglycerides test	
85007	Manual differential WBC	
85018	Hemoglobin	
85651	Erythrocyte sedimentation rate--non-auto	
86580	TB Mantoux test	
87072	Culture by commercial kit, nonurine...	
87076	Culture, anaerobic isolate	
87077	Bacterial culture, aerobic isolate	
87086	Urine culture and colony count	
87430	Strep test	
87880	Direct streptococcus screen	

INJECTIONS

90471	Immunization administration	
90703	Tetanus injection	
90772	Injection	
92516	Facial nerve function studies	
93000	Electrocardiogram--ECG with interpretation	
93015	Treadmill stress test, with physician...	
96900	Ultraviolet light treatment	
99070	Supplies and materials provided	

FAMILY CARE CENTER
286 Stephenson Blvd.
Stephenson, OH 60089
614-555-0000

- ☒ DANA BANU, M.D.
- ☐ ROBERT BEACH, M.D.
- ☐ PATRICIA MCGRATH, M.D.
- ☐ JESSICA RUDNER, M.D.
- ☐ JOHN RUDNER, M.D.
- ☐ KATHERINE YAN, M.D.

NOTES

REFERRING PHYSICIAN	NPI	AUTHORIZATION #

DIAGNOSIS
455.6 Hemorrhoids

PAYMENT AMOUNT
$20 copay, check 3119

FAMILY CARE CENTER
285 Stephenson Boulevard
Stephenson, OH 60089-4000
614-555-0000

PATIENT INFORMATION FORM

Patient				
Last Name Robertson	First Name Stewart	MI	Sex _X_ M __ F	Date of Birth 12/ 21/ 1969
Address 109 West Central Ave.	City Stephenson	State OH	Zip 60089	

Home Ph # (614) 022-3111 Cell Ph # (614) 022-3279   Marital Status Divorced   Student Status

SS# 920-39-4567	Email srobertson@abc.com	Allergies	
Employment Status Full-time	Employer Name Nichols Hardware	Work Ph # (614) 789-0200	Primary Insurance ID# 920394567 Group 63W
Employer Address 12 Central Ave.	City Stephenson	State OH	Zip 60089

Referred By
Dr. Janet Wood   Ph # of Referral (614) 459-3700

Responsible Party (Complete this section if the person responsible for the bill is not the patient)

Last Name	First Name	MI	Sex __ M __ F	Date of Birth / /
Address	City	State Zip	SS#	

Relation to Patient __ Spouse __ Parent __ Other	Employer Name	Work Phone # ( )

Spouse, or Parent (if minor):   Home Phone # (   )

Insurance (If you have multiple coverage, supply information from both carriers)

Primary Carrier Name OhioCare HMO	Secondary Carrier Name
Name of the Insured (Name on ID Card) Stewart Robertson	Name of the Insured (Name on ID Card)
Patient's relationship to the insured _X_ Self __ Spouse __ Child	Patient's relationship to the insured __ Self __ Spouse __ Child
Insured ID # 920394567	Insured ID #
Group # or Company Name Group 63W	Group # or Company Name
Insurance Address 147 Central Ave., Halevile, OH 60890	Insurance Address

Phone # 614-555-0101	Copay $ 20	Phone #	Copay $
	Deductible $		Deductible $

Other Information   Routine Physical

Is patient's condition related to: Reason for visit:

__ Employment   __ Auto Accident (if yes, state in which accident occurred: ___)   __ Other Accident

Date of Accident: / /   Date of First Symptom of Illness: / /

Financial Agreement and Authorization for Treatment

I authorize treatment and agree to pay all fees and charges for the person named above. I agree to pay all charges shown by statements, promptly upon their presentation, unless credit arrangements are agreed upon in writing.

I authorize payment directly to FAMILY CARE CENTER of insurance benefits otherwise payable to me. I hereby authorize the release of any medical information necessary in order to process a claim for payment in my behalf.

Signed: Stewart Robertson   Date: 12/10/2010

ENCOUNTER FORM

12/18/2010	8:00 am
DATE	TIME
Stewart Robertson	ROBERST0
PATIENT NAME	CHART #

OFFICE VISITS - SYMPTOMATIC		
NEW		
99201	OF--New Patient Minimal	
99202	OF--New Patient Low	
99203	OF--New Patient Detailed	
99204	OF--New Patient Moderate	
99205	OF--New Patient High	
ESTABLISHED		
99211	OF--Established Patient Minimal	
99212	OF--Established Patient Low	
99213	OF--Established Patient Detailed	
99214	OF--Established Patient Moderate	
99215	OF--Established Patient High	
PREVENTIVE VISITS		
NEW		
99381	Under 1 Year	
99382	1 - 4 Years	
99383	5 - 11 Years	
99384	12 - 17 Years	
99385	18 - 39 Years	
99386	40 - 64 Years	X
99387	65 Years & Up	
ESTABLISHED		
99391	Under 1 Year	
99392	1 - 4 Years	
99393	5 - 11 Years	
99394	12 - 17 Years	
99395	18 - 39 Years	
99396	40 - 64 Years	
99397	65 Years & Up	
PROCEDURES		
12011	Simple suture--face--local anes.	
29125	App. of short arm splint; static	
29425	App. of short leg cast, walking	
50390	Aspiration of renal cyst by needle	
71010	Chest x-ray, single view, frontal	

PROCEDURES		
71020	Chest x-ray, two views, frontal & lateral	
71030	Chest x-ray, complete, four views	
73070	Elbow x-ray, AP & lateral views	
73090	Forearm x-ray, AP & lateral views	
73100	Wrist x-ray, AP & lateral views	
73510	Hip x-ray, complete, two views	
73600	Ankle x-ray, AP & lateral views	
LABORATORY		
80019	19 clinical chemistry tests	
80048	Basic metabolic panel	
80061	Lipid panel	
82270	Blood screening, occult; feces	
82947	Glucose screening--quantitative	
82951	Glucose tolerance test, three specimens	
83718	HDL cholesterol	
84478	Triglycerides test	
85007	Manual differential WBC	
85018	Hemoglobin	
85651	Erythrocyte sedimentation rate--non-auto	
86580	TB Mantoux test	
87072	Culture by commercial kit, nonurine...	
87076	Culture, anaerobic isolate	
87077	Bacterial culture, aerobic isolate	
87086	Urine culture and colony count	
87430	Strep test	
87880	Direct streptococcus screen	
INJECTIONS		
90471	Immunization administration	
90703	Tetanus injection	
90772	Injection	
92516	Facial nerve function studies	
93000	Electrocardiogram--ECG with interpretation	X
93015	Treadmill stress test, with physician...	
96900	Ultraviolet light treatment	
99070	Supplies and materials provided	

FAMILY CARE CENTER
286 Stephenson Blvd.
Stephenson, OH 60089
614-555-0000

☐ DANA BANU, M.D.
☒ ROBERT BEACH, M.D.
☐ PATRICIA MCGRATH, M.D.

☐ JESSICA RUDNER, M.D.
☐ JOHN RUDNER, M.D.
☐ KATHERINE YAN, M.D.

NOTES

REFERRING PHYSICIAN
Janet Wood, M.D.

NPI

AUTHORIZATION #

DIAGNOSIS
v70.0

PAYMENT AMOUNT
$20 copay, check 416

ENCOUNTER FORM

12/18/2010
DATE

4:00 pm
TIME

Michael Syzmanski
PATIENT NAME

SYZMAMI0
CHART #

OFFICE VISITS - SYMPTOMATIC		
NEW		
99201	OF--New Patient Minimal	
99202	OF--New Patient Low	
99203	OF--New Patient Detailed	
99204	OF--New Patient Moderate	
99205	OF--New Patient High	
ESTABLISHED		
99211	OF--Established Patient Minimal	
99212	OF--Established Patient Low	X
99213	OF--Established Patient Detailed	
99214	OF--Established Patient Moderate	
99215	OF--Established Patient High	
PREVENTIVE VISITS		
NEW		
99381	Under 1 Year	
99382	1 - 4 Years	
99383	5 - 11 Years	
99384	12 - 17 Years	
99385	18 - 39 Years	
99386	40 - 64 Years	
99387	65 Years & Up	
ESTABLISHED		
99391	Under 1 Year	
99392	1 - 4 Years	
99393	5 - 11 Years	
99394	12 - 17 Years	
99395	18 - 39 Years	
99396	40 - 64 Years	
99397	65 Years & Up	
PROCEDURES		
12011	Simple suture--face--local anes.	X
29125	App. of short arm splint; static	
29425	App. of short leg cast, walking	
50390	Aspiration of renal cyst by needle	
71010	Chest x-ray, single view, frontal	

PROCEDURES		
71020	Chest x-ray, two views, frontal & lateral	
71030	Chest x-ray, complete, four views	
73070	Elbow x-ray, AP & lateral views	
73090	Forearm x-ray, AP & lateral views	
73100	Wrist x-ray, AP & lateral views	
73510	Hip x-ray, complete, two views	
73600	Ankle x-ray, AP & lateral views	
LABORATORY		
80019	19 clinical chemistry tests	
80048	Basic metabolic panel	
80061	Lipid panel	
82270	Blood screening, occult; feces	
82947	Glucose screening--quantitative	
82951	Glucose tolerance test, three specimens	
83718	HDL cholesterol	
84478	Triglycerides test	
85007	Manual differential WBC	
85018	Hemoglobin	
85651	Erythrocyte sedimentation rate--non-auto	
86580	TB Mantoux test	
87072	Culture by commercial kit, nonurine...	
87076	Culture, anerobic isolate	
87077	Bacterial culture, aerobic isolate	
87086	Urine culture and colony count	
87430	Strep test	
87880	Direct streptococcus screen	
INJECTIONS		
90471	Immunization administration	
90703	Tetanus injection	
90772	Injection	
92516	Facial nerve function studies	
93000	Electrocardiogram--ECG with interpretation	
93015	Treadmill stress test, with physician...	
96900	Ultraviolet light treatment	
99070	Supplies and materials provided	

FAMILY CARE CENTER
286 Stephenson Blvd.
Stephenson, OH 60089
614-555-0000

☐ DANA BANU, M.D.
☐ ROBERT BEACH, M.D.
☒ PATRICIA MCGRATH, M.D.

☐ JESSICA RUDNER, M.D.
☐ JOHN RUDNER, M.D.
☐ KATHERINE YAN, M.D.

NOTES

REFERRING PHYSICIAN

NPI

AUTHORIZATION #

DIAGNOSIS
870.8

PAYMENT AMOUNT
$20 copay, check# 3139

ENCOUNTER FORM

1/5/2011	9:00 am
DATE	TIME
Luther Jackson	JACKSLU0
PATIENT NAME	CHART #

OFFICE VISITS - SYMPTOMATIC		
NEW		
99201	OF--New Patient Minimal	
99202	OF--New Patient Low	
99203	OF--New Patient Detailed	
99204	OF--New Patient Moderate	
99205	OF--New Patient High	
ESTABLISHED		
99211	OF--Established Patient Minimal	
99212	OF--Established Patient Low	X
99213	OF--Established Patient Detailed	
99214	OF--Established Patient Moderate	
99215	OF--Established Patient High	
PREVENTIVE VISITS		
NEW		
99381	Under 1 Year	
99382	1 - 4 Years	
99383	5 - 11 Years	
99384	12 - 17 Years	
99385	18 - 39 Years	
99386	40 - 64 Years	
99387	65 Years & Up	
ESTABLISHED		
99391	Under 1 Year	
99392	1 - 4 Years	
99393	5 - 11 Years	
99394	12 - 17 Years	
99395	18 - 39 Years	
99396	40 - 64 Years	
99397	65 Years & Up	
PROCEDURES		
12011	Simple suture--face--local anes.	
29125	App. of short arm splint; static	
29425	App. of short leg cast, walking	
50390	Aspiration of renal cyst by needle	
71010	Chest x-ray, single view, frontal	

PROCEDURES		
71020	Chest x-ray, two views, frontal & lateral	
71030	Chest x-ray, complete, four views	
73070	Elbow x-ray, AP & lateral views	
73090	Forearm x-ray, AP & lateral views	
73100	Wrist x-ray, AP & lateral views	
73510	Hip x-ray, complete, two views	
73600	Ankle x-ray, AP & lateral views	
LABORATORY		
80019	19 clinical chemistry tests	
80048	Basic metabolic panel	
80061	Lipid panel	
82270	Blood screening, occult; feces	
82947	Glucose screening--quantitative	
82951	Glucose tolerance test, three specimens	
83718	HDL cholesterol	
84478	Triglycerides test	
85007	Manual differential WBC	
85018	Hemoglobin	
85651	Erythrocyte sedimentation rate--non-auto	
86580	TB Mantoux test	
87072	Culture by commercial kit, nonurine...	
87076	Culture, anaerobic isolate	
87077	Bacterial culture, aerobic isolate	
87086	Urine culture and colony count	
87430	Strep test	
87880	Direct streptococcus screen	
INJECTIONS		
90471	Immunization administration	
90703	Tetanus injection	
90772	Injection	
92516	Facial nerve function studies	
93000	Electrocardiogram--ECG with interpretation	
93015	Treadmill stress test, with physician...	
96900	Ultraviolet light treatment	
99070	Supplies and materials provided	

FAMILY CARE CENTER
286 Stephenson Blvd.
Stephenson, OH 60089
614-555-0000

☒ DANA BANU, M.D.
☐ ROBERT BEACH, M.D.
☐ PATRICIA MCGRATH, M.D.

☐ JESSICA RUDNER, M.D.
☐ JOHN RUDNER, M.D.
☐ KATHERINE YAN, M.D.

NOTES

REFERRING PHYSICIAN	NPI	AUTHORIZATION #

DIAGNOSIS
485 bronchopneumonia

PAYMENT AMOUNT
$20 copay, check# 1291

ENCOUNTER FORM

1/5/2011
DATE

9:00 am
TIME

Jill Simmons
PATIENT NAME

SIMMOJI0
CHART #

OFFICE VISITS - SYMPTOMATIC		
NEW		
99201	OF--New Patient Minimal	
99202	OF--New Patient Low	
99203	OF--New Patient Detailed	
99204	OF--New Patient Moderate	
99205	OF--New Patient High	
ESTABLISHED		
99211	OF--Established Patient Minimal	X
99212	OF--Established Patient Low	
99213	OF--Established Patient Detailed	
99214	OF--Established Patient Moderate	
99215	OF--Established Patient High	
PREVENTIVE VISITS		
NEW		
99381	Under 1 Year	
99382	1 - 4 Years	
99383	5 - 11 Years	
99384	12 - 17 Years	
99385	18 - 39 Years	
99386	40 - 64 Years	
99387	65 Years & Up	
ESTABLISHED		
99391	Under 1 Year	
99392	1 - 4 Years	
99393	5 - 11 Years	
99394	12 - 17 Years	
99395	18 - 39 Years	
99396	40 - 64 Years	
99397	65 Years & Up	
PROCEDURES		
12011	Simple suture--face--local anes.	
29125	App. of short arm splint; static	
29425	App. of short leg cast, walking	
50390	Aspiration of renal cyst by needle	
71010	Chest x-ray, single view, frontal	

PROCEDURES		
71020	Chest x-ray, two views, frontal & lateral	
71030	Chest x-ray, complete, four views	
73070	Elbow x-ray, AP & lateral views	
73090	Forearm x-ray, AP & lateral views	
73100	Wrist x-ray, AP & lateral views	
73510	Hip x-ray, complete, two views	
73600	Ankle x-ray, AP & lateral views	
LABORATORY		
80019	19 clinical chemistry tests	
80048	Basic metabolic panel	
80061	Lipid panel	
82270	Blood screening, occult; feces	
82947	Glucose screening--quantitative	
82951	Glucose tolerance test, three specimens	
83718	HDL cholesterol	
84478	Triglycerides test	
85007	Manual differential WBC	
85018	Hemoglobin	
85651	Erythrocyte sedimentation rate--non-auto	
86580	TB Mantoux test	
87072	Culture by commercial kit, nonurine...	
87076	Culture, anerobic isolate	
87077	Bacterial culture, aerobic isolate	
87086	Urine culture and colony count	
87430	Strep test	X
87880	Direct streptococcus screen	
INJECTIONS		
90471	Immunization administration	
90703	Tetanus injection	
90772	Injection	
92516	Facial nerve function studies	
93000	Electrocardiogram--ECG with interpretation	
93015	Treadmill stress test, with physician...	
96900	Ultraviolet light treatment	
99070	Supplies and materials provided	

FAMILY CARE CENTER
286 Stephenson Blvd.
Stephenson, OH 60089
614-555-0000

☐ DANA BANU, M.D.
☒ ROBERT BEACH, M.D.
☐ PATRICIA MCGRATH, M.D.

☐ JESSICA RUDNER, M.D.
☐ JOHN RUDNER, M.D.
☐ KATHERINE YAN, M.D.

NOTES

REFERRING PHYSICIAN

NPI

AUTHORIZATION #

DIAGNOSIS
034.0 strep sore throat

PAYMENT AMOUNT

ENCOUNTER FORM

1/5/2011	**9:30 am**
DATE	TIME
Nancy Stern	**STERNNA0**
PATIENT NAME	CHART #

OFFICE VISITS - SYMPTOMATIC
NEW

99201	OF--New Patient Minimal	
99202	OF--New Patient Low	
99203	OF--New Patient Detailed	
99204	OF--New Patient Moderate	
99205	OF--New Patient High	

ESTABLISHED

99211	OF--Established Patient Minimal	
99212	OF--Established Patient Low	
99213	OF--Established Patient Detailed	
99214	OF--Established Patient Moderate	
99215	OF--Established Patient High	

PREVENTIVE VISITS
NEW

99381	Under 1 Year	
99382	1 - 4 Years	
99383	5 - 11 Years	
99384	12 - 17 Years	
99385	18 - 39 Years	
99386	40 - 64 Years	
99387	65 Years & Up	

ESTABLISHED

99391	Under 1 Year	
99392	1 - 4 Years	
99393	5 - 11 Years	
99394	12 - 17 Years	
99395	18 - 39 Years	
99396	40 - 64 Years	X
99397	65 Years & Up	

PROCEDURES

12011	Simple suture--face--local anes.	
29125	App. of short arm splint; static	
29425	App. of short leg cast, walking	
50390	Aspiration of renal cyst by needle	
71010	Chest x-ray, single view, frontal	

PROCEDURES

71020	Chest x-ray, two views, frontal & lateral	
71030	Chest x-ray, complete, four views	
73070	Elbow x-ray, AP & lateral views	
73090	Forearm x-ray, AP & lateral views	
73100	Wrist x-ray, AP & lateral views	
73510	Hip x-ray, complete, two views	
73600	Ankle x-ray, AP & lateral views	

LABORATORY

80019	19 clinical chemistry tests	
80048	Basic metabolic panel	
80061	Lipid panel	
82270	Blood screening, occult; feces	
82947	Glucose screening--quantitative	
82951	Glucose tolerance test, three specimens	
83718	HDL cholesterol	X
84478	Triglycerides test	
85007	Manual differential WBC	X
85018	Hemoglobin	
85651	Erythrocyte sedimentation rate--non-auto	
86580	TB Mantoux test	
87072	Culture by commercial kit, nonurine...	
87076	Culture, anerobic isolate	
87077	Bacterial culture, aerobic isolate	
87086	Urine culture and colony count	X
87430	Strep test	
87880	Direct streptococcus screen	

INJECTIONS

90471	Immunization administration	
90703	Tetanus injection	
90772	Injection	
92516	Facial nerve function studies	
93000	Electrocardiogram--ECG with interpretation	X
93015	Treadmill stress test, with physician...	
96900	Ultraviolet light treatment	
99070	Supplies and materials provided	

FAMILY CARE CENTER
286 Stephenson Blvd.
Stephenson, OH 60089
614-555-0000

- ☐ DANA BANU, M.D.
- ☐ ROBERT BEACH, M.D.
- ☒ PATRICIA MCGRATH, M.D.
- ☐ JESSICA RUDNER, M.D.
- ☐ JOHN RUDNER, M.D.
- ☐ KATHERINE YAN, M.D.

NOTES

REFERRING PHYSICIAN	NPI	AUTHORIZATION #

DIAGNOSIS
v70.0 routine physical examination

PAYMENT AMOUNT
$20 copay, check# 1022

ENCOUNTER FORM

1/5/2011	9:30 am
DATE	TIME
Debra Syzmanski	**SYZMADE0**
PATIENT NAME	CHART #

OFFICE VISITS - SYMPTOMATIC
NEW

99201	OF--New Patient Minimal	
99202	OF--New Patient Low	
99203	OF--New Patient Detailed	
99204	OF--New Patient Moderate	
99205	OF--New Patient High	

ESTABLISHED

99211	OF--Established Patient Minimal	
99212	OF--Established Patient Low	
99213	OF--Established Patient Detailed	
99214	OF--Established Patient Moderate	
99215	OF--Established Patient High	

PREVENTIVE VISITS
NEW

99381	Under 1 Year	
99382	1 - 4 Years	
99383	5 - 11 Years	
99384	12 - 17 Years	
99385	18 - 39 Years	
99386	40 - 64 Years	
99387	65 Years & Up	

ESTABLISHED

99391	Under 1 Year	
99392	1 - 4 Years	
99393	5 - 11 Years	
99394	12 - 17 Years	
99395	18 - 39 Years	
99396	40 - 64 Years	X
99397	65 Years & Up	

PROCEDURES

12011	Simple suture--face--local anes.	
29125	App. of short arm splint; static	
29425	App. of short leg cast, walking	
50390	Aspiration of renal cyst by needle	
71010	Chest x-ray, single view, frontal	

PROCEDURES

71020	Chest x-ray, two views, frontal & lateral	
71030	Chest x-ray, complete, four views	
73070	Elbow x-ray, AP & lateral views	
73090	Forearm x-ray, AP & lateral views	
73100	Wrist x-ray, AP & lateral views	
73510	Hip x-ray, complete, two views	
73600	Ankle x-ray, AP & lateral views	

LABORATORY

80019	19 clinical chemistry tests	
80048	Basic metabolic panel	
80061	Lipid panel	
82270	Blood screening, occult; feces	
82947	Glucose screening--quantitative	
82951	Glucose tolerance test, three specimens	
83718	HDL cholesterol	X
84478	Triglycerides test	
85007	Manual differential WBC	X
85018	Hemoglobin	
85651	Erythrocyte sedimentation rate--non-auto	
86580	TB Mantoux test	
87072	Culture by commercial kit, nonurine...	
87076	Culture, anaerobic isolate	
87077	Bacterial culture, aerobic isolate	
87086	Urine culture and colony count	X
87430	Strep test	
87880	Direct streptococcus screen	

INJECTIONS

90471	Immunization administration	
90703	Tetanus injection	
90772	Injection	
92516	Facial nerve function studies	
93000	Electrocardiogram--ECG with interpretation	X
93015	Treadmill stress test, with physician...	
96900	Ultraviolet light treatment	
99070	Supplies and materials provided	

FAMILY CARE CENTER
286 Stephenson Blvd.
Stephenson, OH 60089
614-555-0000

☒ DANA BANU, M.D.
☐ ROBERT BEACH, M.D.
☐ PATRICIA MCGRATH, M.D.

☐ JESSICA RUDNER, M.D.
☐ JOHN RUDNER, M.D.
☐ KATHERINE YAN, M.D.

NOTES

REFERRING PHYSICIAN	NPI	AUTHORIZATION #

DIAGNOSIS
v70.0 routine physical examination

PAYMENT AMOUNT
$20 copay, check# 3219

ENCOUNTER FORM

1/5/2011
DATE

10:15 am
TIME

Sheila Giles
PATIENT NAME

GILESSH0
CHART #

OFFICE VISITS - SYMPTOMATIC

NEW

99201	OF--New Patient Minimal	
99202	OF--New Patient Low	
99203	OF--New Patient Detailed	
99204	OF--New Patient Moderate	
99205	OF--New Patient High	

ESTABLISHED

99211	OF--Established Patient Minimal	X
99212	OF--Established Patient Low	
99213	OF--Established Patient Detailed	
99214	OF--Established Patient Moderate	
99215	OF--Established Patient High	

PREVENTIVE VISITS

NEW

99381	Under 1 Year	
99382	1 - 4 Years	
99383	5 - 11 Years	
99384	12 - 17 Years	
99385	18 - 39 Years	
99386	40 - 64 Years	
99387	65 Years & Up	

ESTABLISHED

99391	Under 1 Year	
99392	1 - 4 Years	
99393	5 - 11 Years	
99394	12 - 17 Years	
99395	18 - 39 Years	
99396	40 - 64 Years	
99397	65 Years & Up	

PROCEDURES

12011	Simple suture--face--local anes.	
29125	App. of short arm splint; static	
29425	App. of short leg cast, walking	
50390	Aspiration of renal cyst by needle	
71010	Chest x-ray, single view, frontal	

PROCEDURES

71020	Chest x-ray, two views, frontal & lateral	
71030	Chest x-ray, complete, four views	
73070	Elbow x-ray, AP & lateral views	
73090	Forearm x-ray, AP & lateral views	
73100	Wrist x-ray, AP & lateral views	
73510	Hip x-ray, complete, two views	
73600	Ankle x-ray, AP & lateral views	

LABORATORY

80019	19 clinical chemistry tests	
80048	Basic metabolic panel	
80061	Lipid panel	
82270	Blood screening, occult; feces	
82947	Glucose screening--quantitative	
82951	Glucose tolerance test, three specimens	
83718	HDL cholesterol	
84478	Triglycerides test	
85007	Manual differential WBC	
85018	Hemoglobin	
85651	Erythrocyte sedimentation rate--non-auto	
86580	TB Mantoux test	
87072	Culture by commercial kit, nonurine...	
87076	Culture, anaerobic isolate	
87077	Bacterial culture, aerobic isolate	
87086	Urine culture and colony count	
87430	Strep test	
87880	Direct streptococcus screen	

INJECTIONS

90471	Immunization administration	X
90703	Tetanus injection	X
90772	Injection	
92516	Facial nerve function studies	
93000	Electrocardiogram--ECG with interpretation	
93015	Treadmill stress test, with physician...	
96900	Ultraviolet light treatment	
99070	Supplies and materials provided	

FAMILY CARE CENTER
286 Stephenson Blvd.
Stephenson, OH 60089
614-555-0000

- ☐ DANA BANU, M.D.
- ☒ ROBERT BEACH, M.D.
- ☐ PATRICIA MCGRATH, M.D.
- ☐ JESSICA RUDNER, M.D.
- ☐ JOHN RUDNER, M.D.
- ☐ KATHERINE YAN, M.D.

NOTES

REFERRING PHYSICIAN

NPI

AUTHORIZATION #

DIAGNOSIS
v03.7 tetanus immunization

PAYMENT AMOUNT

ENCOUNTER FORM

1/5/2011	10:30 am
DATE	TIME
Pauline Battistuta	BATTIPA0
PATIENT NAME	CHART #

OFFICE VISITS - SYMPTOMATIC

NEW

99201	OF--New Patient Minimal	
99202	OF--New Patient Low	
99203	OF--New Patient Detailed	
99204	OF--New Patient Moderate	
99205	OF--New Patient High	

ESTABLISHED

99211	OF--Established Patient Minimal	X
99212	OF--Established Patient Low	
99213	OF--Established Patient Detailed	
99214	OF--Established Patient Moderate	
99215	OF--Established Patient High	

PREVENTIVE VISITS

NEW

99381	Under 1 Year	
99382	1 - 4 Years	
99383	5 - 11 Years	
99384	12 - 17 Years	
99385	18 - 39 Years	
99386	40 - 64 Years	
99387	65 Years & Up	

ESTABLISHED

99391	Under 1 Year	
99392	1 - 4 Years	
99393	5 - 11 Years	
99394	12 - 17 Years	
99395	18 - 39 Years	
99396	40 - 64 Years	
99397	65 Years & Up	

PROCEDURES

12011	Simple suture--face--local anes.	
29125	App. of short arm splint; static	
29425	App. of short leg cast, walking	
50390	Aspiration of renal cyst by needle	
71010	Chest x-ray, single view, frontal	

PROCEDURES

71020	Chest x-ray, two views, frontal & lateral	
71030	Chest x-ray, complete, four views	
73070	Elbow x-ray, AP & lateral views	
73090	Forearm x-ray, AP & lateral views	
73100	Wrist x-ray, AP & lateral views	
73510	Hip x-ray, complete, two views	
73600	Ankle x-ray, AP & lateral views	

LABORATORY

80019	19 clinical chemistry tests	
80048	Basic metabolic panel	
80061	Lipid panel	
82270	Blood screening, occult; feces	
82947	Glucose screening--quantitative	
82951	Glucose tolerance test, three specimens	
83718	HDL cholesterol	
84478	Triglycerides test	
85007	Manual differential WBC	
85018	Hemoglobin	
85651	Erythrocyte sedimentation rate--non-auto	
86580	TB Mantoux test	
87072	Culture by commercial kit, nonurine...	
87076	Culture, anaerobic isolate	
87077	Bacterial culture, aerobic isolate	
87086	Urine culture and colony count	
87430	Strep test	
87880	Direct streptococcus screen	

INJECTIONS

90471	Immunization administration	
90703	Tetanus injection	
90772	Injection	
92516	Facial nerve function studies	
93000	Electrocardiogram--ECG with interpretation	
93015	Treadmill stress test, with physician...	
96900	Ultraviolet light treatment	
99070	Supplies and materials provided	

FAMILY CARE CENTER
286 Stephenson Blvd.
Stephenson, OH 60089
614-555-0000

- ☐ DANA BANU, M.D.
- ☐ ROBERT BEACH, M.D.
- ☒ PATRICIA MCGRATH, M.D.
- ☐ JESSICA RUDNER, M.D.
- ☐ JOHN RUDNER, M.D.
- ☐ KATHERINE YAN, M.D.

NOTES

upper respiratory infection

REFERRING PHYSICIAN	NPI	AUTHORIZATION #

DIAGNOSIS
465.9

PAYMENT AMOUNT

MEDICARE
246 WEST MAIN ST.
CLEVELAND, OH 60120

PROVIDER REMITTANCE
THIS IS NOT A BILL
A PAYMENT SUMMARY AND AN EXPLANATION OF
CODES ARE AT THE END OF THIS STATEMENT

FAMILY CARE CENTER
285 STEPHENSON BLVD.
STEPHENSON, OH 60089-4000

PAGE:	1 OF 1
DATE:	12/31/2010
ID NUMBER:	3470629

PROVIDER: PATRICIA MCGRATH, M.D.

PATIENT: BATTISTUTA ANTHONY   CLAIM: 234567890

FROM DATE	THRU DATE	PROC CODE	UNITS	AMOUNT BILLED	AMOUNT ALLOWED	DEDUCT	COPAY/ COINS	PROV PAID	REASON CODE
10/28/10	10/28/10	99212	1	54.00	37.36	.00	.00	29.89	
10/28/10	10/28/10	82947	1	25.00	5.48	.00	.00	4.38	
	CLAIM TOTALS			79.00	42.84	.00	.00	34.27	

PATIENT: BATTISTUTA ANTHONY   CLAIM: 234567891

FROM DATE	THRU DATE	PROC CODE	UNITS	AMOUNT BILLED	AMOUNT ALLOWED	DEDUCT	COPAY/ COINS	PROV PAID	REASON CODE
11/12/10	11/12/10	99212	1	54.00	37.36	.00	.00	29.89	
11/12/10	11/12/10	82951	1	63.00	16.12	.00	.00	12.90	
11/12/10	11/12/10	87086	1	51.00	11.28	.00	.00	9.02	
	CLAIM TOTALS			168.00	64.76	.00	.00	51.81	

PROVIDER: KATHERINE YAN, M.D.

PATIENT: JONES ELIZABETH   CLAIM: 234567892

FROM DATE	THRU DATE	PROC CODE	UNITS	AMOUNT BILLED	AMOUNT ALLOWED	DEDUCT	COPAY/ COINS	PROV PAID	REASON CODE
10/4/10	10/4/10	99213	1	72.00	51.03	.00	.00	40.82	
	CLAIM TOTALS			72.00	51.03	.00	.00	40.82	

PAYMENT SUMMARY		TOTAL ALL CLAIMS		EFT INFORMATION	
TOTAL AMOUNT PAID	126.90	AMOUNT CHARGED	319.00	NUMBER	3470629
PRIOR CREDIT BALANCE	.00	AMOUNT ALLOWED	158.63	DATE	12/31/10
CURRENT CREDIT DEFERRED	.00	DEDUCTIBLE	.00	AMOUNT	126.90
PRIOR CREDIT APPLIED	.00	COPAY	.00		
NEW CREDIT BALANCE	.00	COINSURANCE	.00		
NET DISBURSED	126.90	AMOUNT APPROVED	158.63		

STATUS CODES:
A - APPROVED   AJ - ADJUSTMENT   IP - IN PROCESS   R - REJECTED   V - VOID

CHAMPVA
240 CENTER ST.
COLUMBUS, OH 60220

PROVIDER REMITTANCE
THIS IS NOT A BILL
A PAYMENT SUMMARY AND AN EXPLANATION OF
CODES ARE AT THE END OF THIS STATEMENT

FAMILY CARE CENTER
285 STEPHENSON BLVD.
STEPHENSON, OH 60089-4000

PAGE: 1 OF 1
DATE: 12/31/2010
ID NUMBER: 76374021

PROVIDER: JOHN RUDNER, M.D.

PATIENT: FITZWILLIAMS JOHN   CLAIM: 123456789

FROM DATE	THRU DATE	PROC CODE	UNITS	AMOUNT BILLED	AMOUNT ALLOWED	DEDUCT	COPAY/ COINS	PROV PAID	REASON CODE
10/4/10	10/4/10	99212	1	54.00	37.36	.00	15.00	22.36	
10/4/10	10/4/10	82270	1	19.00	4.54	.00	.00	4.54	
	CLAIM TOTALS			73.00	41.90	.00	15.00	26.90	

******************** CHECK #76374021 IN THE AMOUNT OF $26.90 IS ATTACHED ********************

PAYMENT SUMMARY		TOTAL ALL CLAIMS	
TOTAL AMOUNT PAID	26.90	AMOUNT CHARGED	73.00
PRIOR CREDIT BALANCE	.00	AMOUNT ALLOWED	41.90
CURRENT CREDIT DEFERRED	.00	DEDUCTIBLE	.00
PRIOR CREDIT APPLIED	.00	COPAY	15.00
NEW CREDIT BALANCE	.00	OTHER REDUCTION	.00
NET DISBURSED	26.90		

STATUS CODES:
AJ - ADJUSTMENT   IP - IN PROCESS   R - REJECTED   V - VOID

MEDICAID
246 WEST MAIN ST.
CLEVELAND, OH 60120

PROVIDER REMITTANCE
THIS IS NOT A BILL
A PAYMENT SUMMARY AND AN EXPLANATION OF
CODES ARE AT THE END OF THIS STATEMENT

FAMILY CARE CENTER
285 STEPHENSON BLVD.
STEPHENSON, OH 60089-4000

PAGE: 1 OF 1
DATE: 12/31/2010
ID NUMBER: 137291449

PROVIDER: ROBERT BEACH, M.D.

PATIENT: PALMER CHRISTOPHER   CLAIM: 56789012

FROM DATE	THRU DATE	PROC CODE	UNITS	AMOUNT BILLED	AMOUNT ALLOWED	DEDUCT	COPAY/ COINS	PROV PAID	REASON CODE
11/12/10	11/12/10	99201	1	66.00	35.58	.00	10.00	25.58	
11/12/10	11/12/10	87430	1	29.00	16.01	.00	.00	16.01	
	CLAIM TOTALS			95.00	51.59	.00	10.00	41.59	

PAYMENT SUMMARY		TOTAL ALL CLAIMS		EFT INFORMATION	
TOTAL AMOUNT PAID	41.59	AMOUNT CHARGED	95.00	NUMBER	137291449
PRIOR CREDIT BALANCE	.00	AMOUNT ALLOWED	51.59	DATE	12/31/10
CURRENT CREDIT DEFERRED	.00	DEDUCTIBLE	.00	AMOUNT	41.59
PRIOR CREDIT APPLIED	.00	COPAY	10.00		
NEW CREDIT BALANCE	.00	OTHER REDUCTION	.00		
NET DISBURSED	41.59				

STATUS CODES:
A - APPROVED   AJ - ADJUSTMENT   IP - IN PROCESS   R - REJECTED   V - VOID

EAST OHIO PPO
10 CENTRAL AVENUE
HALEVILLE, OH 60890

PROVIDER REMITTANCE
THIS IS NOT A BILL
A PAYMENT SUMMARY AND AN EXPLANATION OF
CODES ARE AT THE END OF THIS STATEMENT

FAMILY CARE CENTER
285 STEPHENSON BLVD.
STEPHENSON, OH 60089-4000

PAGE: 1 OF 1
DATE: 12/31/2010
ID NUMBER: 376490713

PROVIDER: DANA BANU, M.D.

PATIENT: SYZMANSKI HANNAH   CLAIM: 78901234

FROM DATE	THRU DATE	PROC CODE	UNITS	AMOUNT BILLED	AMOUNT ALLOWED	DEDUCT	COPAY/ COINS	PROV PAID	REASON CODE
11/12/10	11/12/10	99383	1	224.00	201.60	.00	20.00	181.60	
	CLAIM TOTALS			224.00	201.60	.00	20.00	181.60	

PATIENT: SYZMANSKI MICHAEL   CLAIM: 89012345

FROM DATE	THRU DATE	PROC CODE	UNITS	AMOUNT BILLED	AMOUNT ALLOWED	DEDUCT	COPAY/ COINS	PROV PAID	REASON CODE
11/15/10	11/15/10	99215	1	163.00	146.70	.00	20.00	126.70	
11/15/10	11/15/10	82270	1	19.00	17.10	.00	.00	17.10	
	CLAIM TOTALS			182.00	163.80	.00	20.00	143.80	

PROVIDER: PATRICIA MCGRATH, M.D.

PATIENT: SYZMANSKI MICHAEL   CLAIM: 901234563

FROM DATE	THRU DATE	PROC CODE	UNITS	AMOUNT BILLED	AMOUNT ALLOWED	DEDUCT	COPAY/ COINS	PROV PAID	REASON CODE
12/18/10	12/18/10	99212	1	54.00	48.60	.00	20.00	28.60	
12/18/10	12/18/10	12011	1	202.00	181.80	.00	.00	181.80	
	CLAIM TOTALS			256.00	230.40	.00	20.00	210.40	

PAYMENT SUMMARY		TOTAL ALL CLAIMS		EFT INFORMATION	
TOTAL AMOUNT PAID	535.80	AMOUNT CHARGED	662.00	NUMBER	376490713
PRIOR CREDIT BALANCE	.00	AMOUNT ALLOWED	595.80	DATE	12/31/10
CURRENT CREDIT DEFERRED	.00	DEDUCTIBLE	.00	AMOUNT	535.80
PRIOR CREDIT APPLIED	.00	COPAY	60.00		
NEW CREDIT BALANCE	.00	COINSURANCE	0.00		
NET DISBURSED	535.80				

REASON CODES:
AJ - ADJUSTMENT   IP - IN PROCESS   R - REJECTED   V - VOID

OHIOCARE HMO
147 CENTRAL AVENUE
HALEVILLE, OH 60890

FAMILY CARE CENTER
285 STEPHENSON BLVD.
STEPHENSON, OH 60089-4000

PAGE: 1 OF 1
DATE: 12/31/2010
ID NUMBER: 767729

OHIOCARE HMO CAPITATION STATEMENT
MONTH OF NOVEMBER 2010

PROVIDERS
BANU DANA
BEACH ROBERT
MCGRATH PATRICIA
RUDNER JESSICA
RUDNER JOHN
YAN KATHERINE

MEMBER NUMBER	MEMBER NAME	CONTRACT NUMBER	CONTRACT STATUS
0003602149	FAMILY CARE CENTER	YG34906	APPROVED

AMOUNT OF PAYMENT $2,500.00
EFT STATUS: SENT 12/31/10 2:46PM
TRANSACTION #767729

Glossary

A

accounting cycle   the flow of financial transactions in a business

accounts receivable (AR)   monies that are flowing into a business

adjudication   series of steps that determine whether a claim should be paid

adjustments   changes to patients' accounts that alter the amount charged or paid

administrative safeguards   administrative policies and procedures designed to protect electronic health information outlined by the HIPAA Security Rule

aging report   a report that lists the amount of money owed to the practice, organized by the amount of time the money has been owed

audit/edit report   a report from a clearinghouse that lists errors to be corrected before a claim can be submitted to the payer

audit trail   a report that traces who has accessed electronic information, when information was accessed, and whether any information was changed

autoposting   an automated process for entering information on a remittance advice (RA) into a computer

B

backup data   a copy of data files made at a specific point in time that can be used to restore data to the system

billing cycle   regular schedule of sending statements to patients

C

capitation   advance payment to a provider that covers each plan member's health care services for a certain period of time

capitation payments   payments made to physicians on a regular basis (such as monthly) for providing services to patients in a managed care insurance plan

case   a grouping of transactions for visits to a physician's office, organized around a condition

charges   amounts a provider bills for the services performed

chart   a folder that contains all records pertaining to a patient

chart number   a unique number that identifies a patient

clearinghouse   a service company that receives electronic or paper claims from the provider, checks and prepares them for processing, and transmits them in HIPAA-compliant format to the correct carriers

coinsurance   part of charges that an insured person must pay for health care services after payment of the deductible amount

collection agency   an outside firm hired to collect on delinquent accounts

collection list   a tool for tracking activities that needs to be completed as part of the collections process

Collection Tracer report   a tool for keeping track of collection letters that were sent

consumer-driven health plan (CDHP)   a type of managed care in which a high-deductible/low-premium insurance plan is combined with a pretax savings account to cover out-of-pocket medical expenses, up to the deductible limit

copayment   A small fixed fee paid by the patient at the time of an office visit.

cycle billing   a type of billing in which patients are divided into groups and statement printing and mailing is staggered throughout the month

D

database   a collection of related bits of information

day sheet   a report that provides information on practice activities for a twenty-four-hour period

diagnosis   physician's opinion of the nature of the patient's illness or injury

diagnosis code   a standardized value that represents a patient's illness, signs, and symptoms

E

electronic data interchange (EDI) the exchange of routine business transactions from one computer to another using publicly available communications protocols

electronic funds transfer (EFT) a system that transfers money electronically

electronic medical record (EMR) electronic collection and management of health data

electronic prescribing the use of computers and handheld devices to write and transmit prescriptions to a pharmacy in a secure digital format

electronic remittance advice (ERA) an electronic document that lists patients, dates of service, charges, and the amount paid or denied by the insurance carrier

encounter form a list of the procedures and charges for a patient's visit

established patient a patient who has been seen by a provider in the practice in the same specialty within three years

explanation of benefits (EOB) paper document from a payer that shows how the amount of a benefit was determined

F

fee-for-service health plan that repays the policyholder for covered medical expenses

fee schedule a document that specifies the amount the provider bills for provided services

filter a condition that data must meet to be selected

G

guarantor an individual who is not a patient of the practice, but who is the insurance policyholder for a patient of the practice

H

health maintenance organization (HMO) a managed health care system in which providers agree to offer health care to the organization's members for fixed periodic payments from the plan

health plan a plan, program, or organization that provides health benefits

HIPAA (Health Insurance Portability and Accountability Act of 1996) federal act that set forth guidelines for standardizing the electronic data interchange of administrative and financial transactions, exposing fraud and abuse in government programs, and protecting the security and privacy of health information.

HIPAA Electronic Transaction and Code Sets standards regulations requiring electronic transactions such as claim transmission to use standardized formats

HIPAA Privacy Rule regulations for protecting individually identifiable information about a patient's past, present, or future physical and mental health and payment for health care that is created or received by a health care provider

HIPAA Security Rule regulations outlining the minimum administrative, technical, and physical safeguards required to prevent unauthorized access to protected health care information

I

information technology (IT) development, management, and support of computer-based hardware/software systems

insurance aging report a report that lists how long a payer has taken to respond to insurance claims

K

knowledge base a collection of up-to-date technical information

M

managed care a type of insurance in which the carrier is responsible for both the financing and the delivery of health care

medical coder a person who analyzes and codes patient diagnoses, procedures, and symptoms

medical necessity treatment provided by a physician to a patient for the purpose of preventing, diagnosing, or treating an illness, injury, or its symptoms in a manner that is appropriate and provided in accordance with generally accepted standards of medical practice

MMDDCCYY format a specific way in which dates must be keyed, in which "MM" stands for the month, "DD" stands for the day, "CC" represents the century, and "YY" stands for the year

modifier a two-digit character that is appended to a CPT code to report special circumstances involved with a procedure or service

MultiLink codes groups of procedure code entries that relate to a single activity

N

National Provider Identifier (NPI) a standard identifier for all health care providers consisting of ten numbers

navigator buttons buttons that simplify the task of moving from one entry to another

new patient a patient who has not received services from the same provider or a provider of the same specialty within the same practice for a period of three years

O

Office Hours break a block of time when a physician is unavailable for appointments with patients

Office Hours schedule a listing of time slots for a particular day for a specific provider

once-a-month billing a type of billing in which statements are mailed to all patients at the same time each month

P

packing data the deletion of vacant slots from the database

patient aging report a report that lists a patient's balance by age, date and amount of the last payment, and telephone number

patient day sheet a summary of patient activity on a given day

patient information form form that includes a patient's personal, employment, and insurance data needed to complete an insurance claim

patient ledger a report that lists the financial activity in each patient's account, including charges, payments, and adjustments

patient statements a list of the amount of money a patient owes, organized by the amount of time the money has been owed, the procedures performed, and the dates the procedures were performed

payer private or government organization that insures or pays for health care on the behalf of beneficiaries

payment day sheet a report that lists all payments received on a particular day, organized by provider

payment plan an agreement between a patient and a practice in which the patient agrees to make regular monthly payments over a specified period of time

payment schedule a document that specifies the amount the payer agrees to pay the provider for a service, based on a contracted rate of reimbursement

payments monies received from patients and insurance carriers

physical safeguards mechanisms required to protect electronic systems, equipment, and data from threats, environmental hazards, and unauthorized intrusion

policyholder a person who buys an insurance plan; the insured

practice analysis report a report that analyzes the revenue of a practice for a specified period of time, usually a month or a year

practice management program (PMP) a software program that automates many of the administrative and financial tasks required to run a medical practice

preferred provider organization (PPO) managed care network of health care providers who agree to perform services for plan members at discounted fees

premium the periodic amount of money the insured pays to a health plan for insurance coverage

procedure medical treatment provided by a physician or other health care provider

procedure code a code that identifies a medical service

procedure day sheet a report that lists all the procedures performed on a particular day, in numerical order

prompt payment laws state laws that mandate a time period within which clean claims must be paid; if they are not, financial penalties are levied against the payer

protected health information (PHI) information about a patient's past, present, or future physical or mental health or payment for health care that can be used to identify the person

purging data the process of deleting files of patients who are no longer seen by a provider in a practice

R

rebuilding indexes a process that checks and verifies data and corrects any internal problems with the data

recalculating balances the process of updating balances to reflect the most recent changes made to the data

record of treatment and progress a physician's notes about a patient's condition and diagnosis

referring provider a physician who recommends that a patient see a specific other physician

remainder statements statements that list only those charges that are not paid in full after all insurance carrier payments have been received

remittance advice (RA) an explanation of benefits transmitted electronically by a payer to a provider

restoring data the process of retrieving data from backup storage devices

S

sponsor   in TRICARE, the active-duty service member

standard statements   statements that show all charges regardless of whether the insurance has paid on the transactions

statement   a list of all services performed for a patient, along with the charges for each service

T

technical safeguards   automated processes used to protect data and control access to data

tickler   a reminder to follow-up on an account

U

uncollectible account   an account that does not respond to collection efforts and is written off the practice's expected accounts receivable

W

walkout statement   a document listing charges and payments that is given to a patient after an office visit

X

X12-837 Health Care Claim (837P)   HIPAA standard format for electronic transmission of a professional claim from a provider to a health plan

Index

A

Accidents, Condition tab, 120
Accounting cycle, 18
Accounts receivable (AR), 18
Account tab, 111–113
Acknowledgment of Receipt of Notice of
    Privacy Practices, 37
Activities menu, 48, 49
Address dialog box, 86–89
Address List dialog box, 86–89
Adjudication, 15–17
Adjustments, 158–160
    defined, 136
    transaction entry, 136, 137, 158–160, 204,
        206, 213–215
    unapplied payment/adjustment
        report, 247
Administrative safeguards, 38
Aging reports:
    defined, 248
    insurance aging report, 248, 249–250
    patient aging applied payment report,
        268–269
    patient aging report, 248–249
American Hospital Association (AHA),
    coding guidelines of, 14
American Medical Association (AMA):
    coding guidelines of, 14
    medical necessity and, 14
    National Uniform Claim Committee
        (NUCC), 168
Analysis reports, 242–248
    billing/payment status report, 242–244
    co-payment report, 247, 248
    facility report, 247
    global coverage report, 248
    insurance analysis, 247
    insurance payment comparison, 247
    outstanding copayment report, 248
    practice analysis report, 244–245
    referral source report, 247
    referring provider report, 247
    unapplied deposit report, 247
    unapplied payment/adjustment
        report, 247
Apply Payments button, 52, 151–153
Appointment(s), 27–28
    deleting, 301–302
    scheduling, 27–28, 291–309. See also
        Office Hours
ASC X12 standards, 33–34, 168, 194–196
Assignment of benefits, 116
Assignment of claim, 193
Attachments, sending with electronic
    claims, 185–186
Audit/edit report, 28, 30, 182
Audit trail, 39
Autoposting, 29

B

Backup data:
    defined, 63
    making file when exiting Medisoft, 63–64
    Medisoft utility for, 63–64
    restoring, 65–66
Billing compliance, 14–15
Billing cycle, 17–18
Billing/payment status report, 242–244
Billing process. See Medical billing process
Breaks, creating schedule, 306–307

C

Calendar, Medisoft, 53–56
Capitated plan, 117
Capitation, 6
Capitation payments, 199, 211–213
Carrier 1 tab, 177–178
Carrier 2 tab, 178
Carrier 3 tab, 178
Case dialog box, 106–129
Cases, 103–129
    Account tab, 111–113
    Cancel button, 110
    command buttons for, 105–108
    Comment tab, 125
    Condition tab, 119–121
    defined, 104
    deleting, 105–106
    Diagnosis tab, 114–115
    EDI tab, 125–129
    editing case information, 105, 129
    entering case information, 106–129
    Medicaid and TRICARE tab, 123–125
    Miscellaneous tab, 122–123
    Personal tab, 108–111
    Policy 1 tab, 115–117
    Policy 2 tab, 118–119
    Policy 3 tab, 119
    saving information on, 110
    setting up new, 104–105
    Transaction Entry dialog box, 138, 139
CHAMPUS. See TRICARE
CHAMPVA (Civilian Health and Medical
    Program), 5–6
Charges, 140–148
    applying payments to, 151–153, 201–206
    defined, 136
    entering, 140–148
    saving, 145–146
Chart(s), 107–108, 136–138, 138
Chart numbers, 80–82
    assigning, 80–81
    in claim creation, 173
    described, 80–81
    selecting, 136–138

Claim(s), insurance, 167–186
    cases and, 103–129. See also Cases
    changing status of, 186
    claim selection, 130, 175–176
    clearinghouses for, 28, 29, 114–115
    creating, 168–176
    editing, 176–178
    electronic claims. See Electronic claims
    entering payments in Medisoft, 197–215
    insurance aging report, 248, 249–250
    preparing and transmitting, 15
    types of insurance plans, 5–7, 192–193
Claim dialog box, 175–179
Claim Management dialog box, 168–176, 213
Claims reports:
    audit/edit report, 28, 30, 182
    claim submission report, 182, 184
    verification report, 181–185
Clearinghouses, 28, 29, 114–115
CLIA number, 126
CMS-1500 (08/05), 34, 168, 169–171
CMS-Centers for Medicare and Medicaid
    Services, 5, 33, 38, 264
Coding. See also CPT-4 codes;
        ICD-9-CM codes
    color, in transaction entry, 146–148, 154
    defined, 10
    reviewing compliance with, 14
Coinsurance, 6
Collection agency, 267
Collection letters, 277–280
Collection List, 269–274
    tickler in, 269, 270, 274–277
    using, 269–274
Collection List dialog box, 269–274
Collection process, 10, 18–19, 263–281
    collection agencies in, 267
    collection letters, 277–280
    importance of, 264
    laws governing patient collections, 266
    laws governing timely payment of
        insurance claims, 268
    medical practice financial policy, 264–266
    payment plans in, 85, 267
    practice management programs,
        268–281
    reports in. See Collection reports
    writing off uncollectible accounts, 267
Collection reports, 250
    collection list, 269–274
    Collection Tracer report, 281
    printing, 248
Color coding, in transaction entry,
    146–148, 154
Command buttons, 105–108
Comment tab:
    for case notes, 125
    in editing claims, 179
    statement, 221

Computers. *See* Information technology (IT)
Condition tab, 119–121
Confidentiality. *See* Privacy
Consumer Credit Protection Act, 267
Consumer-driven health plan (CDHP), 7
Copayment, 7, 10, 117
Copayment report, 247, 248
Copy Address button, 81
Copy feature, Copy Case button, 106
CPT-4 codes. *See also* Procedure codes
   described, 47
   development of, 12
   MultiLink codes, 144–145
   sample, 13
   as standards, 34
   in Transaction Entry dialog box,
      141–142, 143
Create Claims dialog box, 172–174
Create Statement dialog box, 218–219
Crossover claims, 119
Current Procedural Terminology (CPT, CPT-4),
   12, 47. *See also* CPT-4 codes
Custom report(s), 253–255
Cycle billing, 224

D

Databases:
   defined, 46
   Medisoft, 46–47
   nature of, 31
Data Selection Questions dialog box, 224,
   233–234
Dates, in Medisoft, 53–56, 140, 234–236
Day sheets, 232–241
   defined, 232
   patient day sheet, 19, 232–238
   payment day sheet, 241
   procedure day sheet, 239–240
Deductible, 117, 203
Delete feature, 58–59
   for appointments in Office Hours,
      301–302
   for cases, 105–106
   purging data, 69–71
   for transaction information, 143–144
Department of Health and Human Services
   (DHHS), 32
Deposit dialog box, 200–201
Deposit List dialog box, 197–215
Diagnosis, 10
Diagnosis codes, 10–12. *See also*
   ICD-9-CM codes
   Diagnosis Code List button, 52
   Diagnosis tab for cases, 114–115
   for entering charges, 142
   in Medisoft database, 47
Dialog boxes. *See specific types of dialog boxes*

E

Early and Periodic Screening,
   Diagnosis, and Treatment (EPSDT),
   123–124, 128
EDI Report, 185–186
EDI tab, 125–129
Edit Case button, 105, 129
Edit feature:
   for appointments in Office Hours,
      301–302
   for case information, 105, 129
   for claims, 179
   for clearinghouse information, 28

   for clearinghouses, 28
   Edit menu, 48, 49
   for information on established patients,
      90, 105, 129
   for insurance claims, 176–178
   for patient statements, 220–221
   for transaction information, 146
Edit Statement dialog box, 220–221
Electronic claims, 180–186
   attachments, sending, 185–186
   audit/edit report, 28, 30, 182
   changing status of claims, 186
   claim submission report, 182, 184
   clearinghouses for, 28, 29, 114–115
   in Medisoft
      creating cases for imported
         transactions, 130
      importing transactions, 130
      transferring patient information, 96–97
   standards for, 33–35, 180
   steps in submitting, 181–183
   transmitting, 185–186
   verification report, 181–185
Electronic data interchange (EDI), 33–34,
   114–115, 180–186
   in cases, 125–129
Electronic funds transfer (EFT), 34
Electronic medical record (EMR), 24–25
Electronic medical record exchange:
   creating cases for imported
      transactions, 130
   importing transactions, 162
   transferring appointment
      information, 311
   transferring patient information, 96–97
   viewing data transfer reports, 259
Electronic prescribing, 25–26
Electronic remittance advice (ERA), 194–196
Emergencies:
   Condition tab, 120
   emergency contact information, 84
Employer Drop-Down List, 84–85
Employer information, 84–85, 86–89, 109–110
EMR (electronic medical record), 24–25
Encounter form, 10, 11, 15, 136
EPSDT (Early and Periodic Screening,
   Diagnosis, and Treatment),
   123–124, 128
Errors:
   common claim, 196
   computers in reduction of, 25, 31
   electronic medical record (EMR) and, 25
Established patients:
   creating new case for, 106
   defined, 79
   editing information on, 90, 105, 129
   searching for patient information, 90–94
Exiting Medisoft, 52, 63–72
Exiting Office Hours, 291
Explanation of benefits (EOB), 15–17

F

F8 function key, 88
Facility report, 247
Fair Debt Collection Practices Act
   of 1977, 266
Fee-for-service plans, 6
Fee schedule:
   defined, 192
   in third-party reimbursement, 192–194
Fields box, 91–92, 94
Field Value box, 93

File maintenance utilities, 66–72
   backing up data, 63–64
   packing data, 68–69
   purging data, 69–71
   rebuilding indexes, 67–68
   recalculating patient balances, 71–72
   restoring backup files, 65–66
File menu, 48, 49
Filters:
   Create Claims dialog box, 173–174
   defined, 173
   selecting, in printing statements, 224–225
Final Enforcement Rule, 38
Finance charges, 266
Follow up payments, 18–19
Form(s):
   X12-270/271 Health Care Eligibility
      Benefit Inquiry and Response, 34
   X12-276/277 Health Care Claim Status
      Request and Response, 34
   X12-278 Health Care Services Review, 34
   X12-835 Claims Payment and Remittance
      Advice, 34, 194–196
   X12-837 Health Care Claim or Equivalent
      Encounter Information (837P), 34, 168
Forms. *See also* Report(s)
   Acknowledgment of Receipt of Notice of
      Privacy Practices, 37
   CMS-1500 (08/05), 34, 168, 169–171
   encounter form, 10, 11, 15, 136
   Notice of Privacy Practices, 35–37
   patient information form, 7–9, 15

G

General tab, 220–221
Global coverage report, 248
Go to Date dialog box, 294
Guarantor (insured), 82–83, 218

H

Health insurance. *See* Medical insurance
Health Insurance Portability and
   Accountability Act of 1996 (HIPAA),
   32–39, 180
Health maintenance organizations (HMOs), 7
Health plans, 5–7, 192–193. *See also*
   Medical insurance
Help feature, 50, 51, 52, 59–62
HIPAA (Health Insurance Portability
   and Accountability Act of 1996),
   32–39, 180
HIPAA Electronic Transaction and Code
   Sets Standards, 33–35, 180
HIPAA Privacy Rule, 35–37, 38, 264
HIPAA Security Rule, 37–39
Home health claims, 128–129
Hospice care, 126

I

ICD-9-CM codes. *See also* Diagnosis codes
   for charges, 142
   described, 47
   development of, 10–12
   sample, 12
   as standards, 34
IDE Number, 113
Indemnity plans, reimbursement
   from, 192
Indexes, rebuilding, 67–68
Indicator code, 123

Information technology (IT), 23–39. *See also* Electronic claims
advantages of computer use, 30–31
cautions concerning, 31–32
defined, 24
HIPAA and, 32–39
medical office applications of, 24–32. *See also* Medisoft; Office Hours
privacy requirements for, 35–37, 38, 264
security requirements for, 37–39
Insurance. *See* Medical insurance
Insurance aging report, 248, 249–250
Insurance analysis report, 247
Insurance carrier database, 46–47
Insurance carrier payments, 197–215
Insurance Coverage Percents by Service Classification box, 117
Insurance identification card, 9–10
Insurance payment comparison report, 247
Insured (guarantor), 82–83, 218
International Classification of Diseases 9th Revision, *Clinical Modification* (ICD-9-CM), 10–12, 47. *See also* ICD-9-CM codes

K

Karnofsky Performance Status Scale, 120
Knowledge base, 60, 62

L

Lab charges, 122–123
Launch Work Administrator, 52
List Only Claims That Match dialog box, 175–176, 213, 214
Lists menu, 49
List Window, 91, 92
Locate buttons option, 93–94

M

Managed care plans:
defined, 6
reimbursement from, 192–193
Medicaid, 5, 32
in cases, 123–124
forgiving/writing off payments, 267
Medical billing process, 3–19. *See also* Payment(s)
billing cycle in, 17–18
checking billing compliance, 14–15
checking in patients, 7–10
checking out patients, 10–14
collections in. *See* Collection process
establishing financial responsibility for visit, 5–7, 270–272
follow up patient payments, 18–19
monitoring payer adjudication, 15–17
overview, 4
practice management program (PMP) in, 28–30. *See also* Medisoft
preparing and transmitting claims, 15. *See also* Claim(s), insurance
preregistering patients in, 4
recording diagnoses in, 47
recording procedures in, 47
reports
billing/payment status report, 242–244
patient statements, 17–18, 217–225
remittance advice (RA), 15–17, 28–29, 34, 194–196
walkout statements/receipts, 28–29, 31, 156–158, 159

reviewing coding compliance in, 14
scheduling appointments in, 27–28, 291–309. *See also* Office Hours
Medical coder, 14
Medical insurance. *See also* Claim(s), insurance
in cases, 104, 115–119
HIPAA Privacy Rule, 35–37, 38, 264
overview, 5–7
payments
capitation payments, 199, 211–213
entering insurance carrier payments, 197–215
insurance aging report, 248, 249–250
insurance payment comparison, 247
reviewing and recording payments, 197–215
unapplied payment/adjustment report, 247
types of, 5–7, 192–193
Medical necessity, 14
Medical records:
Acknowledgment of Receipt of Notice of Privacy Practices, 37
diagnosis codes in, 10–12, 47
electronic medical record (EMR), 24–25
encounter form, 10, 11, 15, 136
procedure codes in, 47, 143, 144
Medicare, 5, 32
in cases, 127
forgiving/writing off payments, 267
Medicare Fee Schedule (MFS), 193
reimbursement from, 193
Medisoft. *See also* Cases; Office Hours
backing up, 63–64
calendar in, 53–56, 140, 234–236
cases in. *See* Cases
claims management, 167–186
claim selection, 136, 175–176
creating claims, 168–176
editing claims, 176–178
entering insurance carrier payments, 197–215
insurance aging report, 248, 249–250
in collection process, 268–281
copying data in, 106
databases, 46–47
dates in, 53–56, 140, 234–236
deleting data in, 58–59, 69–71, 143–144
described, 46
EDI Report, 185–186
electronic medical record exchange. *See* Electronic medical record exchange
entering and editing data in, 146
changing program date, 53–56, 140
established patient information, 90, 105, 129
new patient information, 79–89, 106–129
entering payments
insurance carrier payments, 197–215
patient payments, 150–153
payments made during office visits, 150–153
exiting, 52, 63–72
Help, 50, 51, 52, 59–62
introduction, 45–72
main window, 48
menu bar, 47–51
organization of patient information, 78–79
overview, 46
Program Date, changing, 53–56, 140
reports in. *See* Report(s)

restoring backup file, 65–66
saving data in, 58, 110, 145–146, 153–155, 206
searching for patient information, 90–94
short cuts in. *See* Short cuts in Medisoft
starting, 47–48
student data template, 47
toolbar buttons, 51–52
utilities, 66–72
Menu bar, Medisoft, 47–51
Miscellaneous tab, 122–123
MMDDCCYY format, 56
Modifiers, 12–13
MultiLink codes, 144–145

N

Name, Address tab, 80–82
National Provider Identifier (NPI), 34–35
National Uniform Claim Committee (NUCC), 168
Navigator buttons, 172, 238
New Appointment Entry dialog box, Office Hours, 292–294
New Case button, 106–129
New claims, 168–176
New patients:
creating new case for, 106–129
defined, 79
entering appointments for, 299
entering basic data for, 79–89
entering case information for, 105
Non-Availability (NA) indicator, 125
Notice of Privacy Practices, 35–37

O

Office Hours, 288–309
changing appointments in, 301–302
creating breaks in, 306–307
deleting appointments in, 301–302
entering, 290–291
entering appointments in, 291–309
looking for future date, 294
for new patients, 299
recall lists, 303–306
repeated appointments, 299–300
searching for available appointment time, 297
exiting, 291
Office Hours break, 306–307
Office Hours schedule, 290
overview, 288–290
previewing schedules, 308–309
printing schedules, 308–309
program options, 290
recall lists in, 303–306
starting, 290–291
toolbar buttons, 289
Office Notes tab, 275–276
Office visits:
checking in patients, 7–10
checking out patients, 10–14
entering payments made during, 150–153, 200–201
applying to charges, 151–153, 201–206
saving payment information, 153–155
walkout statements/receipts, 28–29, 31, 156–158, 159

establishing financial responsibility for, 5–7
preregistering patients, 4
scheduling appointments for, 27–28, 291–309. *See also* Office Hours
walkout statements/receipts, 28–29, 31, 156–158, 159
Once-a-month billing, 224
Open Report dialog box, 223, 253–254
Other information tab, 82–85, 86–89
Outstanding copayment report, 248

P

Packing data, 68–69
Partial payment, 10
Patient/Account Information, 136–140
case, 138
charge tab, 140
chart, 136–138
totals tab, 138–139
Patient aging applied payment report, 268–269
Patient aging report, 248–249
Patient data, 28. *See also* Cases
checking in patients, 7–10
checking out patients, 10–14
in collections. *See* Collection process
editing, in Medisoft, 90, 105, 129
electronic medical record (EMR), 24–25
entering, in Medisoft, 79–89
for established patients. *See* Established patients
HIPAA Privacy Rule, 35–37, 38, 264
insurance identification card, 9–10
for new patients. *See* New patients
organization of, in Medisoft, 78–79
patient database, 46
payment information. *See* Payment(s)
preregistering patients, 4
saving, in Office Visits, 153–155
searching for, in Medisoft, 90–94
Patient day sheet, 19, 232–238
Patient/Guarantor dialog box, 79–89
editing patient information, 90
Name, Address tab, 80–82
Other Information tab, 82–85, 86–89
Payment Plan tab, 85
Patient information form, 7–9, 15
Patient ledger, 251–252
Patient List dialog box, 78–79
accessing, 78
case information and, 105–129
closing, 106
search feature and, 90–94
Patient payments, follow up, 18–19
Patient Recall List dialog box, Office Hours, 303–306
Patient statements, 217–225
creating, 17–18, 217–225
defined, 217
editing, 220–221
printing, 206, 222–225
sample, 18
walkout statements/receipts, 28–29, 31, 156–158, 159
Payer(s):
defined, 6
monitoring payer adjudication, 15–17
Payment(s), 149–158. *See also* Medical billing process
capitation payments, 199, 211–213
copayments, 7, 10, 117
deductible, 117, 203

defined, 136
entering in Medisoft, 150–153
insurance carrier payments, 197–215
patient payments made during office visits, 150–153
patient information form and, 7–9, 15
payment day sheet, 241
recalculating patient balances, 71–72
reports
billing/payment status report, 242–244
insurance aging report, 248, 249–250
patient aging applied payment report, 268–269
patient aging report, 248–249
patient ledger, 251–252
patient statements, 217–225
walkout statements/receipts, 28–29, 31, 156–158, 159
reviewing and recording, 197–215
Payment day sheet, 241
Payment plans, 85, 267
Payment Plan tab, 85
Payment schedule, 192
Personal tab, 108–111
Physical safeguards, 38
PIN (provider identification number) box, 34–35
Place of service (POS) box, 142–143
Policy 1 tab, 115–117
Policy 2 tab, 118–119
Policy 3 tab, 119
Policyholders, 5
POS (Place of Service) box, 142–143
Practice analysis report, 244–245
Practice management program (PMP), 13–14, 26–32. *See also* Medisoft; Office Hours
advantages of computer use, 30–31
for appointments, 27–28, 291–309. *See also* Office Hours
claims and billing in, 28, 268–281
in collection process, 268–281
reimbursement in, 28–30
Preferred provider organizations (PPOs), 6
Premiums, 5
Preregistering patients, 4
Prescribing, electronic, 25–26
Preview feature:
in Medisoft, 237
in Office Hours, 308–309
Primary insurance carrier, 115, 173–174
Print Grid button, 106
Printing in Medisoft, 231–255. *See also* Report(s)
collection reports, 248
co-payment report, 247
custom reports, 253–255
facility report, 247
filters in, 224–225
global coverage report, 248
insurance aging report, 249–250
insurance analysis, 247
insurance payment comparison, 247
outstanding copayment report, 248
patient aging applied payment report, 268–269
patient aging report, 248–249
patient day sheet, 19, 232–238
patient ledger, 251–252
patient statements, 206, 222–225
payment day sheet, 241
practice analysis report, 244–245
procedure day sheet, 239–240

referral source report, 247
referring provider report, 247
standard patient lists, 252–253
unapplied deposit report, 247
unapplied payment/adjustment report, 247
walkout statements/receipts, 156–158, 159
Printing in Office Hours, schedules, 308–309
Print Report Where? dialog box, 223
Print/Send Statements dialog box, 222–225
Prior authorization number, 123
Privacy:
Acknowledgment of Receipt of Notice of Privacy Practices, 37
electronic medical record (EMR) and, 25
HIPAA Privacy Rule, 35–37, 38, 264
Notice of Privacy Practices, 35–37
Procedure(s), 10
Procedure codes, 12–14. *See also* CPT-4 codes
in checking billing compliance, 14–15
for entering charges, 144
in Medisoft database, 47
MultiLink codes, 144–145
in Transaction Entry dialog box, 141–142, 143
Procedure day sheet, 239–240
Program date, changing, 53–56, 140
Prompt payment laws, 268
Protected health information (PHI), 35–37
Provider database, 46
Purging data, 69–71

Q

Quick Balance button, 52
Quick Ledger button, 52

R

Rebuilding indexes, 67–68
Recalculating balances, 71–72
Recall lists, Office Hours, 303–306
adding patients to, 304–306
creating, 303–304
Record of treatment and progress, 107–108
Referral source report, 247
Referring provider, 111
Referring provider report, 247
Remainder statements, 219, 225
Remittance advice (RA), 15–17, 28–29, 34, 194–196
described, 194–196
sample, 195
steps for processing, 196
Repeated appointments, booking, 299–300
Report(s), 231–255, 268–281. *See also* Forms; Printing in Medisoft; Printing in Office Hours, schedules
aging reports, 248–250, 268–269
analysis reports. *See* Analysis reports
billing/payments status report, 242–244
claims reports, 28, 30, 181–185
collection reports, 248, 269–274, 281
co-payment report, 247, 248
custom reports, 253–255
day sheets, 19, 232–241
electronic medical record (EMR) and, 25
facility report, 247
global coverage report, 248
insurance analysis, 247
insurance payment comparison, 247
in Office Hours, 308–309

outstanding copayment report, 248
patient aging applied payment report, 268–269
patient aging report, 248–249
patient ledger, 251–252
patient statements, 217–225
practice analysis report, 244–245
referral source report, 247
referring provider report, 247
Report Designer, 253, 255
Reports menu, 49–50
reviewing, 18
standard patient lists, 252–253
unapplied deposit report, 247
unapplied payment/adjustment report, 247
walkout statements/receipts, 28–29, 31, 156–158, 159
Report Designer, 253, 255
Responsible party, 5–7, 270–272
Restoring data, 65–66

S

Save feature:
for cases, 110
for charges, 145–146
Medisoft, 58
for patient information, 153–155
for payments/adjustments, 206
Savings accounts, medical, 7
Scheduling. *See also* Office Hours
of appointments, 27–28, 291–309
of breaks, 306–307
Search feature, 90–94
Field box, 91–92
Locate buttons option, 93–94
in Office Hours, 297
patient information, 90–94
Search For box, 91–92
Security of information:
electronic medical record (EMR) and, 25
HIPAA Security Rule, 37–39
HIPAA Transaction and Code Sets Standards, 33–35, 180
Service authorization exception code, 124
Services menu, 50, 51
Short cuts in Medisoft:
Copy Address button, 81
creating new case for established patient, 106
F8 function key, 88
Locate window, 94
opening cases, 78, 105
printing custom reports, 254
Signature Date, 84
Signature on File, 84
Sponsor, 125

Standard(s). *See also* CPT-4 codes; ICD-9-CM codes
HIPAA Electronic Transaction and Code Sets Standards, 33–35, 180
Standard patient lists, 252–253
Standard statements, 219
Starting Medisoft, 47–48
Starting Office Hours, 290–291
Statement(s). *See* Patient statements
Statement Management dialog box, 217–225
Status drop-down list, 85
Student data template, 47
Superbills (encounter forms), 10, 11, 15, 136
Supervising provider, 112

T

Technical safeguards, 38
Telephone Consumer Protection Act of 1991, 266
Third-party payers. *See also* Collection process
claims disputes, 264
defined, 6
laws governing timely payment of insurance claims, 268
reimbursement from, 192–206
Tickler Item dialog box, 274–277
Ticklers:
in collection list, 269, 270, 274–277
current balance for, 277
defined, 269
entering, 274–276
Tickler tab, 275
Toolbar:
Medisoft, 51–52
Office Hours, 289
Tools menu, 50
TOS (type of service) box, 143
Transaction data, 28
Transaction entry. *See also* Transaction Entry dialog box
adjustments, 136, 137, 158–160, 204, 206, 213–215
billing/reimbursement. *See* Medical billing process
charges, 136, 140–148
collections. *See* Collection process
deleting, 143–144
editing, 146
overview, 136
payments. *See* Payment(s)
transactions database, 47
Transaction Entry dialog box, 135–160
buttons in charges area, 143–145
case, 138, 139

charge transactions, 137, 140–148
chart, 136–138
color coding in transaction entry, 146–148, 154
patient/account information, 136–140
payment/adjustment transactions, 136, 137, 149–160, 204, 206, 213–215
recalculating patient balances, 71–72
Transaction Entry save warning dialog box, 58
Transactions tab, 178–179, 221
TRICARE, 5
in cases, 125
Truth in Lending Act, 267
Type of service (TOS) box, 143

U

Unapplied deposit report, 247
Unapplied payment/adjustment report, 247
Uncollectible accounts, 267
Utilities, Medisoft, 66–72
backing up data, 63–64
file maintenance, 66–72
packing data, 68–69
purging data, 69–71
rebuilding indexes, 67–68
recalculating patient balances, 71–72
restoring data, 65–66

V

Verification report, 181–185
Vision claims, 128

W

Walkout statements/receipts, 28–29, 31, 156–158, 159
Window menu, 50
Workers' compensation, 6, 121
Work Phone and Extension, 85

X

X12-270/271 Health Care Eligibility Benefit Inquiry and Response, 34
X12-276/277 Health Care Claim Status Request and Response, 34
X12-278 Health Care Services Review, 34
X12-835 Claims Payment and Remittance Advice, 34, 194–196
X12-837 Health Care Claim or Equivalent Encounter Information (837P), 34, 168